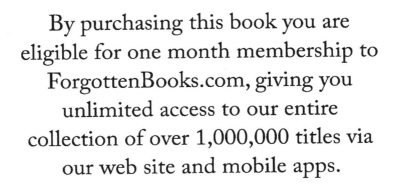

ISBN 978-0-484-61296-8
PIBN 10696120

Vol. XXIV—No. 1   JUNE, 1919   No. 227

ARCHIVES OF RADIOLOGY AND ELECTROTHERAPY

THE OFFICIAL ORGAN OF THE
BRITISH ASSOCIATION RADIOLOGY AND PHYSIOTHERAPY

Editors.

ROBERT KNOX, M.D., Hon. Radiographer, King's College Hospital.
E. P. CUMBERBATCH, B.M., M.R.C.P., Medical Officer in Charge, 'Electrical Department, St. Bartholomew's Hospital.
SIDNEY RUSS, D.Sc., Physicist to the Middlesex Hospital.

IN COLLABORATION WITH

A. E. BARCLAY (Manchester); BELOT (Paris); H. MARTIN BERRY (London); W. H. BRAGG (London); N. BURKE (Woodhall Spa); J. BURNET (Edinburgh); W. J. S. BYTHELL (Manchester); J. T. CASE (Battle Creek, U.S.A.); A. ST. GEORGE CAULFEILD (London); H. A. COLWELL (London); FOVEAU DE COURMELLES (Paris); GUNZBURG (Antwerp); HALL-EDWARDS (Birmingham); HARET (Paris); HAUCHAMPS (Brussels); F. HERNAMAN-JOHNSON (London); W. F. HIGGINS (Teddington); THURSTAN HOLLAND (Liverpool); HURST (London); KLYNENS (Antwerp); LAQUERRIERE (Paris); LAZARUS-BARLOW (London); LEDUC (Nantes); ALEXANDER MACKAY (Edinburgh); REGINALD MORTON (London); HARRISON ORTON (London); W. OVEREND (St. Leonards-on-Sea); PFAHLER (Philadelphia); C. E. S. PHILLIPS (London); GEORGE PIRIE (Dundee); HOWARD PIRIE (Montreal); A. W. PORTER (London); R. W. A. SALMOND (London); WERTHEIM SALOMONSON (Amsterdam); S. SLOAN (Glasgow); SOMERVILLE (Glasgow); W. C. STEVENSON (Dublin); W. J. TURRELL (Oxford); HUGH WALSHAM (London); ROBT. WILSON (Montreal).

SOME BIOLOGICAL EFFECTS OF SMALL QUANTITIES OF RADIUM.

By W. S. LAZARUS-BARLOW, M.D., F.R.C.P.

Director of the Cancer Research Laboratories of The Middlesex Hospital.

IN the early days of any branch of science its literature is characterised by the accumulation of a heterogeneous mass of isolated details and observations, and the new subject of radio-pathology is no exception to the rule. Colwell and Russ's book on "Radium, X rays and The Living Cell," has done much to collect and systematise a large mass of material that is of fundamental importance to the Röntgen Society, and I do not anticipate that I shall be able to add largely thereto in the remarks which I have the honour to make before you to-night.

I have selected the subject of the biological action of small quantities of radium because a large part of my own experimental work, during the past twelve or fourteen years, has been connected therewith. Looking back over that time one is saddened to think of the small progress one has made, but in justice it ought to be remembered how great is the wrench that drags a man out of pure biological studies into a field, not only of a physical nature (itself a primary difficulty to the biologist), but even more into a field in physics which is *terra nova* to the physicists themselves. . To appreciate what it means, I can only appeal to the physicists among you to recall their feelings when stress of circumstances forced them to merge their cleanly branch of learning in that inchoate conglomeration of Brobdignagian molecules which is the subject matter of biology, and is termed "Protein."

When one considers the enormous energy that is set free in the disruption of the radium atom, it is intelligible that the injurious effects of· radium radiations upon animal cells should have been early recognised. It is now known that, under certain conditions, the response of the animal cell to radiations is in the direction of stimulation. This fact, which to the biologist appeared, *a priori*, most probable from his general knowledge of the behaviour of animal tissues to reagents of different kinds, was not established without difficulty. Beckton and I[1] found that the alpha rays of radium in quantities of the order of 5×10^{-7} mgr. acting on the ova of Ascaris megalocephala in the resting stage, for a continuous period of about 30 hours at 0°C, lead to a definite stimulation of the processes of division, in that the irradiated cells pass sooner into the two-celled stage than the controls. The actual amount of stimulation that is induced in these cells is small, so that we obtained statistical confirmation of our conclusion. Greenwood[2] on examination of our results considered that, from a statistical point of view, there was a thirty to one chance in favour of our conclusion being right. As to the question itself of stimulation of growth in tissues that have been treated therapeutically with radium, clinical evidence is so strong that it was already prepared for evidence derived from the laboratory. Curiously, though the evidence in favour of stimulation was so difficult to get in the case of Ascaris ova (Beckton and I counted some half million ova in that research), the following investigation upon which I was engaged afforded evidence that was impossible to ignore. In this case large quantities of radium were being used, it is true, but at a distance from the maximum action of the gamma rays that were employed there was well-marked evidence of increased cell division. The rectal mucosa of the rat was under investigation,[3] and tubes composed of ·5 mm. platinum and containing either 92 or 38 mgr. of the bromide were employed. Here the occurrence of stimulation was shown by a sevenfold increase in the number of columnar cells undergoing mitosis, whereas in the case of the Ascaris ova the increase was only one of about 4 per cent. These two experiments have shown the stimulating effects of alpha and of gamma radiation. The effect of beta radiation Beckton and I showed to obtain in the case of Ascaris ova, when the amount of radium used was about one hundred times as great as that necessary when alpha radiation was used.

The experiments mentioned offer the suggestion that different varieties of cells require exposure to different amounts of radium or for different lengths of time, or both, in order that stimulation may be manifested. I have no definite evidence that this is the case, though it is probably true. On the other hand, when dealing with quantities of radium sufficiently large to induce marked degenerative changes in cells, the following experiment [4] shows that the reaction of different varieties of cells to one and the same dose of radiations is not identical. It was determined electroscopically that the total ionisation produced by the tube containing 92 mgr. during 108 minutes was the same as that produced by the tube containing 38 mgr. during 240 minutes. These tubes were then introduced through the anus of rats in such a way that half of the tube acted upon the columnar cell mucosa of the rectum, and the external half upon the squamous cell skin of the under surface of the tail. The tubes were left *in situ* for the corresponding lengths of time. Though the total bombardment to which the tissues were exposed was the same, the behaviour of the cells shows a marked difference. The smaller quantity acting for the longer time produced the maximum effect upon the

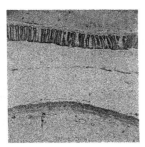

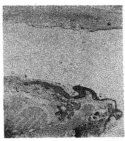

FIG. 1.   FIG. 2.

FIG. 1.—Rectal mucous membranes of two rats, showing the different effects of quantity and time in calculating " radium dose." Estimated electroscopically the ionisation was the same in both cases. The upper of the two specimens (92 mgr. for 108 minutes) shows a still persisting mucous membrane, the lower (38 mgr. for 240 minutes) shows complete desquamation. Compare with Fig. 2.

FIG. 2.—Squamous epithelium of under surface of tail of the same two rats as in Fig. 1. The effects on squamous epithelium are exactly opposite to those on columnar epithelium ; 92 mgr. for 108 minutes (upper) has led to complete desquamation ; 38 mgr. for 240 minutes (lower) has not. Compare with Fig. 1.

columnar cells (Fig. 1), the larger quantity acting for the shorter time produced the maximum effect upon the squamous epithelium (Fig. 2). It follows that in treatment, *undesirable* damage to columnar cells is best avoided by using relatively large amounts of radium for a short time, undesirable damage to squamous cells by using relatively small amounts for a long time.

The experiments hitherto described are of an anatomical character. On the physiological side I cannot recall any definite work (other than observations upon motility of various lower organisms) beyond that to which I wish now to draw your attention.

In 1913, Dunbar and I [5] published a series of observations upon the effect of radium radiations upon the muscle-nerve preparation of the frog. We chose this because we had here the muscle and nerve in one of their simplest combinations, and could differentiate the various components of a muscular contraction occasioned by a single electrical stimulus. I need not go into the details of the experiments, but, speaking generally, they consisted in exposing the entire muscle-nerve preparation to the rays from 7 mgr. of $RaBr_2$ continuously, and determining the minimal induced electrical stimulus which, applied to the nerve, called forth a contraction of the muscle. By suitable means, the nerve and nerve endings were cut out so that we were able to conclude that exposure to the alpha rays was accompanied by a better maintenance of neuro-muscular irritability than is the case with a non-irradiated control, and that this beneficial or stimulative effect is exerted upon the nerve and to some degree upon the muscle, but that the nerve endings are apparently unaffected. We were unable to detect any effects of the beta and gamma rays acting alone up to a period of nine hours.

Although they were never published, we then went on to make experiments on the action of radium upon the isolated, beating frog's heart. We found that alpha rays produce their effects more rapidly, and that a smaller quantity of radium must be used in order to obtain evidence of stimulation. When one considers the musculo-neural mechanisms of the heart and of the gastrocnemius, the greater "sensitiveness" or "vulnerability" of the heart under alpha radiation is not surprising. What we actually found was that, soon after the rays began to be applied, the diastolic excursion of the ventricle and the output of the heart were increased, and therefore that the heart did more work in unit time, but that it became exhausted more rapidly than the non-irradiated organ and ceased to beat earlier.

You will have noticed that the evidence of stimulation by the rays, though real, is subtle. Deleterious effects are so evident at the margins of the picture that, unless the happy moment be seized, the light of the landscape is blotted out by the encroaching shadows. This, indeed, is but an evidence for the extraordinary potency of the rays, and has its counterpart in many experiences of ordinary biological life. I will only cite here the contrast that obtains in the early and in the late stages of such a condition as streptococcal septicæmia. You will recall the mental brilliancy of the patient when, as yet, he is under the influence of a minute dose of the virulent streptotoxin, and will contrast that with the hebetude supervening as the dose of toxin increases within his body. This very characteristic makes all work upon the stimulative action of radium the more difficult, for no sooner has a bombardment with rays sufficient to bring about stimulative phenomena taken place, than the continued impact sets about inducing the destructive action. If a minute tube containing a fraction of a milligramme of radium be placed beneath the skin of an animal and watched from day to day, there is noticed at first a focus of hypertrophied skin immediately over the tube, but this soon gives place to degeneration and the formation of an ever-widening ulcer surrounded by an ever-widening ring of skin-hypertrophy until an equilibrium is produced. As might be supposed, the superficial area of the ulcer and the distance of the ring of hypertrophy from its centre are functions of the amount of radium, the time, the depth at which the tube is placed, and so forth. Nevertheless, wherever the ring of hypertrophy may be placed in reference to the radium, its actual width differs but little in different cases. This is as might be expected, since the animal cell will respond by increased growth to a limited amount of bombardment. Under less than this the cell will not react in any recognisable way, and under more than this it will not be able to resist degenerative changes and ultimate death.

Although the passing stimulation and the definitive degeneration and death to which I have referred is the obvious cycle, and the one with which the radium therapist is well acquainted, particularly on its degenerative side, it is conceivable that under certain circumstances the action of the rays should never go beyond the stimulative stage. If, for example, the quantity of radium in action were gradually reduced, stimulation of cell growth would be kept up after its initiation for an indefinite length of time, the growing and dividing cells would accumulate, and we should not be far from that "habit of growth" which Adami has pointed out is characteristic of the cancer cell, if indeed an actual cancer were not produced. This is the simplest possible way of looking at the question, but one may be practically certain that the problem of the cause of cancer is not solved by Nature after this fashion. The biologist has been taught by bitter experience that the probable truth of any given biological explanation varies inversely as the nth power of its simplicity.

For the purpose of all investigations into the treatment of cancer, it is eminently desirable that we should be able to produce the disease at will in lower animals, and for several years my attention has been turned in this direction.

That there is some close association between rays and cancer appears to me to admit of no doubt ; the occurrence of X-ray cancer; the fact that I have found small quantities of radium present in cancerous tissue, whereas it is absent or practically absent from non-cancerous tissue;[6] the fact that whereas gall stones unassociated with cancer of the gall bladder, contain no radium, or at most traces but little outside the range of experimental detection, gall stones associated with primary carcinoma of the gall bladder always contain relatively large amounts of radium,[7] all support the view. I confess that I have not been able to produce a condition fatal to the animals in the same way as we know cancer to be fatal in man, but I submit that the histological changes I have been able to produce by means of small quantities of radium would, if they had occurred in man, have been regarded as cancer, or, at the very least, so suspiciously like cancer that they would have called for surgical removal.

The experiments in question[8] were conducted as follows: In one, series, minute glass tubes, of radium in quantities varying between 10^{-8} mgr. and 10^{-1} mgr. were placed beneath the skin of rats; in the other series, radium of the order of 10^{-6} mgr. was artificially introduced into the centres of a number of small human gall stones, and these were then introduced into the gall bladders of rabbits. Controls were, of course, carried out in all cases.

Skin of rat experiments.—No obvious effect was produced with radium in quantities of less than about 10^{-4} mgr., even though the radium tube remained *in situ* for many weeks, but with quantities of the order mentioned there was seen, after a time, an alteration of the hair which ended in its shedding.   It was difficult to be certain as to the actual series of changes, as the skin over the tube seemed to be the seat of irritation and led to scratching on the part of the animal.   With quantities of the order 10^{-3} to 10^{-1} mgr. were produced stimulative and degenerative changes in skin and its appendages, subcutaneous connective tissue, and even, when the quantity was large and the time was several weeks, degenerative changes in the subjacent cartilage or bone.   Microscopic sections and silhouettes were prepared of the seats of maximum stimulation of skin in order of "radium dose," *i.e.*, the product of the quantity of radium used in the particular case, and the number of days it was allowed to remain *in situ*.   It was seen that the amount of squamous cell overgrowth, roughly speaking, varies directly as the radium dose.

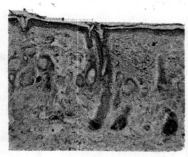

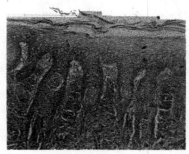

FIG. 3.   FIG. 4.

FIG. 3.—Skin of rat (nearly normal, but showing some hypertrophy of superficial epidermal layers). Hair follicles and sebaceous glands are present, and the absence of downward prolongations of the superficial epithelial layers is to be noted.   The specimen was 0·5 cm. distant from that figured in Fig. 4.

FIG. 4.—Skin of rat acted upon by the beta and gamma rays of 0 14 mgr. of Ra. element for 54 days. Note the absence of hair follicles and sebaceous glands, the invasion of the subcutaneous tissue by irregular down giowths of greatly hypertrophied epithelium, and the existence of " cell nests." The microscopical appearances are those of a commencing squamous cell carcinoma.

When the altered tissue is examined microscopically, it is seen that the normal orderly thin layer of skin, with its numerous hair follicles, is completely changed.   Instead of consisting of not more than two or three superposed layers of cells it consists of many, and instead of a remarkable absence of epithelial processes into the subcutaneous tissues, irregular spurs of proliferated epithelial cells project into the depth though they do not pass beyond the muscular layer.   Here and there, in the middle of the epithelial processes, are to be found veritable " cell nests," so that the resemblance to an early squamous cell carcinoma is exact.   Hair follicles are wanting, and in the majority of cases even the last traces of them have disappeared.   The subcutaneous connective tissue has become more collagenous in character and there is a remarkable absence of lymphocytes, polynuclear leucocytes, or plasma cells (Figs. 3 and 4).

Gall bladder of rabbit experiments.—In these cases the controls differed remarkably from the experimental animals. In the controls (Fig. 6) the presence of a non-radium gall stone led to a thickening of the gall bladder wall such as might naturally be associated with the presence of an aseptic, innocuous foreign body; the connective tissue was enormously increased in thickness and of great density, fibroblasts and connective tissue cells were conspicuously absent, there were no polynuclear cells nor lymphocytes, the lining layer of columnar epithelial cells persisted; and in places there was a small amount of epithelial proliferation, which however in no case invaded the thickened bladder wall. The appearances were simply those of encapsulation of a foreign body. On the other hand the gall bladders of rabbits into which radium-containing gall stones had been introduced (Fig. 7) showed a more or less extensive, irregular proliferation of the columnar epithelium which invaded the surrounding thickened bladder wall. The number of

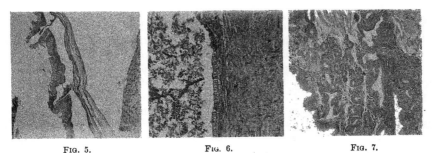

FIG. 5.   FIG. 6.   FIG. 7.

FIG. 5.—Gall bladder of rabbit (normal). To the extreme right is liver substance, in the middle is the thin, loose connective tissue of the gall bladder wall, and further to the left the lining columnar epithelium. High power.

FIG. 6.—Gall bladder of rabbit into which a non-radium containing gall stone was introduced experimentally. The animal lived 38 months. In the middle is seen a single layer of columnar epithelium, with dense fibrous tissue constituting the thickened gall bladder wall on the right, and, on the left, intra-vesicular débris. High power.

FIG. 7.—Gall bladder of rabbit into which a gall stone containing radium of the order 10^{-6} mgr. was introduced experimentally. The animal lived 12 months after operation. Note the irregular proliferation of columnar epithelium which manifests itself by the invasion of the connective tissue of the gall bladder wall, and the presence of numerous irregular tubules lined with columnar epithelium that are cut in all directions. The animal showed a metastatic nodule with similar microscopical appearances at a distant part of the liver. The appearances are those of columnar cell carcinoma. High power.

polynuclear leucocytes varied in different cases, but a characteristic feature was the presence of a zone of lymphocytes in advance of the invading irregular tubules. In one instance a focus was found in a far distant part of the liver, which consisted of irregular tubules reproducing the picture met with in the gall bladder itself; it was totally unconnected with the primary mass, totally unlike any constituent of the liver, and, I think, can only be looked upon as a metastatic nodule. The control animals lived two months to thirty-eight months after the operation; the experimental animals lived twelve months to forty-eight months after operation. Alpha ray electroscopic examination of the gall stones, after death of the animals, showed the absence of recognisable quantities of radium in the case of the control animals, its presence in the case of the experimental animals. One is, therefore, justified in directly associating the peculiar changes of epithelium in the gall bladder, to which I have drawn your attention, with the presence of the small quantities of radium in the gall stones.

It will have appeared already that the inter-relationship between the stimulative and the degenerative effects of radium action, the inter-relationship between the time factor and the quantity factor in forming the " radium dose," the influence of mass and of essential nature of the biological tissue upon which the radium is allowed to act, render the expression " small quantities " used in the title of this communication one of the greatest uncertainty. Deleterious effects produced by small quantities are seen in the destruction of leucocytes in shed blood, and in the escape of hæmoglobin from red blood corpuscles as the result of bombardment by alpha rays that have been described by Chambers and Russ,[9] in the lethal effects of radium, whether alpha, beta or gamma radiation, upon the cells of rat sarcoma, or of mouse carcinoma by Russ in conjunction with Chambers, and with Wedd in the respective cases,[10, 11] in the lethal effects of beta and gamma rays upon tadpoles by Beckton,[12] and, no doubt, by many other authors. It cannot be said, baldly, that stimulative effects are produced by the action of small quantities, whereas deleterious effects are produced by the action of large, though no small modicum of truth would be contained therein. Nevertheless, one may fairly argue, when a given quantity of radium acting for a given length of time on a given mass of a given variety of cells has been observed to be followed by degenerative changes, that a sufficient reduction of the quantity of radium, or of the length of time during which it is allowed to act, will induce a stimulative or beneficial effect.

In the case of stimulated overgrowth of cells, such as occurs in some of the instances mentioned above, one cannot doubt, on general grounds, that the nucleus of the cell is the subject of, at all events, part of the altered metabolism induced by the irradiation. We have no experimental evidence on this point. On the other hand, when deleterious effects are produced by radium, it has clearly been shown that the nucleus is specifically affected. Thus, Paula Hertwig showed in the case of the tadpole that the centrosomes and spindles were unaltered, but that the chromatin was profoundly altered and the chromosomes were broken up.[13] Similiar changes were demonstrated by Mottram to occur in the cells of the growing root-tip of the bean and the ova of Ascaris, and this author added the important observation that nuclei in active mitosis are eight times as vulnerable to the rays as nuclei in the resting stage.[14] That part of growth which consists in actual enlargement of the cell, apart from division of its nucleus, he did not find to be influenced by radium. A remarkable instance of the differentiation between the nucleus and the cytoplasm under the influence of radium was shown by Prime.[15]

Using *in vitro* plasma cultures of embryo chick heart, he found that the nuclei of the muscle fibres were modified to such a degree that they no longer showed the presence of mitoses in sub-cultures, although the fragment of cardiac muscle still continued to pulsate.

This brings us to the more strictly chemical portion of our subject, and I regret that there is but little solid information to present. The bio-chemist is still *rara avis in terra*, and bio-chemists who have devoted attention to the effects of irradiation upon the chemistry of the cell are almost, if not quite, wanting. Work has been done upon the effects of irradiation upon the enzymes, pepsin, trypsin, amylopsin, rennin, diastase, autolysins, erepsin, but the results are most contradictory. It is likely that this depends in part upon the complicated series of changes involved in the passage of the prozymogen, through the zymogen stage, into the enzyme. Opsonin and hæmolytic complement have been shown by Chambers and Russ[16] to be destroyed by alpha radiation, though beta and gamma rays appear to have no effect. Other isolated observations of this nature are to be found scattered throughout literature. I will not trouble you with them, but it is clear that the type of research which they exemplify is at the root of our further advance in radio-pathology.

The foregoing short account of some of the effects of radium action may be of general scientific interest, but there is a practical side to the question, and to this I should like to direct your attention.

You will have noticed that I have made no mention of X rays, and no doubt the idea has passed through your minds that the close relation between radium rays and X rays must mean that the changes which I have mentioned as occurring as the result of radium action must also occur as the result of X-ray action. It is a general belief at the present time that whatever can be effected by radium can also be effected by X rays, and *vice versa*, so that the only essential difference between the two agents, considered from a therapeutic point of view, is that of the relative sizes of the tube of radium and the X-ray bulb for convenience of application of the rays. I am not quite sure that this attitude is justifiable. When one is dealing with the animal cell and the complex products of its metabolism, and recognises, as one is bound to recognise, the wide range covered by the spectrum between ultra-violet light and the hardest gamma rays of radium, on the one hand, and the narrow range separating stimulation and degeneration of the animal cell and analogous changes of their chemical metabolic products, on the other, and when one remembers that however carefully the rays may be filtered, it is in all instances a composite bundle of different wave lengths that is being used in treatment, one wonders whether X-ray therapy and radium therapy can ever be regarded as convertible terms. In a rough fashion, no doubt they can, but just as a composite prescription of medicinal drugs will often act better than, or in a different way from, its individual components, so it is possible that further knowledge of ray therapy will teach us that in order to get a particular kind of reaction on the part of a particular variety of cells we have to use combinations or selections of wave lengths which we can most easily get by using radium rays in one instance and X rays in another. I am treading on very uncertain ground, but I can give you, I think, a simple illustration for the idea that is passing through my mind. Sodium and potassium are very similar chemically and physically, but in respect of the animal cell they differ so fundamentally that neither will replace the other and both are indispensable for the due exercise of cell function.

With this reservation I will pass to consider certain theoretical questions of treatment that are beginning to assume importance.

In the past, and, to a large extent, even at the present time, the destructive side of ray therapy has been the one on which most attention has been fixed. This is most clearly the case in regard to the treatment of cancer by inserting a tube of radium into the centre of the growth. In a more modified fashion it applies to the treatment of uterine fibro-myomata by deep X-ray therapy. Here the desire is not to produce a definite necrobiosis, but to induce such changes in the cells of the tumour that their absorption is brought about by the action of the tissue fluids in a gradual way, so that at no time actually dead tissue is present. So far as I am aware this method of treatment assumes that the body fluids which are to carry out the absorption of the tumour are normal. Somewhat similar is the method of treating contracted scars and cheloids, but here ionisation methods indicate the prevalence of an idea that the cells and tissues which it is sought to influence may be acted upon by inducing a chemical difference in them and in the fluids by which they are bathed. Yet another extension of the twin idea of acting upon the abnormal material, and at the same time upon the body fluids by which it is bathed, is seen in that method of treating tuberculosis (especially of the lungs) which has recently been advocated by Fraenkel.[17] He recommends the combined use of massive doses locally upon the tuberculous focus and stimulative doses over the spleen or thyroid, or, where there is anæmia, over the ovarian region. In the latter instance his idea is to stimulate hæmopoiesis, in the case of the thyroid and spleen he would stimulate, because these tissues have been shown to play some part in immunity actions. This is particularly the case with the spleen, and there is some, as yet undetermined, relationship between the number of lymphocytes and the occurrence of immunity. Thus, the numbers of lymphocytes in the circulating blood may be reduced over lengthened periods by the action of a *large* dose of X rays, and a rat, immune to inoculation with Jensen's rat sarcoma, may be made susceptible to inoculation by the same means, whereas, on the contrary, it is possible by means of repeated *small* doses of X rays to increase the numbers of circulating lymphocytes, or to confer an immunity towards inoculation with rat sarcoma upon a normal susceptible animal. These results have largely been obtained by Murphy and others working in the Rockefeller Institute,[18] and Russ and others working in the Cancer Research Laboratories of the Middlesex Hospital.

With the object of inducing stimulative effects, Fraenkel advises the administration of thorium-X, but, on the basis of my results after introducing small quantities of radium into the animal body, and of the general relationship which, in my opinion, obtains between radiation and cancer, I consider this procedure to be deprecated. Internal administration of any radio-active substance, in view of the difficulty of its elimination and the extremely minute quantities which are necessary to produce marked results, seems to me to be a very dangerous procedure.

On the other hand, administration of X rays or of radium rays by external application, or by internal application of radium in a hermetically sealed tube, seems to be a line of treatment by means of which stimulative radiation might be given, and for which there is a great future. In this connection it is possible that radium emanation water may be employed. Much of the effect that has been ascribed to the action of emanation water is doubtless fictitious, and where benefit has followed upon its use, a part of such benefit is probably explicable on psychical lines. But it would be foolish to deny entirely all power to emanation water when one knows that competent authorities have asserted its value in conditions like rheumatoid arthritis, where all other known medicinal agents are apt to fail. Here, again, it is probably a question of learning how to apply a potent agent in the proper manner. Stevenson's method of treating contracted scar tissue with emanation tubes [20] is essentially one of stimulation by small doses, and one could imagine that it might be extended, for example, to the treatment of stricture of the urethra, and to stenoses of the œsophagus after swallowing of corrosive fluids, to the treatment of adhesions in the body cavities and in joints, while the treatment of interstitial keratitis, and of those inflammatory changes occurring in the heart valves which terminate in the pitiable condition of chronic valvular disease by means of stimulative doses of rays does not appear to be an altogether unreasonable hope for the future. Whether they could be beneficially applied in the treatment of interstitial nephritis and cirrhosis of the liver is a different question. Great though the destructive power of radium and X-radiations have shown themselves to be when these agents are applied in large, or relatively large doses, I submit that there is a far more extensive field for exploration when they are applied in small doses. When we have learned how to control the radiations and the responses made by the various kinds of cells to stimulation with different varieties of wave length and different combinations of varying wave lengths, we shall be able to control the processes of health and disease in a manner undreamt of at the present time.

REFERENCES.

1. *Archives Middlesex Hospital*, Twelfth Cancer Report, 1913, p. 68.
2. *Ibid.*, Twelfth Cancer Report, 1913, p. 72.
3. *Ibid.*, Thirteenth Cancer Report, 1914, pp. 47-49.
4. *Ibid.*, Thirteenth Cancer Report, 1914, p. 54.
5. *Ibid.*, Twelfth Cancer Report, 1913, p. 1.
6. *Ibid.*, Eleventh Cancer Report, 1912, p. 91; *British Medical Journal*, May 9th, 1914.

7. *Ibid.*, Eleventh Cancer Report, 1912, p. 108 ; Twelfth Cancer Report, 1913, p. 87 ;
    British Medical Journal, May 9th, 1914.
8. *Proceedings of the Royal Society of Medicine*, 1918, Vol. XI. (Section of Pathology), p. 1.
9. *Archives Middlesex Hospital*, Tenth Cancer Report, 1911, p. 110.
10. *Ibid.*, Twelfth Cancer Report, 1913, p. 120.
11. *Ibid.*, Eleventh Cancer Report, 1912, p. 50.
12. *Ibid.*, Thirteenth Cancer Report, 1914, p. 124.
13. *Arch. f. mikros. Anat.*, 1911, pp. 77, 301.
14. *Archives Middlesex Hospital*, Twelfth Cancer Report, 1913, p. 110.
15. *Journal of Cancer Research*, Baltimore, U.S.A., 1917, pp. 2, 107.
16. *Archives Middlesex Hospital*, Tenth Cancer Report, 1911, pp. 127-132.
17. *Fortschr. a. d. Geb. d. Röntgenstrahlen*, 1918, pp. 26-43.
18. *Journ. Exp. Med.*, Jan., 1919.
19. *Lancet*, April 26th, 1919.
20. *Lancet*, March 23rd, 1918 ; *Medical Press*, Jan. 8th, 1919.

OSSEOUS ABNORMALITIES OF THE FOOT WHICH CAUSE NO DISCOMFORT.

By Geo. A. Pirie, M.D., Radiologist to Dundee Royal Infirmary.

The article by Lieut.-Col. Dennis, in the January number of the Archives, reminds me of two similar cases which I have met with lately.

A gentleman wished me to examine his right foot because of rheumatic pains which troubled him. On screening the foot I was surprised to notice the scaphoid apparently in two fragments. There was no history of accident, so I examined the other foot and found a similar condition. But the fragments were rounded ; there was no pain on pressure, and the discomfort complained of was more in front and to the outer side. Thus, the condition was evidently congenital. The skiagram (Fig. 1) shows that the scaphoid of each foot has been developed from two centres, and the parts have remained distinct.

In the other case, a lady had sprained her ankle, and wished it examined. The tibia and fibula were seen to be normal, but on screening the foot I found the scaphoid presented a very peculiar appearance. It was narrow externally and broad and prominent internally. Probably, here also the bone had developed from two centres, but the parts had coalesced and formed this irregular shape.

In neither case did the condition cause any discomfort, and it must be rare. Out of 25,000 cases examined during the past twenty years, I do not remember meeting with any other in which the scaphoid was abnormally developed.

Not unfrequently the os calcis develops a spike from its under surface. This is usually blamed for causing pain in walking, and no doubt sometimes with reason. But in other cases the spike may be present and cause no discomfort. For example, in Fig. 2, a well marked spike is shown. It was discovered accidentally, but no complaint was made about the heel. There was general weakness and discomfort in the foot, due to deficient circulation of blood through the calcareous arteries.

Sesamoid bones are often noted in unusual localities, *e.g.*, on outer side of

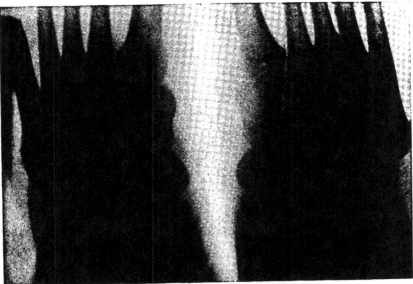

FIG. 1.—Scaphoid developed from two centres in each foot.

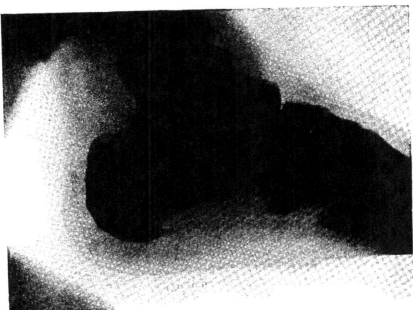

FIG. 2.—Os calcis with spike that caused no discomfort.

the cuboid and on the inner side of the scaphoid ; and one or both of the sesamoids in the ball of the great toe may be in two parts, but these do not cause any discomfort.

It has been my custom to screen every case before taking the skiagram, and in this way any abnormality may be detected and examined from different angles and the best view chosen.

AN UNUSUAL CASE OF TORTICOLLIS.

By R. W. A. SALMOND, M.D.

THIS was the case of a man who was grazed on the back of the shoulder by a piece of shrapnel. A typical and well marked torticollis at once developed, lasted for a week, and then gradually passed off completely.

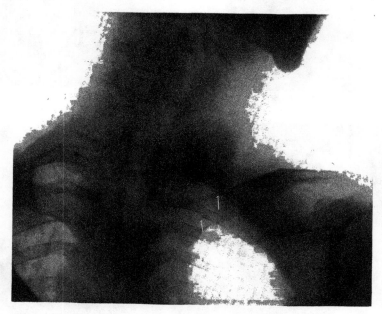

On X-ray examination, the second and third ribs were found to be fractured near their vertebral articulations (see radiogram), the seat of the fracture in the second rib corresponding to the attachment of the scalenus posticus muscle.

The torticollis was, no doubt, due to the head and neck being involuntarily held in the position of greatest rest to the scalenus posticus muscle, and perhaps, in a lesser degree, to one or other of the deep seated muscles of the back, and its extension into the neck ; in other words, it was Nature's method of keeping the fracture at rest while it was uniting.

MOBILE X-RAY WAGGON UNIT.

By Howard *C*. Head.

AMONG the many special productions called for by the requirements of the armies in the field, and at home, none can be more interesting than the Mobile X-ray Unit. Its design opens up great possibilities for the inventive genius of the automobile engineer, the electrical engineer, and the radiologist, but to take advantage of all the suggestions, and to incorporate those of value in the construction of a practical plant, whilst omitting, without offence, the impracticable, I say it with all modesty, requires the exercise of a good deal of ingenuity.

There are many initial difficulties to overcome before one can proceed to carry out the preconceived ideas of the completed unit. The automobile engineer has very strong views on departing from the standard chassis, and it is with great difficulty that he can be persuaded to alter or make any modification of design to arrange, for example, for the direct drive of the generator by the engine of the car.

The power electrical engineer does not appreciate the fact that the generator must be of special design to deal with the oscillatory high-tension load, and, as you will well understand, it is also not easy to incorporate all the requirements of the up-to-date radiologist. So one starts off by taking things as one finds them, and constructing the equipment out of the materials to hand.

Therefore, in describing this Mobile X-ray Unit to you I do not present it as my conception of the perfect X-ray waggon, but as a unit which is a development of previous attempts, and at the same time I may be able to indicate some original improvements which can be elaborated in future outfits, and this, considering the difficulties from a manufacturing point of view at the present time, is all one can hope to accomplish.

The value of these motor X-ray units has been much criticised, but there is no doubt that they are of great practical utility, and may remain of special value after the war. By their means it has become possible to have the X-ray apparatus and its power unit taken to its work instead of the work having to be brought to some centre where there is an established plant, and this without any loss of power or output. At the same time there may be a considerable saving to the patient, and further, the question of distance and the difficulties and risks to be negotiated are frequently such as to make the undertaking impracticable.

In the alleviation of suffering the chief consideration, without doubt, is promptness in the application of the necessary treatment. With the phenomenal increase in the variety of death-dealing instruments which characterise modern warfare, there has been a corresponding increase in the numbers of wounded, and, as a consequence, the evacuation has had to be speeded up to an extent hitherto thought impossible.

The employment of such a unit has helped considerably to that most desired end.

It is of interest to mention that some years prior to the war the Central Powers had attached to each of their army divisions a horse-drawn X-ray unit, but these were comparatively of an inconvenient and cumbersome type (Fig. 1).

As an engineer, in these days of motor vehicles, it is most incongruous to consider a horse-drawn waggon for this purpose.

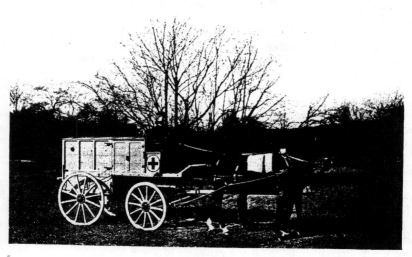

FIG. 1.

There is naturally very little literature available as to what developments have taken place, but I believe the German army is provided with a number of Roentgen war automobiles, and that Prof. Brauer and Dr. Haemisch have designed a special type.

This type consists of two cars, each of about 30/50 h.p. The apparatus is mounted in the cars and occupies the whole of the interiors, and has to be entirely removed and built up outside and independent of the cars. The outfit consists of a separate engine of 15 h.p., and dynamo capable of generating 8-9 k.w., mounted up as one unit, with petrol tank and switch-board attached, but with a separate water tank. The X-ray generator is a rotating high-tension apparatus, of 5 k.v.a., provided with a switch-table and a rotary converter of 200 volts.   The equipment includes an elaborate screening stand, provided with an adjustable chair and arranged with rails for 2-metre work. The X-ray table is of the most primitive type, consisting of a simple top on four legs, with a folding flap for the extremities of the patient, and all examinations from below are made with the tube in a heavy cumbersome metal tube stand.   The table is mounted on casters, and the table and patient are moved together in a restricted area over the tube box.

It appears to me that better use might have been made of the bodies of the cars instead of for packing purposes only, and one of the car engines coupled to an alternator, and the rectifier provided with a synchronous motor, instead of supplying a separate engine and dynamo and rotary converter. It also seems as if an over-elaborate screening stand has been provided at the expense and neglect of the X-ray table, as one would hardly expect to undertake heart examination or orthodiagraphic work on the field, omitting the necessary apparatus for the efficient localisation, and radiographie and radioscopie examinations with the tube below the couch.

The first serious point for consideration was the selection of the type of chassis most suitable and convenient for the work, but this, in spite of the great variety of most excellent makes, was not so difficult, because the model of the Austin Motor Company offered, in addition to its general excellence, the special feature that the loading line was much lower and nearer the ground than any other type employed. being practically equal to an underslung type of car.

This is most important for the following reasons :—

1. The induction coil and its fittings, the distribution switch-board and the control board. can be all manipulated from the car, because the controls come within the reach of a man of average height, so that none of these pieces of apparatus require moving into the portable X-ray theatre.

2. As the body of the car is so near the ground, only one step is necessary instead of four or five, as with an ordinary chassis, and this is a great advantage in loading and unloading the plant, or, if necessity should arise. getting patients in and out of the vehicle.

3. It enables all the weight to be kept low, and there is less tendency for such a car to overturn, even when at a considerable angle, and, owing to its low centre of gravity, it is practically immune from side-slip.

It is unnecessary for me to give a detailed description of the chassis. as this is best obtained from the maker's catalogue, but one or two points are of interest.   The model is a 2-3 ton chassis, and fitted with an engine with four separate cylinders. but that which is of special importance to us in the present case is the differential box, the rear axle, and the frame.

The drive is distributed through substantial bevel wheels by a propeller shaft to each rear wheel.   This special arrangement enables a light back axle to be provided without any massive parts in the centre; consequently such an axle will run on rough roads without the wheels losing contact with the ground, as the springs are not subject to reaction through the inertia of heavy central axle parts.

The bevel wheel of the drive is mounted upon a short sleeve, which carries the rear wheel itself, and the two drives are connected by an axle, giving all the advantages of a dead axle combined with a live bevel drive. It is owing to this construction that a specially designed frame, built on the lattice girder principle, can be utilised to obtain the low loading line or low body which is such a valuable advantage for this particular work.

The change speed is operated through a gate, which is carried direct on

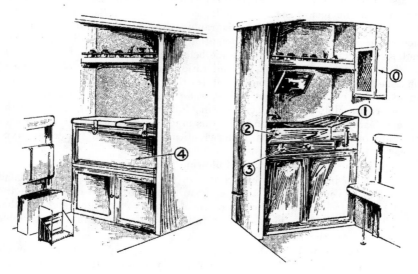

FIG. 3   FIG. 2.

the top of the gear box cover, with the control handle to the left of the driver. This enables speeds to be changed with facility even on the roughest roads.

One of the first equipments produced with this type of chassis was built in July, 1915, and has since been in use near Paris, and many of its shortcomings have been eliminated. The present outfit is fitted with a panelled teak body, not only elegant in appearance, but very practical for use in such climates as Mesopotamia, where this car is destined for.

The size of the body is 12ft. 9in. long, 7ft. wide, and 7ft. high, and this is divided into two compartments: 1, the photographic dark room: and 2, the room containing the X-ray apparatus.

The photographic dark room measures 3ft. 4in. long by 7ft. wide, and is practically a tabloid studio, but fitted with every arrangement to facilitate the work (Figs. 2 and 3). It is partially lead lined, that is, on the side towards the portable X-ray theatre, to protect the plates, etc., from the radiation of the tube. Water is obtained from a 30-gallon storage tank underneath, and this is pumped as required by a hand pump into a second smaller tank (0) fitted above the sink on one side. The sink (2) is fitted with a removable cover arranged to form a rocking table. Immediately under this a light-tight drawer (3) is provided, in which a partially developed or unfixed plate may be temporarily housed in the event of the operator having to open the door for any purpose. A special safe-light is provided above the sink, with easily adjusted control for either daylight or electric light. On the opposite side of the room are several bins (4) for chemicals and plates, and the top of these form a printing and plate-changing bench, also provided with a duplicated safe-light. Draining racks, nests for measuring glasses, and other necessary apparatus and racks for bottles are fitted round the walls. A folding seat is provided for the operator, and last, but not least, an electrically driven fan, fitted to a special flue, is provided to draw off tainted air from the room, fresh air being drawn in through special vents near the floor.

The apparatus room is 9ft. long by 7ft. wide, and the apparatus is so arranged in this room that radiography of the extremities can be carried out with a tube stand, and it is even possible, should the emergency occur, to erect the couch and radiograph the patient on the same. but I must admit that this latter is not working under ideal conditions. Every piece of apparatus has a special fitting to which it is secured by clamps and thumb buttons, but for additional safety a leather strap and metal buckle is fastened round each article, so that, however rough the travelling may be, the apparatus cannot suffer.

In addition there is the portable X-ray theatre. This measures 12ft. 9in. long by 10ft. 6in. deep by 9ft. high at back, and 6ft. 8in. high at front. A framework of poles and tie-rods is erected on the near side when the caravan is on the road, and these, together with the cover, are stored upon the roof. Having the poles erected, the tent canvas roof and sides are placed in position. The portion forming the roof and front is rolled down over the poles after the ends, which are provided, with openings have been attached to the frame. The canvas covering is of special material, 3-ply, and so thick and close in texture that light and water are absolutely excluded. In addition, a second light waterproofed canvas covering is provided for tropical climates. The theatre is lit by an electric lamp, which may be connected, if desired, to the foot switch. The material used for forming the cover of this tent is so efficient that X-ray work can be carried on inside even when there is brilliant sunshine outside.

I will now draw your attention to the electrical equipment.

The generator, which is situated on the exhaust side of the engine, is of special construction, and is driven by means of a Westinghouse noise rocker chain coupled to the main shaft of the engine, and is designed to give an output of 3 kilowatt or 20 amperes at 150 volts when the engine is running at 1,700 r.p.m. The rocker chain is disconnected when the car is running on the road, and is only connected when the generator is to be used, either for charging the battery of accumulators, or running the X-ray plant direct. When the engine is driving the generator the whole of the starting, running, and stopping can be carried out from the position of the main distribution board at the rear of the car. The generator is of light design, having a laminated field. It is provided with special protection against dust and dirt, and in addition has a fan on the shaft of the armature for cooling purposes. The windings are also protected by a condenser and lamp in

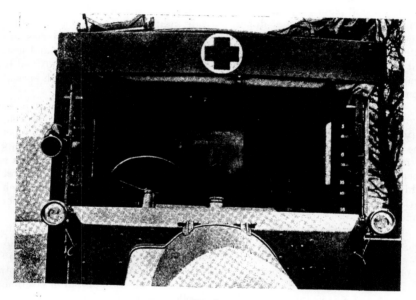

Fig. 4.

parallel to one another to prevent high-frequency surgings getting back to the machine.

A special battery of accumulators is fitted in two special cupboards at the back of the driver's cab (Fig. 4), and the doors of these cupboards are fitted with louvres to ensure perfect ventilation; by this arrangement no acid fumes can enter the car, and the whole battery is most accessible should it be necessary to give it attention. The battery is built up in special ebonite composition boxes, these being superior to celluloid because the latter material decomposes under the influence of heat; further, as the boxes chosen are unbreakable under ordinary conditions of handling, they are preferable to ebonite, and lead lined wood cases are prohibited on account of weight. Each cell is fitted with a float to indicate the level of the electrolyte. The accumulator battery consists of 38 2-compartment 4 volt units, making 76 cells in all of the sealed-in type. The capacity of each cell is 80 ampere hours (intermittent), or 10 amperes for 2½ hours, or 30 amperes for 5 minutes.

Therefore, the X-ray operator is provided with a supply of energy capable of undertaking the quickest work and the most difficult cases, for he has at his command 20 amperes at 150 volts from his generator, 30 amperes at 150 volts for 5 minutes from his battery of accumulators, or 50 amperes at 150 volts when running with generator and accumulators in parallel.

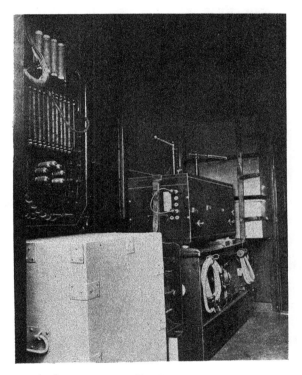

FIG. 5.

Now, so far as the X-ray outfit itself is concerned, this I consider may be open to a certain amount of criticism, not that it is inefficient in any way, but individual tastes vary in the selection of apparatus, and, as this outfit is for use at the front, it has been thought expedient to adopt in several instances, such as the couch, stereoscope, etc., the standard War Office equipment for field service, so that in case of necessity spares or renewals could be obtained locally.

Apart from this, the outfit is provided with a 16in. spark heavy discharge induction coil, built up in box form and fitted with a variable primary winding. The coil is mounted on a table on pneumatic buffers to provide against mechanical shock, and beneath the table are fitted three interrupters, a dipper mercury interrupter, a centrifugal mercury interrupter, and an electrolytic interrupter, together with the condenser, speed regulators, and a small interrupter selector switch-board. (Fig. 5.)

In order that the coil may be operated without moving it into the portable

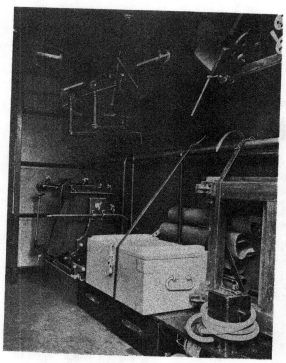

FIG. 6.

X-ray theatre, a portion of the side of the car is made to hinge upwards, and a distribution shelf for the valve tubes, milliammeter, spark gap, and rheophors is attached, and connection is established to the X-ray couch. Next to the coil is the Coolidge control outfit, fitted with a 12 volt accumulator of very large capacity. A further use has been made of this battery, and that is, for supplying the necessary current for the head, side, and tail lamps of the car, through a switch-board mounted on the dash. To change over from the lamps to the Coolidge connection, or to put the battery in series with the main one for charging, is the work of a moment.

On the same side of the car, at the end, is the switch-gear; this consists of a main distribution switch-board and a control switch-board for the primary circuit of the coil. The latter is provided with a transport case. The former is mounted on an iron pillar, on which it rotates, so that it can be manipulated either from inside the car or from the portable theatre. In the latter case a door at the side of the car is opened, when both switch-boards can face into the portable theatre with the Coolidge control to the left hand. So that up to the present all the apparatus remains and is used in the car. The only portions of the equipment that it is necessary to bring into the portable theatre are the couch, foot switch, and of course the tube, screen, etc., but none of the heavy gear.

On the opposite side of the room containing the apparatus is fitted the portable field service couch, a tube stand, and all the other necessary adjuncts for carrying out the best work, including localizers by screen and plate, protection aprons, gloves, face masks, etc., plate-holders, fluorescent and intensifying screens, plate recorders, in fact it is extraordinary how much one can pack away in a small space (Fig. 6).

At the end of the apparatus room are tube boxes in racks, for the equipment includes, in addition to the Coolidge tube, six tungsten target tubes and three valve tubes. On the inside of the roof is fitted the stereoscope, which can be used inverted in this position, and in addition a small portable viewing box is provided.

As one of the functions of this type of plant is to provide a powerful apparatus for use in any temporary hospital, or house, a means must be found for accomplishing this with the least amount of trouble. The plant has, therefore, been so arranged that the minimum number of pieces of apparatus are carried out into the building which is serving as the temporary hospital. It is only necessary to take the induction coil and its fittings, together with a trestle table, which is carried on the door of the car, the couch, and the small control switch-board; all the other apparatus, including the interrupters, remain in the car, and connection is established from the car to the temporary X-ray room in the hospital by special cable, which is wound on cable drums carried by the chauffeur's cab. One can, therefore, undertake radiography and radioscopy, and for that matter therapeutic treatment, as well, in the car itself, in the portable X-ray theatre, or in any hospital, house, or temporary building.

I should now like to mention how the plant is operated from the main distribution board (Fig. 7). The engine may be started by using the battery of accumulators for motoring the generator, in the same way as a self-starter on a motor car, and this is carried out by closing the D.P. switch on the left-hand side and the S.P. switch at the bottom, and slowly switching on the starter or automatic cut-out. The speed of the engine is controlled by a Bowden wire throttle control mounted beside the main switch-board, and below, near the floor, is an "on" and "off" switch for earthing the primary of the magneto and thereby stopping the engine, so that there is no necessity to leave the portable X-ray theatre, or in fact the vicinity of the switch-board, to start up the plant, to operate it, or to shut it down. The row of fuses on the top of the board control the interior and tent lights and ventilating fans, as well as the motors of the mechanical interrupters, and these are all supplied with energy by the accumulators. In the case of the interrupters this is very important in order that the speed may remain constant.

To charge the main accumulator battery, after ascertaining by means of a voltmeter switch that the voltage for charging is the correct one, close the S.P. switch at the bottom, the D.P. switch on the left hand side, and the

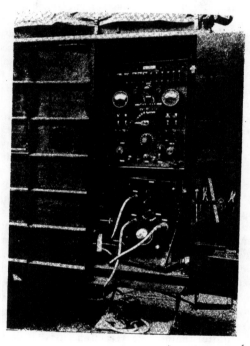

Fig. 7.

automatic cut-out. Beneath the automatic cut-out is a shunt regulator for regulating the output of the generator.

A regulator is provided for controlling the lights of the interior of the car, situated underneath the row of fuses.

When it is desired to operate the X-ray apparatus from the accumulators entirely, the left hand D.P. switch is closed, and the niphan socket on the left is connected to its plug, which is attached to the cable hanging behind the switch-board, but if the coil circuit is to be operated from the generator, then both D.P. switches are closed and the niphan socket on the right hand side is used.

Again, should it be desirable to parallel the generator and accumulator battery, then all switches must be closed and the automatic cut-out as well.

When paralleling generator and battery, care must be taken to keep the voltages equal under all conditions of load.

It will now be obvious that with this switch-board and plant one can obtain current in the following ways:—

1. Running the X-ray apparatus direct from the generator.

2. Running the X-ray apparatus direct from the accumulator battery.

3. Running the X-ray apparatus direct with the generator and accumulators in parallel.

4. Running the X-ray apparatus direct from the generator and at the same time charging the accumulator battery.

5. Running the generator for charging the accumulator battery only.

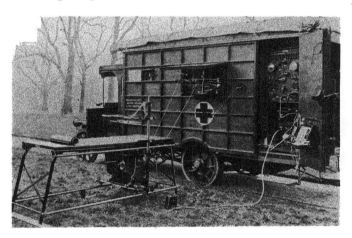

Fig. 8.

I have already mentioned that the Coolidge tube battery can be charged with the main battery, and there is provided at the side of the switch-board a small switch for cutting in or out these extra cells.

The connecting up of the various parts of the apparatus is next proceeded with, and this is carried out by means of the special cables provided. The induction coil and the foot switch are each connected by their respective plugs to the sockets on the control board, and the foot switch and main switch on the control board are in parallel, so that either can be used irrespective of the other. The other socket on the control board is connected by means of a triphan plug to the small distribution board for the interrupter.

There is, in addition, a regulating resistance in series with the primary of the induction coil, and an amperemeter. As has been previously mentioned, the induction coil is provided with a variable self-induction, and this can be altered by means of a plug contact in order to obtain the most suitable self-induction for the interrupter selected.

The small switch-board for the interrupters is provided so that the operator can change from one to another by simply changing over two switches, one controlling the motor circuits, and the other the coil circuits. All the plug connections are made non-reversible, with the exception of one on the control board, and this is left reversible, in order that the polarity of the primary and secondary circuits can be changed instantly if occasion requires.

This completes the primary connections, and the secondary or tube circuit is assembled by placing the high-tension distributing bracket in front of the coil, and connecting up the coil to the milliammeter, valve tube, and spark gap,

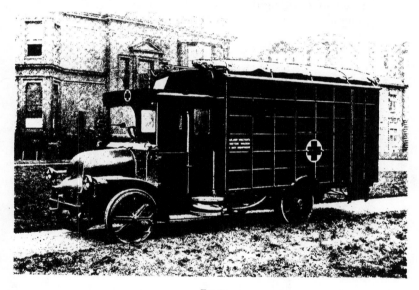

Fig. 9.

care being taken that the pole of the coil adjacent to the switch-boards is negative. This is somewhat important, as the Coolidge tube control is on this side.

The couch is erected in the portable theatre, a tube inserted in the tube box, and connected to the distributing bracket by the spring rheophors (Fig. 8).

If desirable, the 3-ply wooden top of the couch can be removed and an ordinary stretcher used in its place.

Everything is now ready to commence work. The engine and generator are running and the accumulator battery is charged. It is now only necessary to close the correct switches for motor and coil circuits, and the tube will then be excited by closing either the foot switch or the control switch. It will be noticed in working that as soon as the load of the induction coil comes on the voltage of the generator will fall; therefore, when regulating the coil rheostat, the shunt regulator should also be adjusted to maintain a constant voltage. In this outfit one great inconvenience is obviated, and that is, the speed of the mercury interrupters is kept constant by always running them from the main battery and not from the generator.

When using the Coolidge tube instead of an ordinary tube, the only alterations that have to be made are in the secondary circuit, and such connections are well known to all workers. These connections, as well as the Coolidge control, have been specially designed to fit in with the other modifications necessary in an outfit of this description.

I think you will agree that such a Mobile X-ray Unit affords exactly similar facilities to those available in the base hospitals, and when one considers the many temporary hospitals established in large private hotels and houses at home here and on all the fronts, without X-ray outfits of their own, its usefulness is at once recognised.

Many wonderful advances have been made on the surgical and medical side in the treatment of the wounded, but these have been more than equalled by the provision of such a vehicle and equipment, and, further, it proves that the ways and means are available in this country to meet any possible requirements of the Army Medical Corps or allied branches.

The possibilities of the utility of such a unit in normal times for mining districts, scattered areas, and so forth, are by no means small, but sufficient is the task which confronts us now, and we can return to the other uses at a more opportune time.

THREE CASES OF INTEREST, INCLUDING SPASTIC PARALYSIS OF DELTOID MUSCLES, LEUCOPLAKIA, and LAGOPHTHALMUS.

By J. Delpratt Harris, M.D., M.R.C.S.

Senior Medical Officer in Charge of the Electrical Department, Royal Devon and Exeter Hospital; Late Surgeon in Charge of Five Sections V.A.D. War Hospitals, as Radiographer.

The following three cases seen of interest as giving hints for treatment. The cases, although hardly rare, do not occur every day. They include—:

A case of spastic paralysis, affecting both deltoid muscles in an infant.

A case of leucoplakia affecting the buccal and labial mucous membrane.

A case of lagophthalmus, ending in cure.

Spastic Paralysis, Affecting both Deltoid Muscles in an Infant.

A child of nine months was brought to the Royal Devon and Exeter Hospital with a very indefinite history. The reason of its being brought was that there was "something the matter" with its arms. Inspection showed that the arms could not be approximated to the trunk without causing pain. This condition, although bilateral, was worst on the right side. Dislocation seemed a likely cause of such a condition, and the case was referred to the Electrical Department for screening, or radiography, if thought necessary.

Screening at such an early age was not found very helpful, and a radiograph was attempted, but the child could not be kept sufficiently still for a good plate, so a second was made under an anaesthetic. It was clear, however, from the second plate that no bony displacement had taken place, and the screen examination agreed.

It was christened a case of congenital deformity of the shoulder joint, possibly akin to rickets.

Before the case had entirely faded from memory, I was fortunate in securing a copy of Duchenne's works, translated by the Sydenham Society. At page 318 a paragraph occurs which in few words seems to put this case in a fresh light, and explain the symptoms recorded.

The paragraph is as follows:—

"*Contracture of the Deltoid.*—The deltoid, it is well known, is the chief elevator of the arm. It separates the arm from the trunk either directly outwards by its middle third, or forwards and inwards by its front third, or backwards and inwards by its hinder third. It is not generally known that an isolated contraction of this muscle may cause a faulty position of the scapula.

"While the upper limb is separated from the trunk by the contraction of the deltoid it weighs upon the outer angle of the scapula, producing in that bone (a) a tilting movement whereby the acromion is depressed, while the lower angle moves up and towards the middle line ; and (b) a rotation of the bone on an imaginary axis passing through the outer angle, so that the spinal edge is separated from the chest wall, and a gutter of varying depth is formed between the edge and the corresponding part of the thorax.

"I have seen one case of contracture *en masse* of the deltoid in which the arm was always out from the trunk and the scapula was in the faulty position just described.

"Without doubt contracture is very seldom limited to the deltoid."

He then relates a case in which the subscapularis shared the contracture with the front third of the deltoid. He next draws attention to the similarity of the posture of the arm in wasting of the serratus magnus. He adds. "however, the two conditions cannot be confounded, for in palsy of the serratus the deformity of the scapula occurs *only when the arm is raised*, while in contracture of the deltoid it is present with the arm at rest, and lessens or vanishes when it is raised."

With these helps to diagnosis it should not be difficult in any future case to come to a right decision. But, although I had the help of the standard works on medicine, I could find no description of a similar condition. And even in Duchenne's description nothing is mentioned of the condition ever being bilateral. Certainly in this case now reported it was practically bilateral, although the right side was more advanced than the left. Duchenne seldom wrote of the pathology of his cases, but one may consider it probable that in such an instance the trouble was in the upper motor neuron on both sides.

The case cannot, at present, be further traced ; but should it be again seen it would be of great interest to observe whether the condition had spread to other muscles.

As Duchenne speaks of the condition being rare, it seems desirable this case should be placed on record, for no other similar case has presented itself at this hospital during ten years.

Buccal and Labial Leucoplakia.

A. C., aged 55, was made an in-patient on December 30th, 1915, for a sore mouth. On inspection, a large proportion of the buccal and labial mucous membrane was found of a whitish colour. The white portions were raised above the general level ; there were outlying portions, and the larger raised parts had filiform papillæ projecting from them. These appearances were mostly confined to the lower lip, from one corner to the other, but those on the buccal mucous membrane extended to the limit of the alveolar reflection. The case was christened leucoplakia, and sent to the Electrical Department. Here the patient was treated with X rays for about five months, for he seemed to be getting better ; but, by May 11th, the progress was so slow it was determined to try the effect of CO_2 snow, and from May 15th till October 26th he received that treatment weekly, for the surface was still so large that it was possible to vary the site of application each time.

He at once began to show distinct signs of improvement, until at last but a small white patch could be found on the buccal mucous membrane on the left side.

He was inspected on January 4th, and treated finally : seen again on February 15th and found cured.

This case seems of interest, for although so many remedies have been suggested to relieve this condition, CO_2 is not among them in such books as I have access to. In this case the result has been so very satisfactory that a second application to a given spot was never required. The principal difficulty was in the application, for the patient's warm breath melted the CO_2 very quickly, also folds of mucous membrane intervened in places.

No doubt the leucoplakia was of a superficial type, and there was no deep seated swelling or tumour to suggest epithelioma. The length of time the CO_2 was applied was forty-five seconds. The man was a smoker, but denied excessive use of it, and gave it up on hearing that his condition was serious.

Lagophthalmus.

In October, 1917, I was consulted by Mrs. H. G. for a condition of lagophthalmus on the left side. The condition had then only lately supervened, and no known cause existed, unless it were neuritis following excision of a sebaceous cyst in the forehead. The condition was fairly complete, and the white of the eye could be seen well above the sclero-corneal junction when looking straight ahead. The electrical reactions showed no alteration in the muscles innervated by the facial, and a very mild application of faradism at the outer commisure of the lids caused complete spasm of both upper and lower muscle-bundles of orbicularis with closure of the lids. The intrinsic muscles of the orbit were all active, with the supposed exception of the levator palpebræ superioris.

As this muscle is innervated by a branch of the third nerve, it would explain why lagophthalmus existed to a marked degree, although the muscles supplied by the facial were in normal condition.

As the patient occupied a prominent position in the town she resided in, naturally she greatly desired relief from a condition that could not fail to attract attention, and became accentuated with any excitement.

I took the opportunity of reading the condition up in works on the eye and general medicine, and, of course, "Quain's Dictionary." But whilst the condition is noted in almost every work, the treatment is dismissed by a sentence to the effect that it must be treated on general principles of paralysed muscles.

But in this case it was not at all certain a paralysed muscle existed. It would explain the symptoms equally well if one suggested a spastic condition of the levator palpebræ superioris, and explain the closing of the lid by the orbicularis overcoming temporarily the spastic contraction, bringing the condition into line with the spastic contraction of internal rectus in hypermetropic strabismus.

With these thoughts in my mind I therefore treated this case for three months with mild galvanism as a sedative.

At the end of that time faradism was commenced. It was noted that the streak of sclerotic above the cornea was certainly narrower when looking straight ahead. It was noted that the patient fancied herself better able to look down after receiving faradism on the closed lid; this attitude was therefore carefully adopted, and persisted in for over one year.

In April, 1919, her condition was eminently satisfactory, and whereas she used to have to remember not to look at things below her line of sight, now, in order to show the lagophthalmus, she has to look down as far as possible, for usually it appears quite all right.

For the future, therefore, our text-books should draw attention to two separate forms of paralysis causing lagophthalmus, namely, paralysis, flaccid in character, affecting the orbicularis supplied by the facial nerve, and spastic paralysis of the levator palpebra superioris, supplied by the third nerve. Also, after a preliminary course of treatment by galvanism, faradism applied through the closed lid may give a most gratifying result.

BRITISH ASSOCIATION OF RADIOLOGY AND PHYSIOTHERAPY.

In the next number of the ARCHIVES will be published the complete list of those who, up to the date of publication, have been elected to membership of the British Association of Radiology and Physiotherapy.

A general meeting of the latter will be held at a later date. At this meeting, the time and place of which will be notified to each member, matters of importance concerning the future of the Association will be discussed.

Below will be found the Report of the Special Board for Medicine, at Cambridge, upon a proposal to establish a Diploma in Medical Radiology and Electrology. This has already been communicated to the Senate.

"Report of the Special Board for Medicine upon a proposal to establish a Diploma in Medical Radiology and Electrology in the University.

20 *May,* 1919,

"The SPECIAL BOARD FOR MEDICINE beg leave to present the following Report to the Vice-Chancellor for communication to the Senate :

"The Board have had under their consideration a memorandum referred to them by the Council of the Senate concerning a proposal for the establishment of a Diploma in Medical Radiology and Electrology in the University. In this Memorandum, sent to the Vice-Chancellor on 26 May, 1917, by Dr. A. E. Barclay of Manchester, on behalf of a Committee composed of some of the leading English radiologists, attention is specially drawn to the lack of teaching in Medical Radiology and Electrology, to the urgent need of sufficient tests of the proficiency of candidates in the subjects, and to the many scientific problems calling for investigation in connection with the diagnosis and treatment of disease in this new but important branch of Medicine. Professorships and Lectureships in Medical Radiology have been established in many Universities abroad, and qualifying examinations in the subject have been held for several years, but in England there is as yet no organised teaching or examination in the subject. The Board are of opinion that the establishment of a Diploma in Medical Radiology and Electrology by the University would not only be of service to the community by raising the standard of practice but would also lead to the advancement of teaching and research in this branch of Medicine.

" The Board are of opinion that, although it would be inadvisable to offer a degree, a diploma, specifying the qualification of the holder for official posts in Radiology and Electrology at home or other parts of the British Empire, might well be awarded to those who undergo a satisfactory course of training, part at least of which should be in this University, and satisfy the examiners either by written, practical, clinical and viva voce examinations, or in the case of qualified medical men by Thesis or Published work, that they have special knowledge of Radiology and Electrology. They are helped to the conclusion that a diploma is preferable by the following considerations: (*a*) The medical curriculum being already overladen it would be impossible to introduce such an important and extensive group of subjects as that under consideration into the fourth or fifth year of study of the medical student; (*b*) that only the trained medical man, relieved of the burden of a 'qualifying' examination, is in a position to derive full benefit from so special a course of study.

" Moreover the Board consider that the above group of subjects can be studied with the most fruitful results by mature students who have already received some preliminary training in Physics, Anatomy, Physiology, Pathology, and other branches of scientific and practical medicine and surgery, and that, whilst much of the purely technical work can well be carried out by skilled photographic and electrotechnical expert assistants, only medical men who have received special training in Physics and Practical Radiology, Electrotherapy, and Electrology generally, are in a position to understand and foresee not only the development of their application to diagnosis and treatment, but also their limitations and dangers. After conferring with the Committee of the British Association of Radiology and Physiotherapy, and in consultation with them, the Board have framed a scheme of instruction and examination for the proposed Diploma, believing, as they do, that Hospital authorities would soon come to recognise such a Diploma as a qualification to be held by all medical men intending to practise Radiology and Electrotherapy, and by candidates for appointments in Public Institutions where these methods of diagnosis and treatment are employed.

" In the present crippled state of the University Treasury, the financial aspect of the question has naturally received the most careful attention of the Board, who have however been enabled to arrive at a favourable decision in this matter by a liberal contribution by one of our medical graduates of the sum of £1000 towards the payment of teaching and examination expenses likely to be incurred during the first five years when the examination may not be self-supporting. With the above reserve it will certainly not be necessary to appeal to the University Chest.

" Having regard to the importance of the subject, to the facilities for instruction and research in Physics, Physiology, Anatomy, Histology and Morbid Anatomy, and to the financial support already assured to the University, the Board feel justified in recommending the University to undertake the work of preparing candidates, and to organise and carry out the examinations for a Diploma in Radiology and Electrology. The University is able to provide instruction in the subjects of Part I and most of those in Part II.

" The Board accordingly recommend:

" 1. That a Diploma in Medical Radiology and Electrology be established.

" 2. That a Committee on Medical Radiology and Electrology, hereinafter called the Committee, be appointed by the State Medicine Syndicate; the Committee to consist of the Regius Professor of Physic, the Cavendish Professor of Experimental Physics and nine other members, of whom not less than six shall be members of the Syndicate; and that of the nine members three retire in rotation on the thirty-first day of December in every year, their places being supplied by three members appointed by the Syndicate before the end of full term in the preceding Michaelmas Term and that four members form a quorum.

" 3. That it be the duty of the Committee to fix the number of Examiners in each year; to nominate them for election by the Senate: to fix and announce to the Senate in the Easter Term of each year the time for the Examination or Examinations in the ensuing academical year; to determine, subject to the approval of the State Medicine Syndicate, the payment to the Examiners; to draw up and publish from time to time schedules defining the range and details of the subjects of the Examination; to recognise courses of study and places for clinical instruction and to perform such other duties as may be assigned to them by the Senate.

" 4.   That the Committee be required to make an annual Report to the State Medicine Syndicate for communication to the Senate.

" 5.   That a candidate for the diploma shall either (a) present himself for examina- tion or (b) submit for the approval of the Special Board for Medicine a dissertation. The dissertation may include or consist of any work already published by the candidate.

" 6.   That an Examination for the Diploma in Medical Radiology and Electrology be held once or, if the State Medicine Syndicate think fit, twice in the year.

" 7.   That the Examination be in two Parts: that the subjects in Part I be (a) Physics and (b) Electrotechnics; in Part II, (a) Radiology (including Radiography and Radiotherapy), and (b) Electrology (including Electrodiagnosis and Electrotherapy); and that in each subject there be at least one paper and a practical or a clinical examination.

" 8·   That Part I be open to candidates who hold a recognised Medical qualification and who produce evidence that after qualification they have for three months at least attended a course of lectures and of practical instruction recognised by the Committee both in Physics and in Electrotechnics: that Part II be open to candidates who are at the time of entering for the Examination duly qualified medical practitioners of not less than one year's standing, have attended a course of lectures on Radiology and Electrology for at least three months and have had at least six months' clinical experience and instruction in the electrical department of a Hospital recognised by the Committee.   The course of lectures may be attended during the period of clinical instruction in the elec- trical department of a 'recognised Hospital.'

" 9.   That a candidate who has passed both Parts of the Examination to the satisfaction of the Examiners be entitled to a Diploma testifying to his knowledge of Radiology and Electrology in the following form:

Know all men by these presents that   hath been duly examined by   the Examiners on that behalf appointed by the Chancellor, Masters and Scholars of the University of Cambridge and hath approved himself to the Examiners by his KNOWLEDGE AND SKILL IN MEDICAL RADIOLOGY AND ELECTROLOGY to wit the diagnosis and treatment of disease by methods founded on clincal observations combined with radiological and electrological research In Testimony whereof the Vice-Chancellor of the said University by the authority of the said Chancellor Masters and Scholars hath hereto set his hand and seal the   day of   one thousand nine hundred and

(LS)   A.B. Vice-Chancellor.

" 10.   That candidates who present themselves for examination be required to pay fees, to be fixed at the discretion of the Committee, subject to the approval of the State Medicine Syndicate.

" 11.   That Candidates for either part of the Examination be required to send in their names to the Registrary, together with the requisite certificates, not less than three weeks before the day fixed for the beginning of the Examination, and that the fee be paid at the same time.

" 12.   That it shall be the duty of the Registrary to examine the certificates and to ascertain that no one is improperly admitted to the Examination.

" 13.   That a candidate who wishes to proceed to the Diploma under Regulation 5 (b) shall be required to send to the Registrary with his dissertation certificates (a) that he has been qualified for not less than ten years as a medical practitioner and (b) has been engaged for not less than five years in the practice of medical radiology and electrology in the Electrical Department of a public Hospital, the nature of such practice to be approved in each case by the Committee.

"14.   That the certificates together with the dissertation submitted by the Candidate shall be sent by the Registrary, in the first instance, to the Special Board for Medicine who shall transmit it to the Committee, who if they approve the nature of the clinical practice required under Regulation 13 (*b*) shall appoint two or more Referees to examine the work submitted by the Candidate, to examine the Candidate, if it be thought necessary, on the subject of his work either orally or otherwise, and to report thereon to the Committee.

"15.   That every candidate on sending in his dissertation shall pay to the Registrary a fee of ten guineas which shall be returned to him if the certificates of clinical practice required under Regulation 13 (*b*) be not approved by the Committee.

"16.   That, if the Committee after considering the reports of the Referees approve the dissertation submitted by the Candidate, they shall recommend to the Special Board of Medicine that the Diploma be granted to him, and shall send with their recommendation the reports of the Referees upon which their recommendation is based.

"17.   That a candidate whose work is approved by the Special Board for Medicine on the recommendation of the Committee shall be entitled to receive a Diploma in the following terms :

Know all men by these presents that   whose dissertation has been duly examined by the Referees in that behalf appointed by the Committee on Radiology and Electrology of the University of Cambridge has approved himself to that Committee and to the Special Board for Medicine of the said University by his KNOWLEDGE OF RADIOLOGY AND ELECTROLOGY and especially in the following branches thereof to wit   In Testimony whereof the Vice-Chancellor of the said University by the authority of the Chancellor Masters and Scholars hath hereto set his hand and seal the   day of   .   one thousand nine hundred and

(LS)

                                                              A.B. Vice-Chancellor.

"18.   That every Candidate before receiving a Diploma under Regulation 5 (*b*) shall deposit in the Library of the Medical School a copy of his dissertation.

"19.   That in the first instance the scheme for the Diploma be established for five years only.

"If the foregoing Regulations for a Diploma in Medical Radiology and Electrology be approved, the Special Board for Medicine are prepared to recommend to the Senate that the number of Members of the State Medicine Syndicate should be increased from fifteen to eighteen.

"This report of the Special Board for Medicine has been considered by the State Medicine Syndicate and has been approved by them.

"G. SIMS WOODHEAD, *Chairman.*	G. H. F. NUTTALL.
"H. K. ANDERSON.	F. G. HOPKINS.
"CLIFFORD ALLBUTT.	GEO. E. WHERRY.
"J. B. BRADBURY.	F. W. DOOTSON.
"L. COBBETT.	T. G. BEDFORD.
"G. S. GRAHAM-SMITH.	S. W. COLE."
"J. N. LANGLEY.	

NOTES AND ABSTRACTS.

Simultaneous Exposure of a Plate and Bromide Paper.—TOUSSAINT (*Jour. de Radiol. et d'Elect.*, Dec., 1918, p. 128).—The method depends on the fact that with a tube (Benoist 6 penetration) the exposure of a plate is the same as bromide paper + an intensifying screen.

All these are put in the casette, the rays passing through the plate before reaching the bromide paper and its intensifying screen.

R. W. A. S.

Method for the Colouring of Lamps.—LAILLY (*Jour. de Radiol. et d'Elect.*, Dec., 1918 p. 127).—The colouring of electric bulbs is obtained by the following formula :—

Alcohol - - - - 100 gram.
Collodion (1 in 100) - - 100 ,,
Colouring matter (methylene
    blue or fuchsin) - - q.s.

If lumpy, add ether ; if too liquid, allow to evaporate a little.   R. W. A. S.

An Electromyographic Study of Chorea.—S. COBB (*Bull. of The Johns Hopkins Hosp.*, Feb., 1919, p. 35, with 4 tracings).—The author's conclusions are as follows :—

Choreiform movements give an electromyogram similar to that of a short, normal, voluntary muscular contraction.

The inability to maintain voluntary contraction is clearly shown in the electromyograms.

Weakness of muscular contraction is shown electromyographically by the lessened electrical discharge.   R. W. A. S.

Congenital Absence of Left Lung.—A. H. TEBBUTT (*Med. Jour. of Australia*, Nov. 23rd, 1918, p. 450).—The condition found at the autopsy was as follows: The right lung was bulky, and had apparently pushed the heart to the left side. There was no vestige of a left lung, the left side of thorax being occupied by the heart, a distended pericardial sac and pericardial adhesions. The upper and middle lobes of the right lung were partially subdivided by vertical furrows and the lower lobe by a transverse furrow.   R. W. A. S.

The Practical Use of the Wheatstone Stereoscope.—H. C. SNOOK (*Amer. Jour. of Roent.*, Jan., 1919, pp. 39-47, with Figs. and table).—The various fallacies in the use of this stereoscope are fully described, and Snook states that the conditions of correct vision for the patient right side up require that the two plates be placed in the view boxes with their glass sides "out," the plate with the right hand shift in the right hand view box, and similarly for the left hand shift, with the eye plate distance the same as the focal plate distance, and with the lines of movement of the tube between exposures on each plate horizontally parallel to each other.

An interesting table is given showing the resulting views obtained by looking at the plates in other combinations than the above.

R. W. A. S.

RADIO-DIAGNOSIS.

The Diagnosis of Ureteral Calculi.—D. N. EISENDRATH (*Surg., Gynec., and Obstet.*, Nov., 1918, pp. 461 to 468, with 17 Figs. and 2 radiographs).—In a paper which contains the notes and findings of several interesting renal and ureter cases, and which shows the difficulties that are met with in many of these cases in making a correct diagnosis, the author states that the clinical history cannot be absolutely relied upon to make a diagnosis of ureteral calculus as there are many other conditions giving rise to ureteral colic which must be excluded.

The presence of a shadow along the course of the ureter does not necessarily mean a calculus. In his opinion, the three best methods to determine whether the shadow lies within or without the ureter are, the X-ray catheter, ureterography, and stereo-radiography, with an opaque catheter *in situ*. The last named he considers to be the most reliable, and should be employed if possible in every case. Kuemmel's method of intensification of a weak shadow, by allowing some of the opaque solution to be deposited on the surface of the calculus, is also warmly recommended in doubtful cases.   R. W. A. S.

PUBLICATIONS RECEIVED.

Book.

United States Army X-ray Manual. Authorised by the Surgeon - General of the Army. Prepared under the Direction of the Division of Roentgenology. London: H. K. Lewis & Co., Ltd. New York: P. B. Hoeber. 18s. net.

Journals.

Archives d'Electricité Médicale et de Physiothérapie, May, 1919.

American Journal of Electrotherapeutics and Radiology, Nov., 1918.

American Journal of Roentgenology, April-May, 1919.

British Journal of Dermatology and Syphilis, Jan.-Mar., 1919.

Bulletin of the Johns Hopkins Hospital, May, 1919.

Bulletin et Memoirs de la Société de Radiologie medicale de France, April-May, 1919.

Gaceta Médica Catalana, April 30th, May 15th, 31st, 1919.

Hospitalstidende, April 23rd, 30th; May 7th, 14th, 21st, 28th, 1919.

Journals—*continued.*

Il Policlinico, May 15th, 1919.

Journal of Cutaneous Diseases, April, 1919.

Journal of the Röntgen Society, April, 1919.

Medical Journal of Australia, Feb. 1st, 15th, 22nd; Mar., 1st, 8th, 22nd; April 5th, 12th, 1919.

Medical World, Mar. 28th, 1919.

Modern Medicine, May, 1919.

New York Medical Journal, April 26th; May 3rd, 10th, 17th, 24th, 1919.

New York State Journal of Medicine, May, 1919.

Norsk Mag. for Læger, April, May, 1919.

Proceedings of the Royal Society of Medicine, April-May., 1919.

Quarterly Journal of Medicine, April, 1919.

Rivista Italiana di Neuropatologia, Psichiatria ed Elettrotherapia, April, 1919.

Surgery, Gynæcology, and Obstetrics, May, 1919.

Ugeskrift for Læger, May 8th, 15th, 22nd, 29th, 1919.

War Medicine, Feb., Mar., 1919.

NOTICES.

ARCHIVES OF RADIOLOGY AND ELECTROTHERAPY is published monthly.

The index for each volume, which ends with the May number, is supplied with the June number of each year.

Communications to the Editors should be addressed to "ROBERT KNOX, M.D., 38, Harley Street, W. 1."

Communications and illustrations from American contributors may be sent to Messrs. REBMAN COMPANY, 141-145, West Thirty-sixth Street, New York City.

All radiographs and photographs must be originals, and must not have been previously published. Drawings should be supplied on separate paper.

Owing to the scarcity of paper the Publishers are reluctantly compelled—as a temporary war measure—to reduce the number of free reprints of Papers to twenty-five.

Annual Subscriptions, payable in advance, 30/- including postage. Single copies, 3/- (postage 2d.) Single numbers and back numbers can be supplied on application.

Vol. XXIV—No. 2   JULY. 1919.   No. 228

ARCHIVES OF RADIOLOGY AND ELECTROTHERAPY

THE OFFICIAL ORGAN OF THE

BRITISH ASSOCIATION OF RADIOLOGY AND PHYSIOTHERAPY

Editors.

ROBERT KNOX, M.D., Hon. Radiographer, King's College Hospital.
E. P. CUMBERBATCH, B.M., M.R.C.P., Medical Officer in Charge. Electrical Department, St. Bartholomew's Hospital.
SIDNEY RUSS, D.Sc., Physicist to the Middlesex Hospital.

IN COLLABORATION WITH

A. E. BARCLAY (Manchester); BELOT (Paris); H. MARTIN BERRY (London); W. H. BRAGG (London): N. BURKE (Woodhall Spa); J. BURNET (Edinburgh); W. J. S. BYTHELL (Manchester); J. T. CASE (Battle Creek, U.S.A.); A. ST. GEORGE CAULFEILD (London); H. A. COLWELL (London); FOVEAU DE COURMELLES (Paris); GUNZBURG (Antwerp); HALL-EDWARDS (Birmingham); HARET (Paris): HAUCHAMPS (Brussels): F. HERNAMAN-JOHNSON (London): W. F. HIGGINS (Teddington); THURSTAN HOLLAND (Liverpool); HURST (London); KLYNENS (Antwerp): LAQUERRIERE (Paris); LAZARUS-BARLOW (London); LEDUC (Nantes); ALEXANDER MACKAY (Edinburgh); REGINALD MORTON (London); HARRISON ORTON (London); W. OVEREND (St. Leonards-on-Sea); PFAHLER (Philadelphia); C. E. S. PHILLIPS (London); GEORGE PIRIE (Dundee): HOWARD PIRIE (Montreal): A. W. PORTER (London); R. W. A. SALMOND (London); WERTHEIM SALOMONSON (Amsterdam); S. SLOAN (Glasgow): SOMERVILLE (Glasgow); W. C. STEVENSON (Dublin); W. J. TURRELL (Oxford): HUGH WALSHAM (London); ROBT. WILSON (Montreal).

THE EXAMINATION OF THE LIVER, GALL BLADDER, AND BILE DUCTS.

By ROBERT KNOX.

(A portion of this paper was read at a meeting of the Electrotherapeutic Section of the Royal Society of Medicine, held in April, 1919, and formed part of a discussion on the Radiography of Gall Stones.)

THE value of a correct diagnosis of the presence of gall stones in the gall bladder or bile ducts is very great. The differential diagnosis between a condition of gall stones and conditions which give rise to similar symptoms is very difficult. In a consideration of lesions on the right side of the upper abdomen, there are so many structures situated in this region which may give rise to perplexing symptoms, that any method of examination likely to aid in the differential diagnosis is worth any trouble its execution may entail. The X-ray examination of the liver and structures in its vicinity is sometimes extremely useful, and if the percentage of accurate diagnoses can be increased, the value of the method will rise proportionally to the increase in the percentage of accuracy. It is, therefore, essential that all steps should be taken to ensure the proper carrying out of the technique.   It is also imperative that the radiologist should be conversant with the anatomy of the region, and that he should have a sound working knowledge of clinical medicine ; with these should be coupled a familiarity with the radiogram and its interpretation.

An exhaustive description of the radiography of the liver, and the differential diagnosis of the conditions met with in the course of the examination of many hundreds of cases, would occupy too great a space.   It is therefore necessary to dismiss this part of the paper with a brief reference only.   The detailed description of lesions of the liver comes in more appropriately in the diagnosis of thoracic and abdominal conditions.   All that is necessary at present is to call attention to the value of radiography in the diagnosis of liver conditions, apart from the lesions involving the gall bladder and bile ducts.

A review of the literature of the radiography of the liver, gall bladder, and bile ducts is instructive ; it reveals a gradual conversion of radiologists from an attitude of almost sceptical indifference to one of overweening confidence in the conviction that gall stones may be diagnosed in a very large percentage of the cases examined.   This percentage rises as high as between 80 to 90 per cent. with a number of workers and falls as low as 5 to 10 per cent. with others.   A diversity so great requires careful consideration before a decision can be arrived at regarding the value of radiography in the diagnosis of the presence of gall stones.

It is obvious that there must be an explanation of this great difference in opinion.   It may be largely explained by a difference in the technique employed by various workers and the importance they attach to the exhibition of doubtful shadows.   The technique is readily standardised, so this should offer no serious obstacle to an understanding of the value in the future. Critical workers refuse to admit a doubtful shadow as having any value in diagnosis; this is too positive a position to assume, since the demonstration of a doubtful shadow may be of considerable value, in that it may lead to further investigation.   It should not be taken as an indication for operation when clinical signs and symptoms do not support the suggested diagnosis. A negative radiographic report is of no value, because it is not possible to demonstrate all cases of gall stones, and we have the authoritative statement of C. H. Mayo "largely to depend upon radiographic evidence, as now developed, would be to step back twelve years in the advance of gall bladder and bile duct surgery and diagnosis."

A careful study of the doubtful shadow is of value if for no other reason than that it encourages research, and stimulates the observer to obtain better results in order that a more positive opinion may be expressed.   The observation of, and the recording of all doubtful shadows must be of value when operative measures are afterwards employed, because then the findings of radiography may be compared with what is found at the operation.   In this way valuable aids to diagnosis may be acquired.   Until quite recently the writer, along with the majority of workers, was sceptical regarding the value of radiography in the diagnosis of gall stones. During many years of observations only a few cases had been met with which could be positively diagnosed as gall stones. The recorded observations of workers in various parts of the world, notably Thurstan Holland in England, Ledoux Lebard in France, Carmen and Miller, Leonard and George and J. T. Case in America, and MacLeod of Shanghai, gave cause for thought, and led to a careful study of the literature of the subject, the technique employed, and a critical examination of the published radiograms. This was followed by experimental work with calculi, comparisons of densities of tissues, absorption of radiations, and particularly an enquiry into the photographic processes employed.

The investigations were carried out under the following headings —

(1) Anatomical considerations.
(2) Pathology of gall stones, classification, and chemical composition.
(3) Experimental investigation on absorption coefficients of gall stones and surrounding tissues.
(4) Radiographic appearance of gall stones.
(5) Technique of the examination.
(6) Situations in which gall stones may be found.
(7) Differential diagnosis.
(8) The pathological gall bladder.
(9) Record of cases.
(10) Résumé of the literature and general conclusions.

Anatomical Considerations.

A survey of the under surface of the liver and the structures in relation to it will be helpful when the exact position and nature of a shadow in the region has to be determined. Cross section plates of anatomical dissections are very valuable, because then it is possible to make out with a fair degree of accuracy the exact position of the gall bladder and the bile ducts, and their depth from the anterior, posterior, or lateral walls. The direction of the ducts, and particularly the common bile duct, will be appreciated when these cross sectional plates are studied. The anatomical descriptions of the gall bladder and bile ducts with the organs in relation to them are given briefly.

The gall bladder is roughly 7 to 10 cm. long by 2 to 5 cm. wide, it is widest at the fundus, and tapers down to about 2 cm. at the neck. It is described as having a fundus, a body, and a neck. The cystic duct is continued downwards from the neck, and passes to join the hepatic ducts; these form the common bile duct.

RELATIONS OF THE GALL BLADDER—The body of the gall bladder is in relation by its upper surface with the liver, by its under surface with the commencement of the transverse colon, and further back with the upper end of the descending portion of the duodenum, but sometimes with the inferior portion of the duodenum or the pyloric end of the stomach.

The fundus is completely invested by peritoneum; it is in relation in front with the abdominal parietes immediately below the ninth costal cartilage, behind with the transverse colon.

The neck is narrow, and curves upon itself like the letter S; at its point of connection with the cystic duct it presents a well marked constriction.

THE CYSTIC DUCT.—The cystic duct, about 4 cm. long, runs backwards and downwards and to the left from the neck of the gall bladder, and joins the hepatic ducts to form the common bile duct.

THE COMMON BILE DUCT is formed by the junction of the cystic and hepatic ducts. It is about 7·5 cm. long and of the diameter of a goose quill. It descends along the right border of the lesser omentum behind the superior portion of the duodenum, in front of the portal vein and to the right of the hepatic artery; it then runs in a groove near the right border of the posterior surface of the head of the pancreas; here it is situated in front of the inferior vena cava and is occasionally completely embedded in the substance of the pancreas. It opens in the medial side of the descending portion of the duodenum, a little below its middle, about 7 to 10 cm. from the pylorus.

The following anatomical figures are given to facilitate the visualisation of the position of the gall bladder and the bile ducts. The source from which they come is acknowledged beneath each figure—the value of a careful study of the figures cannot be over-estimated.

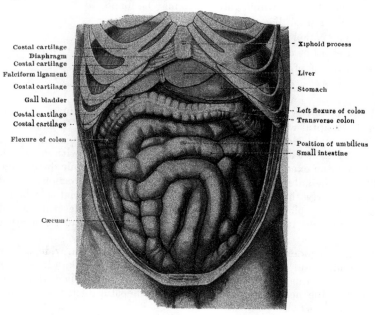

(*Cunningham's Anatomy*)

FIG. 1.—The abdominal viscera, after removal of the great omentum. Note the position of the gall bladder and its relationship to surrounding structures, and the very small superficial area presented in the normal subject.

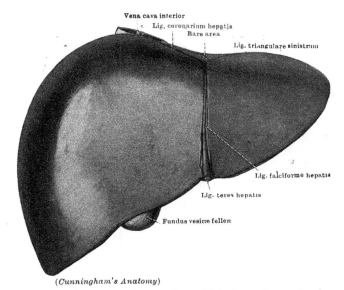

Vena cava inferior

Lig. coronarium hepatis

Bare area

Lig. triangulare sinistrum

Lig. falciforme hepatis

Lig. teres hepatis

Fundus vesicæ felleæ

(*Cunningham's Anatomy*)

Fig. 2.—The liver viewed from the front. Note the small area of surface presented by the gall bladder below the liver border.

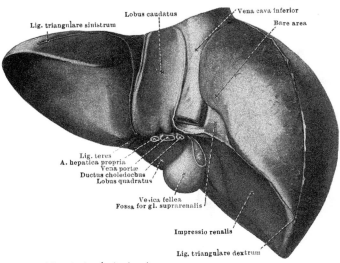

Lobus caudatus

Vena cava inferior

Bare area

Lig. triangulare sinistrum

Lig. teres

A. hepatica propria

Vena portæ

Ductus choledochus

Lobus quadratus

Vesica fellea

Fossa for gl. suprarenalis

Impressio renalis

Lig. triangulare dextrum

(*Cunningham's Anatomy*)

Fig. 3.—The liver viewed from behind, showing the position of the gall bladdeer and the area it occupies on the under surface of the liver. The figure shows clearly the relative positions of the gall bladder and the ducts.

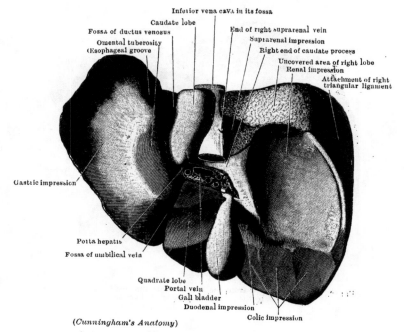

(*Cunningham's Anatomy*)

FIG. 4.—Inferior surface of the liver.

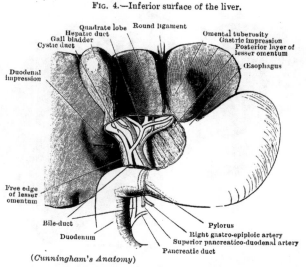

(*Cunningham's Anatomy*)

FIG. 5.—Structures between the layers of the lesser omentum, showing the relations of the gall bladder, cystic, hepatic and common bile duct to the duodenum, etc.

* Gall Stones (Biliary Calculi).

These are of frequent occurrence, especially in people past middle age, and in those of sedentary habits, but they may occur at any age. They occur more frequently in the female, and are formed in the gall bladder either by a process of crystallisation or merely by a deposition of some substances contained in the bile or produced by its decomposition. They are composed of cholesterin, bile pigments, altered mucus, and salts of lime and magnesia, in varying proportions—some being almost pure cholesterin; the majority, however, being composed of a mixture of this substance with bile pigments.

The cause of their formation is obscure, some authors attributing it to the action of bacteria. Stagnation of the bile is no doubt an important predisposing cause, and catarrh of the gall bladder may also play an important part by supplying, as it were, a "nucleus" of mucus and shed epithelium, round and in which the bile pigment, etc., may collect. The calculi occur singly or in numbers.

Of solitary gall stones there are two principal varieties:—

(a) Oval, somewhat translucent masses, smooth or slightly irregular on the surface, and measuring, perhaps, from a half to three quarters of an inch in diameter. These are easily cut or broken, and, on section, do not show lamination. They are composed almost entirely of cholesterin.

(b) Acorn-like masses, from, it may be, one inch to one and three-quarters inches or more in length, and having a smooth surface which is covered with mucus. These are often dark in colour, and, on section, show distinct concentric lamination. They are composed of cholesterin, bile pigments, etc.

Multiple gall stones are much more common. There may be two, three or more of these, or the numbers may reach hundreds. If few, they are, as a rule, comparatively large; if numerous, they are small. They are usually faceted, and the gall bladder may be completely filled with them. They are brownish-yellow in colour, have a smooth surface, and on section present a central darkish nucleus surrounded by more or less regular layers of different colours—the lighter-coloured layers being usually cholesterin, the others combinations of bile pigment with lime salts. Extremely small calculi, composed almost entirely of bile pigment—biliary sand or gravel—may occur in enormous numbers. Small, soft masses—putty-like in consistence and usually dark in colour—are of frequent occurrence in the gall bladder. They probably represent an early stage in the process of calculus formation.

Adami gives the following classification of gall stones:—

(i) Pure (or almost pure cholesterin), most often single and of oval shape, of white or yellowish colour, consisting of 95 to 98 per cent. of cholesterin. There is a minimal amount of associated calcium present.

* The description is largely a quotation from Beattie and Dickson's Pathology.

(ii) Laminated cholesterin, also solitary, often of large size, white or yellowish in colour, differing from group one in containing a larger percentage of calcium.

(iii) Common gall stones, single or numerous, deep brown, reddish brown, or green in colour. There is a nucleus or central portion which may be a cavity. The cavity is due to the drying of a soft nucleus. One section, the calculus, shows a characteristic concentric structure consisting of successive layers. The main constituents are, cholesterin, bilirubin calcium, with small quantities of copper and iron. Calcium carbonate is not uncommon, and is laid down in minute nodules, more rarely in considerable quantities. Calcium sulphide and phosphates have been detected.

(iv) Pure bilirubin calcium, often occurring as bile gravel and consisting almost entirely of calcium salts.

(v) Pure calcium carbonate. These are generally small and very dense in structure.

Experimental Investigation on the Absorption Coefficient of the Various Constituents of Gall Stones and Comparisons with Tissues around the Gall Bladder Area.

The property possessed by all organic and inorganic bodies of absorbing radiations is an important one in regard to the demonstration of gall stones by X rays. This property varies with the density of the body in direct ratio to the density. It has been generally understood that gall stones are not opaque enough to offer sufficient obstruction to the radiations, and that the rays in a large percentage of the cases examined pass through the gall stones leaving no trace of their presence upon the photographic plate. That this is not so can easily be demonstrated. A number of gall stones of varying size and density placed upon a photographic plate and submitted to X rays all gave a clear impression upon the plate, and in no instance did the rays fail to make an impression on the plate. Rays of varying penetration were used, from $\frac{1}{2}$ in. spark gap up to $9\frac{1}{2}$ in. The less penetrating rays with a long exposure gave negatives richer in contrast and full of detail ; the very penetrating ray gave negatives with less contrast but good detail in all parts ; the moderately penetrating rays gave thin negatives, largely because the exposure was much under that necessary to blacken the plate ; longer exposures gave greater contrast. The value of a short exposure is great when radiographing stones in the living subject, because when a long exposure is given, movements on the part of the patient during respiration lead to a loss of sharpness in the shadows of objects in the radiogram. In attempting to differentiate these shadows when very thin negatives are obtained, it is essential that the shadows be sharp, since blurring of the edge of these shadows may prevent the observer from appreciating their presence.

In the living subject the difficulty is to differentiate between the shadow of the gall stone and that given by tissues in front of or behind it. When the density of a gall stone and liver tissue or muscular tissue is equal, it may be impossible to differentiate between them. The absorption equivalent of cholesterin, for example, may be equal to or nearly equal to that of liver tissue. Fortunately, however, very few gall stones are entirely composed of cholesterin ; most have a proportion of lime salts somewhere in their structure. Lime salts, when in any quantity, give shadows which approximate to those of bone structure ; the shadow cast by the lime salt may even equal that of bone itself. A gall stone with lime salt deposited on its periphery will give a definite outline of the salt, hence a ring-like shadow or a triangular one may be all the indication given of the presence of a gall stone. Should the shadow be super-imposed by bone, such as a rib or a transverse process of a vertebra, the gall stone shadow may readily be overlooked.

The density of the gall stone and that of the liver may be equal; it may be assumed that in this circumstance no shadow of the gall stone will be obtained, the one negativing the other. Experience proves the contrary to be the case. In an experiment with gall stones and a piece of liver, the shadows of the gall stones covered by the liver are more intense than those not so covered. This is an instance of the value of adding two densities to get an accentuation of shadow.

In all examinations· for gall stones it should be a routine practice to expose several plates to the radiation of tubes of different penetration, and to develop the plate to give the maximum of ·contrast. For this purpose it is probable that tubes of moderate vacuum will give negatives showing greater contrast than those with a very high vacuum. The Coolidge tube may be used, when it is only necessary to vary the heating current to obtain rays of varying penetration. To increase the contrast with short exposures intensifying screens will be useful; a double coated film with two screens, one on the back and the other on the front of the film, will give a negative full of contrast and very fine detail. The double coated film and two intensifying screens may be used to great advantage when it is necessary to obtain a lateral view of the kidney or gall bladder region, because then it is possible to greatly shorten the exposure. Negatives obtained in this way will give a better opportunity for differentiation.

It should be possible to work out the absorption coefficient of cholesterin, bile, calcium and other constituents of gall stones ; thus, taking the layers of the gall stone in order and submitting them to chemical analysis it should be possible to clearly define the constituent parts. The coefficient value of the tissues and gall stones will be dealt with at a later date when experimental work already in hand has been completed.

Radiographic Appearance of Gall Stones after Removal from the Gall Bladder or Bile Ducts.

To facilitate a ready appreciation of the X-ray appearances of gall stones, a number of these have been radiographed, together with a number of kidney stones. Practically all varieties of gall stones have been so treated. To aid in an appreciation of the penetration required a penetration gauge was used.

It is interesting to note the great variation in the density of these stones when X-rayed under the same conditions. One point is impressed upon the mind, and that is the fact that in no instance have the rays actually failed to make an impression of the gall stone upon the plate. The stones, which are presumably largely composed of cholesterin, give faint shadows. The comparison between the density of pure cholesterin stones and that of liver tissue is interesting; the shadows closely approximate in density, and it is clearly shown that when these structures become super-imposed in the living subject it may be impossible to detect a stone. That this actually happens in practice is proved over and over again. However, even when the gall stone is composed of pure cholesterin—a somewhat rare occurrence—it may be possible in the future to devise a method of differentiation. The suggestions that occur to the mind are the improvement of the photographic emulsion, rendering it more sensitive to finer variations in density. A variation in the exposure may also be helpful, and the taking of a number of radiograms with a tube of varying penetrative power. This suggestion is based on the assumption that even a slight variation between the densities of the two substances may be shown upon the plate if the variation in the conditions are such as will allow of any differentiation.

Details of Experiments and Photographic Records of Gall Stones and Kidney Stones, showing the Variations in Density with Exposures from Tubes of Different Vacuum.

A penetration gauge has been used when possible on each plate ; this gives the penetration value of the rays in each experiment, and shows the degree of penetration with which good detail is obtained in the different varieties of gall stone. A good deal of experimental work has been done on these lines in the endeavour to ascertain the best possible condition of the X-ray tube for the production of negatives of diagnostic value. The experiments are elaborated in the hope that the results may be useful to other workers, and above all in the belief that if more care is devoted to the examination for the detection of gall stones greater accuracy will ensue. The attitude of mind brought to bear upon the subject by the observer plays an important part in the investigation. Too many of us in the past have been prone to approach the subject in a sceptical mood, and perhaps even a negative one. It should be evident that the proper frame of mind to adopt is that it is possible to demonstrate the presence of gall stones in a fairly large percentage of the cases ; perfunctory examinations will then disappear and greater attention will be paid to the technique; the result will be gratifying in a number of cases. If, after a thorough examination, a negative result is obtained the observer will be satisfied that he has done all that is possible to show the gall stone, and if he has failed it is because in the particular instance differentiation is impossible.

The experiments are given in order in the following illustrations, with explanatory notes added where necessary. These experiments were carried out to ascertain the absorption equivalents of each group. The group of small biliary calculi and those of the mixed gall stones were placed in finger stalls and radiographed under varying conditions; these are given in detail below —:

Experiments with dried calculi of various kinds:—

    1. (FIG. 6) A plate showing nine groups of stones chiefly gall and urinary stones; figure shows these printed to show the greatest detail in the smaller and least opaque calculi. The plate was obtained with a tube of low vacuum; the detail of the wooden box could clearly be seen in the negative.

    2. (FIG. 7) Six groups of calculi printed from the same negative as preceding figure; each group has been printed to show the maximum detail obtainable.

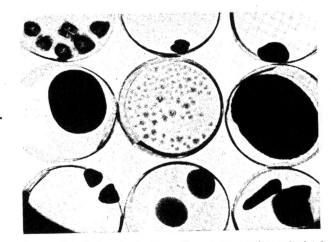

FIG. 6.—Calculi of varying densities radiographed on one plate and printed to show detail in those of least density.

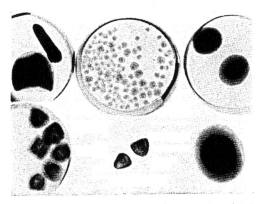

FIG. 7.—From same plate as preceding figure, but printed to give the best detail for each variety of calculus.

Exposures with varying conditions of tube and duration of exposure:—

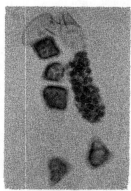

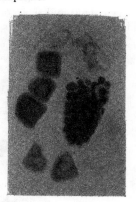

FIG. 8.—Experiment with gall stones. Exposure 2 minutes, 20 milliamperes, 1½-inch spark gap. Shows good detail in gall stones.

    Two groups of gall stones, each contained in a rubber finger stall; the two lower figures show one of the larger gall stones split in two to show the internal structure. Note the outline of the finger stall.

FIG. 9. — Exposure $\frac{1}{10}$ of a second; 5 inch spark, 2-3 milliamperes.

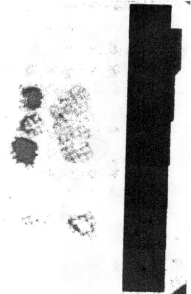

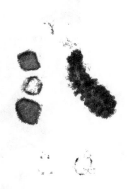

FIG. 11.—Exposure $\frac{1}{10}$ of a second, 8-inch spark gap.

    This figure shows an under exposure, yet good detail is shown.

FIG. 10.—Experiment with gall stones and penetrometer. Conditions: 4 milliamperes, 1 second exposure. Bauer Qualimeter, 6½.

    The effect upon the plate is less than in the next figure, although the exposure was ten times as long the penetration is less.

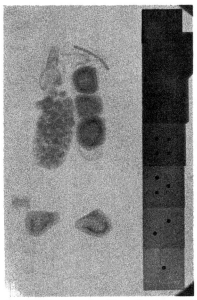

FIG. 12.—Experiment with gall stones and penetrometer scale. Conditions: Exposure $\frac{1}{10}$ of a second, 9-spark gap, 6 milliamperes. Bauer Qualimeter, 8¾.

The penetration value is high, the lead spots are clearly seen in division five of the gauge, 16 mm. of aluminium. Faint shadows of the spots are seen in the division above =- 32 mm. aluminium.

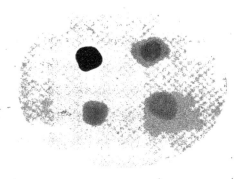

Radiogram by Dr. Salmond.

FIG. 13.—Gall stones showing the great range of density, according to chemical composition.

(1) Nearly pure calcium.
(2) Calcium with cholesterin.
(3) Cholesterin.
(4) Mixed.

Experiment to demonstrate the differentiation of cholesterin stones with a piece of liver placed over the calculi. Note how the thicker portion of liver approximates in density to the shadow of the gall stones.

FIG. 14. — Cholesterin gall stones radiographed along with a portion of liver cut to give varying thickness for purposes of comparison.

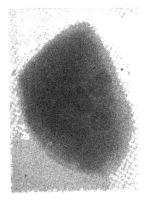

Radiogram by Dr. Salmond.

A   B

Radiogram by Dr. Salmond.

FIG. 15.—A small piece of liver tissue radiographed with a small cholesterin gall stone. Note how closely the shadows approximate in density.

A Liver.   B Cholesterin gall stone.

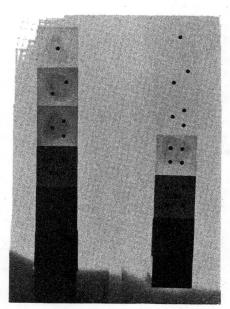

FIG. 16.—Mixed biliary calculi placed upon the steps of an aluminium penetrometer and radiographed. Same conditions of tube in the two exposures. B received twice the exposure of A. The steps of the penetrometer equal 1, 2, 4, 8, 16, 32, and 64 mm. Detail of the calculi is well seen. Sixteen mm. of aluminium and faintly 32 mm. = a pure calcium calculus gives detail, through a greater thickness of aluminium. It can be seen clearly through 32 mm. of the metal.

Experiments with a pentrometer scale and gall stones, to show the effect of an intensifying screen and the influence of an interposed filter of aluminium (9 mm. in thickness).

Three plates with gall stones and penetrometer. Plate without screen = exposure 1 second; 20 milliamperes; 6-inch spark gap. The plate shows a full exposure with the structures fully developed. There is distinct over-exposure with a good penetrative value.

(b) Plate with one intensifying screen—same conditions greatly over-exposed. Penetration very good.

(c) Intensifying screen used under same conditions, with the addition of 9 mm. of aluminium between the objects and the tube. It is assumed that 1 mm. of aluminium is equal to 1 cm. of tissue, so the 9 mm. represent 9 cm. of tissue.

The plate is under-exposed, but it shows good detail and very good penetrative value. This is the type of plate obtained in barium and gall stone work.

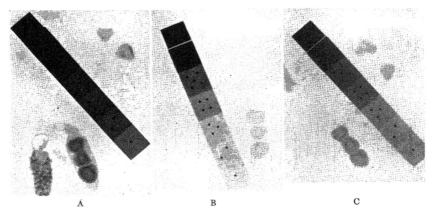

A   B   C

FIG. 17.—Three plates exposed under conditions generally employed in opaque meal examinations namely, distance between anticathode and surface of the plate 20 in., 20 milliamperes secondary current, 6-inch spark gap, exposure 1 second. A, ordinary double wrapped plate. B, with intensifying screen. C, with intensifying screen of and 9 mm. aluminium between the tube and the plate. A shows a full exposure. B an over exposure and a consequent failure to print out fully. C shows an under exposure with shadows approximating to those obtained in opaque meal examination in an average subject.

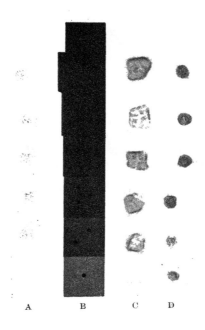

FIG. 18.—Experiment with penetrometer scale and gall stones of different composition. A long exposure with a very "soft" tube on a process plate. Good detail is obtained in all of the calculi, those containing a large percentage of calcium give the denser shadows. A, cholesterin calculi. B, penetrometer. C, mixed calculi. D, calculi, chiefly calcium salts.

A   B   C   D

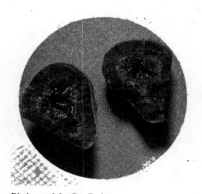

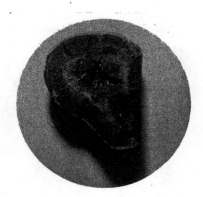

Photograph by Dr. Rodman.

FIG. 19.—A mixed gall stone cut longitudinally
to show internal structure.
This calculus was taken from the group of
mixed calculi used in the detailed experiments.

Photograph by Dr. Rodman.

FIG. 20.—Photograph one-half (enlarged to
show detail) of a gall stone cut longitudinally to show internal structure.

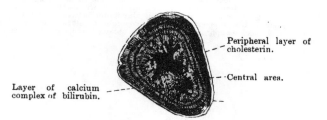

Peripheral layer of
cholesterin.

Central area.

Layer of calcium
complex of bilirubin.

FIG. 21.

The writer is indebted to Dr. Drummond for an analysis of this calculus.
"It is of the type known as a mixed gall stone. It consists largely of
cholesterin, probably 70-80 per cent. of the dry weight. The brown pigment
is calcium complex of bilirubin. Accordingly the colouration is directly
proportional to the amount of the calcium complex present."

(To be continued.)

AN INTERESTING CASE OF DOUBLE SHADOW CAUSED BY ONE STONE IN THE KIDNEY.

By T. Garfield Evans, M.D. Lond., Capt. R.A.M.C., Officer in charge X-ray Dept.

Pte. E.——was sent up for examination on August 7th, 1918, with stone (?) in the left kidney.

An X-ray report was returned stating that two large stones were detected in the right kidney, one in the lower pole and the other in the pelvis. It was also suggested that the kidney was slightly enlarged.

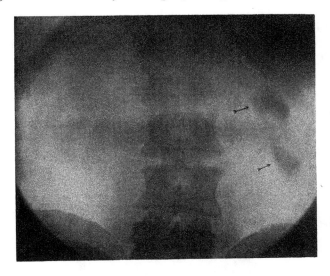

On August 14th, 1918, the patient was operated on, and only one stone was detected and removed from the pelvis of the kidney. It was noticed at the operation that the kidney moved at least 2 in. during respiration, with long pauses at the end of inspiration and expiration. There were early signs of hydro-nephrosis and the stone was freely movable in a much dilated pelvis.

Undoubtedly the double shadow caused by the stone was due to its movement, with pauses at the end of inspiration and especially expiration. The shadow between the points of maximum movement was very slight, and at the time it was not appreciated that this fine shadow was due to the movement of a single stone.

We have detected numerous stones in the kidneys which have simply shown the irregular border due to movement, but have seen no sign of a double shadow.

The apparatus used was a Butt's field apparatus, as supplied to general hospitals, with a Coolidge tube, and the exposure was 240 milliampere seconds.

The tube was placed above, the patient lying on his back, and a cylindrical compressor was used.

The exact diagnosis could, of course, have been made by screening the case at the start, but so many cases are sent up for diagnosis, and the plate method being more reliable we adopt the practical method of "plating" every case.

We have looked up the literature on the subject, and cannot find an instance where a mistake in diagnosis was made by two distinct and separate shadows caused by the movement of a single stone, which may have been exaggerated by the kidney slipping up and down under the compressor.

The case was examined after operation and no stone detected.

A photograph of this case is attached. This photograph was taken by Pte. Beattie, R.A.M.C.

I am grateful to Lt.-Col. Maturin, Officer Commanding, for kind permission to publish this case.

NOTES ON THE OSSIFICATION OF THE COSTAL CARTILAGES.

By R. W. A. SALMOND, M.D.

ON the whole, the younger the patient, the less ossification there is, but cases under twenty years of age showing ossification are frequently met with. The ossification is very symmetrical on the two sides.

FIG. 1.

The first cartilage is by far the most often affected. In nearly every case showing any ossification, it is involved. This is probably to be accounted for by the smaller range of respiratory movement the first rib has in comparison with the others.

The usual type of ossification of the first cartilage appears to be different from the rest. In the first, it generally starts in the form of whorls towards the inferior border, and proceeds from the costal to the sternal end (Fig. 1).

At the others, it generally commences as a thin, well-defined margin on both the upper and the lower borders of the cartilage, and also at the costo-chondral

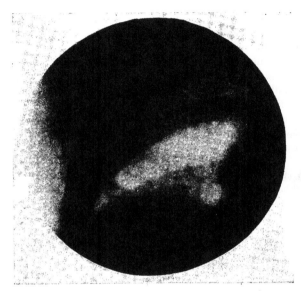

Fig. 2.

junction, and proceeds along the edges from the costal to the sternal or free end (Fig. 2). Later on, while the margins are showing progressing ossification, the interior of the cartilage becomes invaded.

THE "COR PENDULUM" OR "DROPPING HEART."

By Dr. H. C. GEUKEN, Apeldoorn (Netherlands).

THE "Cor pendulum" or "Dropping Heart" is, as is generally known, a constitutional anomaly, in which the heart is abnormally narrow, lengthened out and placed medianly.

With normal individuals the heart is situated so that one fourth of its breadth lies to the right, and three fourths of it are lying to the left of the median line.   With the " cor pendulum," on the contrary, the heart is lying totally, or nearly totally, in the median line, whilst sometimes the left ventricle part is turned to the right (front side); the heart is not resting on the diaphragm, as in normal cases, but is hanging down like a drop, and so at its contraction is deprived of the supporting influence of the diaphragm, which want of support will be especially unfavourable to the contraction of the heart at the inspiratory movement of the diaphragm.

Not always, but very frequently, this anomaly is accompanied with little development and insufficient growth of the entire body, together with a general habitus anomaly, and we often meet with a general enteroptose and a more or less depressive character of the psyche.

The accompanying radiographs have been taken from a seventeen years old boy, who shows the symptoms both of a " cor pendulum " and an ulcerous process of the pylorus part of the stomach.   The patient was sent to me for examination of the stomach on account of stomach complaints.   He was small, cyanotic, and seemed to be not only bodily but also physically undeveloped. Upon examination the ictus cordis was not to be seen, nor palpable, though the boy was a very lean individual, and on percussion there were not to be observed any outlines of the heart.

On Fig. 1, taken in dorso-ventral direction, the heart is situated medianly, and makes one think of dextrocardie.

Fig. 2, in first diagonal direction, shows distinctly that the heart is hanging down like a drop, and does not rest on the diaphragm when in inspiration attitude (position), but is a good deal removed from it.

Fig. 3.   The stomach immediately after the bi-meal is lengthened out with spastic contraction opposite to the lower third part of the little curvature, the pylorus is visible somewhat to the left and below the navel.   The position of the stomach is too low, though not so low as might be expected from the stomach complaints, on account of the frequently coinciding of general enteroptose with cor pendulum, whilst the presence of ulcus ventriculi or duodeni before the examination seemed to be very improbable, the patient being only seventeen years of age.

Fig. 4 has been taken six hours after the bi-meal, and shows a considerable retention with symptoms of an ulcerous process and adhesions of the pylorus.

Fig. 5, fifty-two hours after the bi-meal.   The stomach has emptied itself, the colon transversum shows a bent $\sqrt{}$, so that in this case we may declare a coloptose.

The conclusion may be drawn that if the stomach had not been fixed by adhesions it would have had a lower position, and the whole of the digestion apparatus would have shown more distinctly the image of enteroptose.

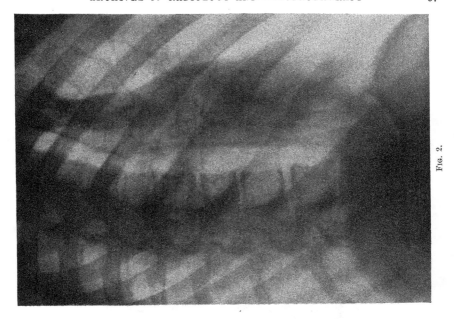

Fig. 2.

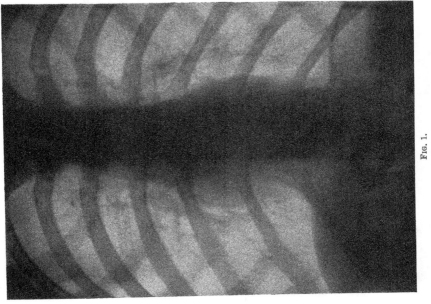

Fig. 1.

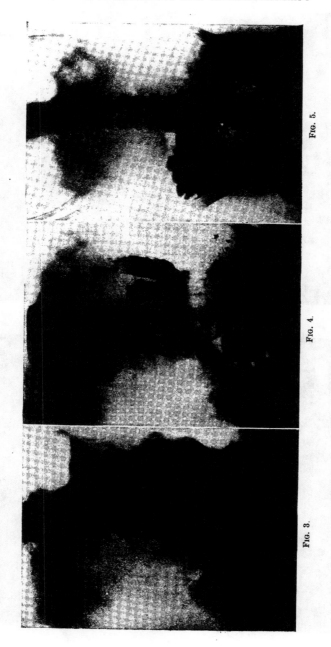

FIG. 5.

FIG. 4.

FIG. 3.

SPLENIC CALCULI.

By WILLIAM MITCHELL, M.B. and C.M. (Edin).

Hon. Phys. Bradford Royal Infirmary, in charge Electrical and Radiological Departments, etc.

IN the bibliography of radiology the spleen occupies a very small place, and that is mainly concerned with the practice of radiotherapy in leukæmic and other conditions. In radiography it is hardly mentioned at all, except in as far as some writers say that its size can be thus determined. I have never seen such a thing as a splenic calculus mentioned in the journals or text books, and yet most experienced radiologists must have observed them occasionally. Personally, the writer has seen four or five clear cases *intra vitam*, and on two occasions has found numerous calculi *post mortem*. It is true calculi in the spleen are not of much importance from the radiologist's point of view, but when single or few in number, in an elongated spleen, they might be mistaken for left renal calculi. It is, therefore, perhaps worth while to place on record the following case and skiagram of the spleen itself showing the very numerous and variously sized and shaped calculi contained. When this spleen was newly removed from the body it was covered on its antero-external surface with many snow-white plaques raised up above the level of the capsule one eighth to one sixteenth of an inch. It struck

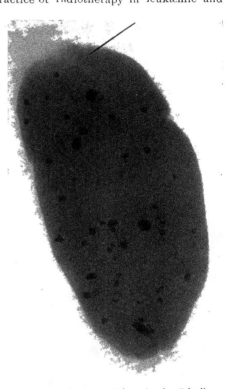

FIG. 1.—Radiogram of Spleen showing Calculi.
(⅔ actual size.)

me these might be calcareous, so I made a skiagram (reproduced) and found numerous dense shadows, readily visible through the whole thickness of the body of a twelve stone man. Not unnaturally I jumped to the conclusion that the shadows, which seemed to coincide with the white plaques, were due to them. Professor Stewart, of Leeds University, kindly examined them for me and reported the condition as being simply thickened capsule, *i.e.*, fibrosis. Examining sections, he found no evidence of calcification or lime salt deposit of any sort, and having seen the skiagram, was surprised at the depth of shadow these plaques apparently gave. I then had the nodules examined by Mr. F. W. Richardson, Bradford City Analyst, and got a report that they contained only "0·9 per cent. mineral matter, consisting largely of potash salts with minute amounts of iron and alumina with scarcely a trace of calcium." Clearly that did not account for the shadows. I took the spleen back to the X-ray room and had another look at it with the fluoroscope. The shadows were there right enough, but on cutting one of the largest plaques off, the shadow still remained in its place. This shadow-producing body I removed under the screen and found it to be a hard calculus firmly embedded in a fibrous capsule. Having removed quite a number, analysis showed them to consist of 67·7 per cent. calcium carbonate. Of their origin or pathology I am ignorant. Possibly they are miliary tuberculous foci which have become healed and calcified. The spleen was from a man 67 years of age, otherwise quite healthy, and who died of internal anthrax.

A NEW GOGGLE FOR USE IN FLUOROSCOPY.

By I. S. TROSTLER, M.D., Roentgenologist to St. Joseph's Hospital, Consulting Roentgenologist to Children's Memorial Hospital, and to the American Hospital, Chicago.

THAT every roentgenologist should protect his eyes by wearing a pair of heavy lead glass goggles or a mask while doing fluoroscopy is admitted by all experienced workers in the field of roentgenology.

It is also acknowledged by busy men in this field, who must frequently go

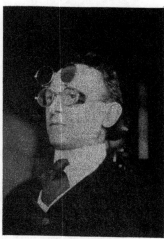

FIG 1.

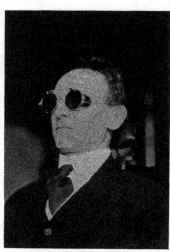

FIG. 2.

from the dark fluoroscopic room into a much more brightly lighted room, that a pair of dark glasses save much time in getting the eyes in a proper condition so as to see well in the dark.

After becoming tired of repeatedly changing glasses many times in a

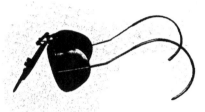

FIG. 3.

morning's work, I devised and constructed what seems to me to be a most practical and convenient combination goggle. I attached, by hinges, a pair of smoked glass goggles in front of my lead glasses. While in the darkened fluoroscopic room I have the smoked glasses raised up against my forehead. When ready to light the room I turn the smoked glasses down in front of the

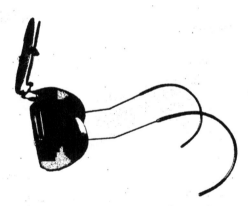

FIG. 4.--Goggles with smoked glass raised.

lead glasses and preserve all the dilatation of the pupils that is needed for quick resumption of fluoroscopy within one minute if desired.

Those needing correcting lenses may have them cemented inside the lead glasses, so that they may have virtually three pairs of glasses in one.

BRITISH ASSOCIATION OF RADIOLOGY AND PHYSIOTHERAPY.

THE undermentioned have been elected members of the British Association of Radiology and Physiotherapy. They are asked by the Hon. Secs. of the Association to receive this notification of their election in place of communication by letter:—

George Alexander, M.B., F.R.C.S. Ed.
Norman Aldridge, M.B.
William Drewitt Armison, M.D.
Martin Berry, M.D.
Frank Brightman, M.R.C.S., L.R.C.P.
William James Storey Bythell, M.D.
Allan Barrett, M.B.
Herbert Charles Buckley, M.R.C.S., L.D.S.
George Beckett Batten, M.D.
Charles Frederick Bailey, M.D., M.R.C.P.
Alfred Ernest Barclay, M.D.
Robert Maitland Beath, M.B.
Ch istian Constance Bernard, L.S.A., L.M.S.S.A.
Elliott Beverley Bird, L.R.C.P.I., L.M., L.R.C.S.I.
Harold Black, M.D.
Noel Michael Hawley Burke, M.R.C.S., L.R.C.P.
Thomas Lowe Bunting, M.D.
Arthur Ambrose Burrell, M.B.
George Edward Bowker, M.D.
Charles Vincent Cotterell, L.D.S.
Andrew Charles, F.R.C.S.I.
William Newlands Clemmy, M.R.C.S., L.R.C.P.
John Alfred Codd, M.D.
Robert Higham Cooper, L.S.A.
John Sandison Crabbe, L.R.C.P., L.R.C S.
Percival Templeton Crymble, F.R.C.S.
Charles Alex. Clark, L.D.S.
Edward Bellis Clayton, M.B.
Thomas Edwyn Cecil Cole, M.D., M.R.C.P.
Frederick Nesfield Cookson, M.D., F.R.C.S.
Elkin Percy Cumberbatch, B.M., M.R.C.P.
Wilfred B. Dight, M.B.
William Dale, M.R.C.S., L.R.C.P.
John Dodd, M.D.
Herbert Annesley Eccles, M.D.
Henry Stuart Elworthy, F.R.C.S.
John Stanley Ellis, M.R.C.S., L.R.C.P.
L. Erasmus Ellis, M.D.
Neville Samuel Finzi, M.B.
Frank Fowler, M.D.
William Hope Fowler, M.B., F.R.C.S. Ed.
William James Foster, F.R.C.S.
Ernest Edward Frazer, M.D.
Edmund Frost, M.D.
Herbe:t Ashley Gaitskell, M.D.

Harold Ernest Gamlen, M.B.
Howard Trevelyan George, M.R.C.S., L.R.C.P.
Lachlan Gilchrist.
Wilfrid Garton, M.R.C.S., L.R.C.P.
John Johnston Grace, F.R.C.S., M.B.
Russell Arthur Green, M.B.
Arthur Herbert Gregson, M.B.
William Alfred Griggs, M.R.C.S., L.R.C.P.
William Geoffrey Harvey, M.D., F.R.C.P.I.
John Owen Harvey, M.D.
William John Hancock, M.R.C.S., L.R.C.P.
Herschel Harris, M.B.
John Delpratt Harris, M.D.
George Harrison, L.R.C.P., L.R.C.S.
William Hampson, L.M.S.S.A.
Frederick Harwood-Hardman, M.D.
Maurice Richard Joseph Hayes, F.R.C.S I.
Frederick James Harlow, B.Sc., A.R.C.Sc., D.I.C.
Francis Hernaman-Johnson, M.D.
Alfred Ernest Wilson Hird, M.R.C.S., L.R.C.P.
John Hall-Edwards, M.D., L.R.C.P.
Charles Hitchcock, M.R.C.S., L.R.C.P.
Charles Thurstan Holland, M.R.C.S.. L.R.C.P.
James F. C. Hossack, F.R.C.S. Ed.
Edmund Henry Howlett, F.R.C.S.
Howard Humphris, M.D., F.R.C.P. Ed.
Graham Hunt, L.D.S.
Arthur Frederick Hurst, D.M., F.R.C.P.
Francis Field Jagger, M.B.
Horace Jefferies, M.R.C.S.
Alfred Jordan, M.D., M.R.C.P.
Christopher Richard Kempster, M.R.C.S., L.R.C.P.
Preston King, M.D.
Robert Knox, M.D.
Cecil Lyster, M.R C.S., L.R.C.P.
Arthur Edward Anthony Lathbury, M.R.C S., L.R.C.P.
Arthur Hill Laird, M.B.
Percy Lambert, M.R.C.S., L.R.C.P.
David Lawson, M.D.
John Reid Levack, M.B.
Charles Arthur Ashton Lever, L.R.C.P.I. and L.M
John E. A. Lynham, M.D.
William Christopher Long, M.R.C.S., L.R.C.P.

John Miller Woodburn Morison, M.B.
Hugh Meyrick Meyrick-Jones, M.D.
Edward McCulloch, M.B.
Archibald Campbell Macrae, M.B.
John McGinn, F.R.C.S.I.
Alastair MacGregor, M.D.
James McKail, M.B.
Andrew Bruce MacLean, M.B.
Neil MacLeod, M.B.
Ethel Mary Magill, M.B.
Douglas Duncan Malpas, M.R.C.S., L.R.C.P.
William Martin, M.A.. M.D., M.S.
Stanley Melville, M.D.
William Mitchell, M.B.
James Douglas Morgan, M.D.
Reginald Morton, M.D., F.R.C.S. Ed.
John Muir, M.B.
David F. Myers, M.B.
George Percy Norman, M.D.
Harry Carew Nott, M.B.
William Harwood Nutt, M.D.
Harold Nuttall, M.D.
H. E. H. Oakeley, B.C.
Walker Overend, M.D.
George Harrison Orton, M.D.
Walter Charles Oram, M.D.
Edmund Price, M.B. C.L.B.
Alfred Ernest Payne, M.B.
George Alexander Pirie, M.D.
Robert Chambers Priestley, M.B.
L. K. Poyntz, M.D.
Francis Stedman Poole, M.R.C.S., L.R.C.P.
William Barrington Prowse, M.R.C.S., L.R.C.P.
Arthur Ernest Rayner, M.D.
William Morton Robson, M.D., M.R.C.P.
May Rathbone, L.M.S.S.A.
Robert Lindsay Rea, M.B.
John Magnus Redding, F.R.C.S.
Ernest William Reed, M.B.
Sir Archibald Douglas Reid, M.R.C.S.,L.R.C.P.

James Herbert Rhodes, M.B., M.R.C.P.
Dalton Richardson, M.D.
James Robertson Riddell, F.R.F.P.S.
Walter Netherwood Rishworth, M.B.
Leonard Alfred Rowden, M.B.
Sidney Russ, D.Sc.
George Herbert Rutter, M.B.
William Stenart, M.R.C.S., L.R.C.P.
Claude William Scott Saberton, M.D.
Robert Williamson Asher Salmond, M.D.
Richard Harvey Sankey, M.B.
Agnes Forbes Savill, M.D., M.R.C.P.I.
Ettie Sayer, M.B.
Francis Shillington Scales, M.D.
Harold Brooke Scargill, M.B.
Sebastian Gilbert Scott, M.R.C.S., L.R.C.P.
Edward Warren Hine Shenton, M.R.C.S., L.R.C.P.
Robert Simpson, L.R.C.P. and L.M.; L.R.C.S.I.
Samuel Sloan, M.D.
Edmund Ivens Spriggs, M.D., F.R.C.P.
Alfred Speight, L.R.C.P., L.R.C.S.
Florence Ada Stoney, M.D.
Edith Stoney, D.Sc.
William Townsend Storrs, M.R.C.S.,L.R.C.P.
Kenneth Vincent Trubshaw, M.B.
Charles Edward Treble, M.D.
Gerald Earl Thornton, M.B.
Walter John Turrell, D.M.
Clement Arthur Webster, M.R.C.S., L.R.C.P.
John Curtis Webb, M.B.
Mathias Wilhelm Eberhard Widegren, M.R.C.S., L.R.C.P.
Justina Wilson, L.M.S.S.A.
J. H. Douglas Webster, M.D.
Eva Muriel White, M.R.C.S., L.R.C.P.
Arthur Benjamin Winder, M.D.
John Hearn Woodroffe, M.D.
John Crossley Wright, M.B.
Alister Cameron Young, M.R.C.S., L.R.C.P.

The following members have made donations to defray the initial expenses of the Association. Further donations from those who have not yet subscribed will be gladly received.

	£	s.	d.		£	s.	d.
Charles Frederick Bailey	5	5	0	Noel Michael Hawley Burke	5	5	0
George Beckett Batten	5	5	0	Charles Alex. Clarke	5	5	0
Christian Constance Bernard	5	5	0	Charles Vincent Cotterell	2	2	0
Martin Berry	5	5	0	John Sandison Crabbe	1	1	0
Harold Black	2	2	0	Elkin Percy Cumberbatch	5	5	0
George Edward Bowker	5	5	0	William Dale	1	1	0
Frank Brightman	1	1	0	Sir James Mackenzie Davidson	100	0	0

	£	s.	d.
Herbert Annesley Eccles -	5	5	0
W. H. Fowler -	1	1	0
Edmund Frost -	5	5	0
Howard Trevelyan George	25	0	0
John Johnston Grace	5	5	0
John Owen Harvey -	5	5	0
Francis Hernaman-Johnson	5	5	0
Sir Charles Thurstan Holland -	5	5	0
James F. C. Hossack	1	1	0
Edmund Henry Howlett	1	1	0
Howard Humphris -	5	5	0
Christopher Richard Kempster	3	3	0
Preston King -	1	1	0
Robert Knox -	5	5	0
Cecil Lyster -	5	5	0
Arthur Hill Laird -	2	2	0
William Christopher Long	1	1	0
John E. A. Lynham	5	5	0
Alastair MacGregor	5	5	0
Andrew Bruce MacLean	1	1	0
Neil MacLeod	2	2	0
Douglas Duncan Malpas	1	1	0
Stanley Melville	5	5	0

	£	s.	d.
William Mitchell -	1	1	0
John Miller Woodburn Morison	3	3	0
Reginald Morton -	3	3	0
George Percy Norman	1	1	0
George Harrison Orton	5	5	0
Edmund Price -	2	2	0
William Barrington Prowse	5	5	0
May Rathbone -	5	5	0
Archibald Douglas Reid -	5	5	0
Dalton Richardson -	10	10	0
James Robertson Riddell	1	1	0
Leonard Alfred Rowden -	3	3	0
George Herbert Rutter	1	1	0
Claude Saberton	5	5	0
Agnes Savill -	1	1	0
Sebastian Gilbert Scott	5	5	0
Samuel Sloan -	1	1	0
Florence Stoney -	5	5	0
Gerald Earl Thornton -	1	1	0
Walter John Turrell -	5	5	0
Eva Muriel White -	1	1	0
Justina Wilson -	2	2	0
Alister Cameron Young	1	1	0

REVIEW.

Chest Radiography at a Casualty Clearing Station, with Atlas. By R. LINDSAY REA, B.Sc., M.B., late Supervising X-Ray Officer, 4th Army. Belfast: Mayne, Boyd and Son, Ltd., 2, Corporation Street. London: H. K. Lewis and Co., Ltd., 136, Gower Street, W.C. 1. 1919. Cr. 4to., pp. viii. + 24; 61 figures. 15s. net.

Dr. Lindsay Rea is to be congratulated on the production of what is an interesting record of this work during the war in the forward areas, and it will, doubtless, appeal to many who have worked under such conditions. As X-ray Supervisor of the 4th Army, Rea experienced all the difficulties which radiologists had to face in the later months of the struggle, when the war became a war of movement affecting the C.C.S.s just as much as the fighting line. The types of portable huts, the apparatus and power supply, and the routine which a wounded man went through from the time of his injury to his examination at the C.C.S. are fully described. The various chest conditions, as seen in war,

are discussed and illustrated, and some original observations made; also the method he used for the localisation of thoracic foreign bodies.

A good deal of the space is devoted to the question of the diaphragmatic curves and movements, and the author puts forward the theory that in an injured lung the vagus nerve, which controls its vitality, can reflexly inhibit the diaphragmatic movement on that side through the phrenic nerve. Attention is not confined to the lungs and diaphragm, but some observations on the heart are also made.

The atlas consists of the skiagrams of a number of various chest conditions, with explanatory notes beneath. Owing to the conditions under which they were done, results with the sharpness of instantaneous radiograms cannot be expected, but at the same time, it is felt that the reproductions are capable of improvement.

The book gives a true and interesting picture of the conditions and problems which were met with in radiology in the forward areas during the war and shows what can be, and has been done, under the circumstances.

NOTES AND ABSTRACTS.

RADIO-DIAGNOSIS.

An Investigation into the Blood Supply of Muscles.—J. CAMPBELL and C. M. PENNE-FATHER (*Lancet*, Feb. 22nd, 1919, pp. 294-6, with 5 radiograms). — These observations were made by injecting the main vessel of the region with a light bismuth salt and then radiographing the excised muscles. Comparing the skiagram with those showing arterial distribution in the brain, heart, and small gut, the writers found that the arrangement is identical in all cases. In none of them are the vessels strictly terminal. In all cases anastomoses are present, but only as very fine ones. Large loops, like those in the mesentery or subcutaneous tissues, are rare.

These observers are able to divide the muscles into three main classes:—

1. Those with a blood supply derived from many different sources, and in which potential anastomoses between the different sources are quite numerous.

2. Those with a blood supply derived from only two or three different sources, but in which the potential anastomoses between these sources are, relatively speaking, few in number.

3. Those with a blood supply derived, for all practical purposes, from only one source, and in which, granted that this main supply is cut off, almost the entire muscle becomes ischæmic, and thus liable to almost complete destruction, owing to the practically complete absence of potential collateral channels.

The practical value of these investigations in their relation to the amount of tissue removed in primary excision of wounds and to the spread of gas gangrene will be communicated later.   R. W. A. S.

A Roentgenologic Contribution to the Possible Cause of Hereditary Optic Atrophy--H. K. PANCOAST (*Amer. Jour. of Roent.*, Jan., 1919, pp. 17-22, with 6 radiograms and 3 Figs.).—Fisher had advanced the theory that hereditary optic atrophy, or Leber's disease, might be due to a transient disorder of the pituitary body with enlargement occurring at definite epochs of sexual life.

X-ray examination appears to be the most certain means of proving or disproving this, provided the enlargements are sufficient and of a necessary prolongation to produce a visible deformity of the sella turcica.

Pancoast's studies of the affected members of two families tend to support such an etiological factor.   R. W. A. S.

"Propeller Fracture."—A. L. JOHNSON (*Lancet*, Feb. 22nd, 1919, pp. 293-4, with 4 radiograms).—Analagous to the type of fracture caused by "back fire" when starting a motor, this writer draws attention to a fracture caused by faulty starting of an aeroplane. This he calls "propeller" fracture, and it is described as a compound fracture of the humerus from one to three inches above the epicondyles.   R. W. A. S.

Orthodiagraphic Observations on the Size of the Heart in Cases of So-called "Irritable Heart."—J. C. MEAKINS and E. B. GUNSON (*Heart*, Vol. VII, No. 1, pp. 1-16, with 4 Figs. and 11 tables).—The heart, in cases of so-called "irritable heart" is, on the average, somewhat smaller (0·7 cm.) than normal.

In cases with a diffuse apical impulse, no enlargement is shown by the orthodiagraph. On the contrary, the average measurement is smaller than the normal, in the same proportion as in those who do not exhibit this sign.

When cases of so-called "irritable heart" rest in bed there is an average increase in the transverse diameter of the heart of 0·7 cm.

After strenuous Swedish exercise in cases having no material symptoms there is a decrease (1 cm.) in the size of the heart, while in cases showing conspicuous symptoms there is, on the average, no appreciable change in the size of the heart.

R. W. A. S.

The Opaque Meal *versus* the Stomach Tube in the Diagnosis of Gastric Hypomotility.—I. H. LEVY (*Amer. Jour. of Med. Sciences*, Dec., 1918, pp. 795-799).—It is well known that stomachs differ in size and rapidity of digestion, and that a number of factors, such as kind of food, size of meal, position, mental state, etc., modify the evacuation time.

The X-ray diagnosis is based on a residue six hours after the taking of an opaque meal. Levy points out, however, that no standard technique has been followed by radiologists and urges that it should be standardized, like the Boas test breakfast.

The author reports on 1,000 cases examined both with the stomach tube and with X rays. In the radiographic examination the six hours residue is observed, and for the stomach tube examination, the residue seven hours after the taking of a meal composed of meat, potato, bread, and some light dessert. From an analysis of the above cases Levy concludes that the seven-hour tube test is superior to the six-hour opaque meal method as practised by radiologists.

The most serious objection to the opaque meal as a test for hypomotility is that barium or bismuth do not enter into the human dietary, and for practical purposes it matters very little how long these substances remain in the stomach. It would seem much more rational to test the motor function by giving the patient a meal he is in the habit of eating.

Levy considers the opaque meal examination as commonly practised is not sufficiently delicate for many clinical purposes.

R. W. A. S.

Remarks on Roentgenographic Pelvimetry.
—W. R. MacKenzie (Brit. Med. Journal, June 1st, 1918, p. 612).—The author's method of pelvimetry is as follows :—

A normal pelvic bone is obtained which is designated the "standard pelvis," and the various diameters are accurately measured. When this bone is radiographed, definite points can be marked on the plate ; the distance between these points will bear a definite ratio to that between the corresponding points measured on the pelvis. This radiograph is taken as the "standard plate."

By radiographing the patient in the same position as the "standard pelvis," having the points of focus the same, the tube at the same angle and same distance from the plate, the author believes that an accurate comparison of the patient's plate with the "standard plate" will be obtained, and therefore of the

patient's pelvis with the "standard" or normal pelvis. When compared to the direct measurements there was an error of 2 mm. only.

To work out mathematically the desired diameter is merely a question in proportion ; for example, if the transverse diameter of the pelvic inlet is wanted, the length of the transverse diameter of the radiograph of the patient is multiplied by the transverse diameter of the standard pelvis and divided by the transverse diameter of the standard plate.

In practice, it is necessary to take the plate in the earlier stages of pregnancy, otherwise the outlines of the pelvis may be more or less obliterated by the presenting part. An accurate comparison between the fœtal skull and the pelvic inlet can be obtained if the radiograph is taken when the head is about to engage in the pelvis.   R. W. A. S.

Osteomalacia, its Roentgenographic Appearance and Classification.—G. W. Holmes (Amer. Jour. of Roent., Nov. 1918, pp. 507-512, with 8 radiograms).—From the point of view of the radiologist it is stated that there are two distinct types of this disease, both of which occur in childhood as well as in adult life, hyper- and hypoplastic malacia.

In the hypoplastic group in children are the cases generally classed as osteogenesis imperfecta or fragilitas ossium. There is a loss of lime salts and thinning of the cortex which produces a diminution in density, but the trabeculæ remain normal. There is no change in the size or shape of the bones unless fractures are present. A large number of cases show multiple fractures with deformity and more or less callous formation.

In the hyperplastic group are the cases occurring in infants and early childhood, sometimes diagnosed as osteogenesis imperfecta and sometimes as osteomalacia. These cases show both destruction and proliferation of the bone, and the trabeculæ are irregular. There is a diminution of lime salts and an increase in the fibrous tissue. The long bones are widened, particularly at the diaphysis, and there is extreme bowing and deformity. The picture resembles rickets, but does not show the characteristic changes along the epiphysial line. Fractures are less common in this type.

The hypoplastic type in adults (commonly called osteomalacia) may be localised or general. There is thinning of the cortex and absorption of lime salts without proliferative changes or deformity.

In the hyperplastic type in adults, multiple fractures are not common. There is proliferation and laying down of new bone along with the destructive process. The trabeculæ are coarse and irregular. The bones are large, bowed and deformed—the picture seen in typical cases of Paget's disease.

The differential diagnosis in children is from rickets and achondroplasia, both of which show their greatest activity along the epiphysial line and in the epiphysis, whereas osteomalacia is a disease of the shaft as well.

In adults, the differentiation is from primary and metastatic malignant diseases, syphilis, and osteomyelitis. The wide extent of the local lesion or the presence of multiple lesions will usually distinguish it from primary malignancy. Differentiation from metastatic malignancy is more difficult.

Syphilis, when general in the bones, is usually periosteal in type, whereas osteomalacia is a disease of the cortex and medullary portion of the bone. In differentiating Paget's disease from syphilis, the absence of involvement of the epiphysis in syphilis and its early involvement in Paget's disease is of help.

Osteomyelitis, while usually a localised process, may involve several bones. Periosteal changes are the rule, while they are generally absent in osteomalacia.

The prognosis as far as cure is concerned is bad. Some cases of the adult hypoplastic type have been benefited by castration—radiotherapy of the ovaries should be considered.

R. W. A. S.

The " Penetrating-Irradiations-Sickness."

—A. Béclère (*Amer. Jour. of Roent.*, Nov., 1918, pp. 498-506).—The author discusses the views of Pfahler, Llewellyn Jones, and Paul Roth, recently published. He states that this condition, produced by either X rays or the gamma rays of radium, is caused chiefly by the adulteration of the blood with toxic substances, resulting from the disintegration of the pathological or normal cellular elements destroyed by these radiations.

The inhalation of a vitiated atmosphere and bad odours play only a secondary part in the production of the symptoms.

The best method of avoiding the condition, or at least of restricting its effects, he suggests, is to limit the use of intensive radiotherapy to those cases where the nature and the course of the disease demand the most rapid type of treatment. In most of the other cases a milder and less rapid treatment would be preferable. R. W. A. S.

Surgical Pathology of the Human Prostate Gland.

—O. S. Lowsley (*Annals of Surg.*, Oct., 1918, pp. 399-415, with 12 Figs.).—In discussing prostatic calculi, the author states that his post-mortem findings lead him to believe that about 20 per cent. of cases showed one or more calculi.

Prostatic calculi are, as a rule, quiescent, and rarely give rise to symptoms, although occasionally a stone may pass after prostatic massage, and abscess arising from or accompanying the condition will cause pain in the perineum. Routine rectal and X-ray examination will reveal many more calculi than has been hitherto suspected. The urinary and sexual symptoms, when present, are those which are usually found in any chronic inflammatory condition of the gland.

In interpreting radiographs of this region, it is important to remember that the large veins on the ventral and lateral surfaces of the prostate are particularly prone to harbour phleboliths.

R. W. A. S.

PUBLICATIONS RECEIVED.
Journals.

American Journal of Roentgenology, June, 1919.

Archives de Medicine et de Pharmacie militaires, Feb., 1919.

Bulletin et Memoirs de la Société de Radiologie medicale de France, May, 1919.

Gaceta Médica Catalana, June 15th, 1919.

International Journal of Orthodontia and Oral Surgery, May, 1919.

Journal of the Röntgen Society, May, 1919.

Journals—*continued*.

Medical Journal of Australia, May, 1919.

New York Medical Journal, May 31st, June 7th, 1919.

Norsk Magazin for Lægevidenskaben, June, 1919.

Policlinico, Il., May 1st, June 1st, 1919.

Proceedings of the Royal Society of Medicine, June, 1919.

Surgery, Gynæcology, and Obstetrics, June, 1919.

Ugeskrift for Læger, June 12th, 1919.

NOTICES.

Archives of Radiology and Electrotherapy is published monthly.

The index for each volume, which ends with the May number, is supplied with the June number of each year.

Communications to the Editors should be addressed to "Robert Knox, M.D., 38, Harley Street, W. 1."

Communications and illustrations from American contributors may be sent to Messrs. Rebman Company, 141-145, West Thirty-sixth Street, New York City.

All radiographs and photographs must be originals, and must not have been previously published. Drawings should be supplied on separate paper.

Owing to the scarcity of paper the Publishers are reluctantly compelled—as a temporary war measure—to reduce the number of free reprints of Papers to twenty-five.

Annual Subscriptions, payable in advance, 30/- including postage. Single copies, 3/- (postage 2d.) Single numbers and back numbers can be supplied on application.

Vol. XXIV—No. 3   AUGUST, 1919   No. 229

ARCHIVES OF RADIOLOGY AND ELECTROTHERAPY

THE OFFICIAL ORGAN OF THE

BRITISH ASSOCIATION OF RADIOLOGY AND PHYSIOTHERAPY

Editors.

ROBERT KNOX, M.D., Hon. Radiographer, King's College Hospital.
E. P. CUMBERBATCH, B.M., M.R.C.P., Medical Officer in Charge, Electrical Department, St. Bartholomew's Hospital.
SIDNEY RUSS, D.Sc., Physicist to the Middlesex Hospital.

IN COLLABORATION WITH

A. E. BARCLAY (Manchester); BELOT (Paris); H. MARTIN BERRY (London); W. H. BRAGG (London), N. BURKE (Woodhall Spa); J. BURNET (Edinburgh); W. J. S. BYTHELL (Manchester); J. T. CASE (Battle Creek, U.S.A.); A. ST. GEORGE CAULFEILD (London); H. A. COLWELL (London); FOVEAU DE COURMELLES (Paris); GUNZBURG (Antwerp); HALL-EDWARDS (Birmingham); HARET (Paris); HAUCHAMPS (Brussels); F. HERNAMAN-JOHNSON (London); W. F. HIGGINS (Teddington); THURSTAN HOLLAND (Liverpool); HURST (London); KLYNENS (Antwerp); LAQUERRIERE (Paris); LAZARUS-BARLOW (London); LEDUC (Nantes); ALEXANDER MACKAY (Edinburgh); REGINALD MORTON (London); HARRISON ORTON (London); W. OVEREND (St. Leonards-on-Sea); PFAHLER (Philadelphia); C. E. S. PHILLIPS (London); GEORGE PIRIE (Dundee); HOWARD PIRIE (Montreal); A. W. PORTER (London); R. W. A. SALMOND (London); WERTHEIM SALOMONSON (Amsterdam); S. SLOAN (Glasgow); SOMERVILLE (Glasgow); W. C. STEVENSON (Dublin); W. J. TURRELL (Oxford); HUGH WALSHAM (London); ROBT. WILSON (Montreal).

AIDS TO DEFINITION IN X-RAY WORK.

By B. T. LANG, F.R.C.S. Eng., Capt. R.A.M.C., Specialist Ophthalmic Surgeon.
Sometime Officer in Charge, No. 2 (Ladies' College, Cheltenham) Mobile X-ray Unit.

IN order to improve definition, diaphragms are used. Two types are recognised.

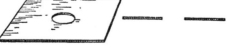

FIG. 1.

1. The ordinary flat disc or plate type, consisting of a piece of material opaque to X rays, in which a central hole has been cut. See Diagram 1.

2. The tube, cylinder, or cone diaphragm, in which, in addition to the
   above, a cylindrical or conical portion of similiar material is attached
   to the edges of the central hole.   See Diagram 2.

Now it is a matter of common knowledge—a point about which every X-ray

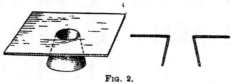

FIG. 2.

worker is agreed—that the definition obtained with a tube diaphragm is
superior to that obtained with a flat one, more particularly when dealing with
thick tissue, such as the head in ophthalmic work or the hip joint.

The only apparent difference between the two types is the ability of the
cone portion of the cone diaphragm to protect the surrounding parts of the
limb from the secondary rays arising from the tube walls.   Now these
secondary rays, when they fall on tissues, set up new rays again, and these
conceivably might influence the definition of the shadows.   This is clearly
shown in Diagrams 3 and 4.

Diagram 3 shows one of these rays, SR, falling on the limb and there

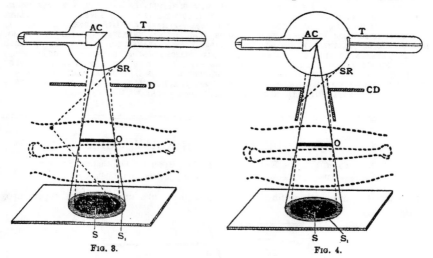

FIG. 3.   FIG. 4.

setting up new rays, which fall on the densely black shadow S and reduce
its blackness.

Diagram 4 shows how the cone part of the cone diaphragm protects the
limb, and, therefore, eliminates the possibility of this disturbing ray arising.

These new rays would obviously have only very slight penetrating power, and their capacity for blurring the shadow seemed doubtful, but I saw no other logical explanation of how the cone diaphragm could act in a manner superior to that of the plane diaphragm D.

To test the point I tried the following experiment :—

I employed a large plane diaphragm, D, made of lead 3 mm. thick—see Diagram 5—and a lead disc, D_1, also 3 mm. thick. This was of such size, and so placed, that no primary X rays fell on the area A. In this part, at P, I placed an X-ray plate P_1, half of which was covered with a piece of lead 3 mm. thick.

I then exposed it for three minutes, with about 4 milliamperes of current passing through a tube of about Benoist 7, the tube being 50 cm. from the plate.

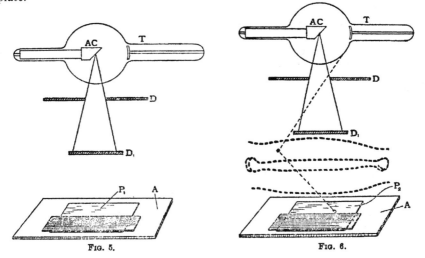

FIG. 5.   FIG. 6.

I next interposed a patient between the disc D_1 and the area A— see Diagram 6—and exposed another plate, P_2, under otherwise similar conditions.

Now, if the theory suggested above be true, the secondary rays arising from the tube walls will fall copiously on the patient's body, and very many new rays will arise, many of which will fall on the plate P_2 and will fog the uncovered half, which on development should be quite dark. While the plate P_1, since there is nothing in this case from which secondary rays can arise, should be entirely free from fog.

The plate, P_1, on development showed slight, very slight fogging of the half uncovered by the lead, while the other half was entirely clear. This showed me that the 3 mm. of lead of D_1 was not enough to cut off all the primary rays, but that 6 mm. (made up by supplementing the 3 mm. of D_1 with the 3 mm. of lead laid on the plate) was ample.

The plate, P_2, was completely free from fog. This showed that the patient's body had made up for the deficiencies of the disc D.1, and that no secondary rays had affected the plate.

The question then arose, what was the peculiar property of the tube diaphragm whereby one was enabled to obtain with it results superior to those obtained with a plane one?

I next started testing the opaqueness of the ordinary X-ray diaphragm for primary X rays. I found that all the plane diaphragms that I tested were incapable of protecting a plate from being fogged by about 240 milliampere seconds exposure with a Benoist 7 tube. These diaphragms were quite capable of screening off all the secondary rays arising from the glass walls of the tube, and some of the softer rays arising from the anticathode, but they were penetrated by the harder rays.

I found that it was only when the rays had to pass the entire length of the cylindrical or conical portion of the cylinder or cone diaphragm that the material was of sufficient thickness to protect the plate, and that it was in this area only that the plate was protected.

If a tube diaphragm of lead glass be placed on a plate so that the normal ray from the X-ray tube passes down its central axis and an exposure be made, it will be found on development that the base of the diaphragm only partially protects the plate, but that there is a clear, entirely fog-free ring corresponding to the tube. With this new fact at my disposal, I started using plane lead diaphragms at least 5 mm. thick, and with them obtained results just as good as those obtained with a tube diaphragm.

So that it would appear that the true explanation of the superior action of the cone diaphragm is, that owing to the fact that it is quite opaque, it entirely protects the surrounding tissues from X rays.

The ordinary diaphragm allows the hard primary X rays to pass through it. These enter the surrounding tissue, and there set up secondary rays which blur the shadow.

Diaphragms are usually mounted close to the tube wall. This is done because for any one given sized pencil of X rays, the nearer the diaphragm is to the tube, the smaller may the hole in the diaphragm be, and the smaller the hole, the less the area of the tube wall uncovered, and, therefore, the less the quantity of secondary rays arising from the wall that can fall on the patient. But, as shown above, the secondary rays arising in this manner are of only the very slightest importance, if of any importance at all. Therefore, this assiduous guarding of the tube wall is quite superfluous.

So long as the tissues are entirely and completely shielded from unnecessary primary X rays, it is of no practical importance where the diaphragm is placed. It may be convenient, on occasion, to place it in contact with the patient.

In order to determine the quantity of the fog produced by secondary rays, I carried out the experiment shown in Diagram 7.

I placed a sheet of lead L, about 8 mm thick, between the tube and the patient, so arranged that it shaded half of the X-ray plate from the primary rays. I then gave an ordinary exposure. On developing the plate, I was able to see, on one half, the ordinary X-ray negative, and on the other, where no primary rays had fallen, a general fog, which was densest where it abutted on to the radiograph and gradually faded off in those parts of the plate that were furthest under the lead screen.

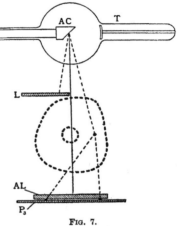

FIG. 7.

These secondary rays are of necessity soft, *i.e.*, of low penetration, and I therefore conceived the idea of filtering them off by means of thin aluminium sheet. In order to determine what thickness would be most suitable, I assembled several sheets, each about half a millimetre thick, in the form of a staircase, as can be seen in Diagram 8. I now placed this between the patient and the plate, as may be seen in Diagram 7, where it is labelled AL. I was thus enabled to determine the effect of screening off various quantities of these secondary rays, both on that part of the plate where the primary rays fell and on the part where there were only secondary rays. I observed, that within limits, small thicknesses of aluminium cut off some of these secondary rays with resulting improvement in the contrast of the negative. In that part where the aluminium was 4 mm thick nearly all the secondary rays were cut off. This thickness naturally also cut off some of the primary rays as well, but the total result gave the effect of enhanced contrast, but detail was wanting, as the negative in this area was under-exposed.

AL

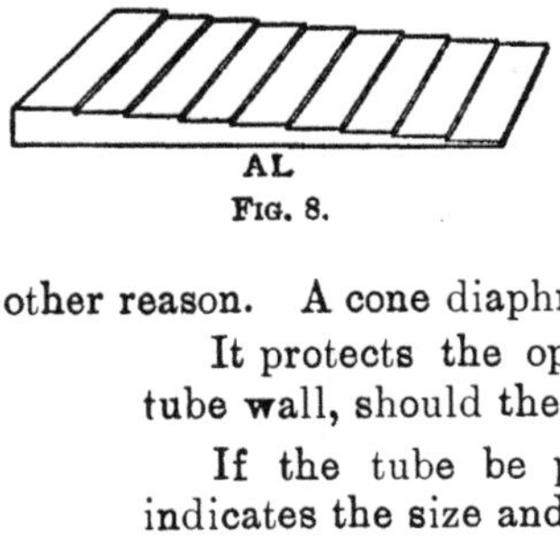

FIG. 8.

In conclusion, a cone diaphragm gives clearer, sharper X-ray negatives, because it is more opaque than the usual plane form, and for no other reason. A cone diaphragm has three other advantages:—

It protects the operator from the secondary rays arising from the tube wall, should the table not be fitted with the usual opaque aprons.

If the tube be properly centered, the cone diaphragm clearly indicates the size and direction of the pencil of X rays, and is then very useful, when working from above, in aiding one to determine what area will be exposed to X rays.

The cone diaphragm can be, and often is, used as a compressor diaphragm, to press the intestines on one side when X-raying the kidney area, for example.

FURTHER EXPERIENCE WITH THE COOLIDGE TUBE RUN ON THE "EARTHED" PRINCIPLE.

By Capt. J. A. SHORTEN, B.A., M.B., I.M.S. ; assisted by Capt. T. W. BARNARD, U.L.

IN the ARCHIVES OF RADIOLOGY AND ELECTROTHERAPY, for August, 1917, in conjunction with Captain Barnard, I described experiments with X-ray coils run with the negative pole earthed, and pointed out the advantages to be derived from running the Coolidge tube on this system. I also suggested that it would now be possible to heat the tungsten spiral of the Coolidge tube direct from the mains—through a suitable resistance in the case of continuous current, or step-down transformer in the case of alternating current. This suggestion has been carried out by Dr. Hernaman-Johnson (ARCHIVES OF RADIOLOGY AND ELECTROTHERAPY, November, 1917). More recently the method has been criticised by Dr. Jordan (ARCHIVES OF RADIOLOGY AND ELECTRO-THERAPY, March, 1918).

Since writing the above quoted paper I have had a year's further experience of this method of running an X-ray set, and have every reason to be satisfied with the results. During this period over 2,000 cases, including a fair number of treatments, have been dealt with. All tubes, both of the Coolidge and ordinary types, have been run in this way, without valve tubes or other rectifying device. During the period in question two coils have been in use, viz., Watson's 16-inch and 12-inch intensified coils. Neither of these coils have shown any sign of deterioration up to date. The expenditure of tubes also has been remarkably low.

From correspondence with other X-ray experts and manufacturers of X-ray apparatus, I understand that there are two main objections to the introduction of my system, viz. :—

1. The danger of increased strain on the coil insulation, leading to breakdown.

2. The danger of shock through contact with the positive wire.

In the present paper I propose to deal with these difficulties.

I. *Danger of Damage to the Coil.*

As explained in my former paper, this resolves itself into danger of break-down in the secondary insulation at the positive end of the coil (I have had no experience with high tension transformers run on this method).

Many coils are still furnished with platinum interrupters and condensers fitted in the base of the coil stand. I shall take such a coil as an example to show how breakdown or damage to insulation may occur. If we refer to Fig. 1

we see that there are three possible paths by which the high tension current leaving the positive end of the secondary winding may reach earth without passing through the tube circuit.

1. *Viâ* the primary winding through a puncture in the vulcanite tube surrounding the primary.

2. *Viâ* the core and platinum break, when the latter is in contact with the core as arranged for running with a mercury interrupter.

3. By surface creeping over the coil to the condenser, primary winding or coil supports.

It will also be noted that since the primary and secondary windings are now directly connected through earth (the insulation of the primary offers

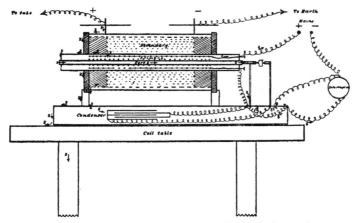

FIG. 1.—Sectional Diagram of Coil to show possible paths of leakage to *earth*.

little resistance to the passage of high tension current), it is only necessary for the vulcanite tube surrounding the primary to puncture at one point instead of two to cause a complete breakdown.

It is obvious that the surface creeping involved in paths 2 and 3 (Fig. 1) would lead to rapid deterioration of the insulation, especially in damp climates.

It should be easy to construct coils with increased insulation around the positive end. In fact, I understand that Messrs. Watson & Son have actually turned out coils on these lines. Such a coil should have the vulcanite tube surrounding the primary of double the ordinary thickness. The core should not reach the end of the primary tube and should be well protected. Platinum interrupters, now obsolete for X-ray work, should be dispensed with; and lastly, the condenser should be mounted independently of the coil, preferably incorporated with the switch and resistance board. It is probable, however, hat coils constructed on these lines would still suffer from surface creeping in damp weather, and in any case it would not help to solve the problem for owners of coils of the old type.

The writer believes he has largely solved the difficulty by a very simple device, viz., by connecting the positive pole of the coil electrically to a lead plate screwed on to the table on which the coil rests, and efficiently insulating the coil table from the earth (Fig. 2). By this means surface creeping to the coil supports is entirely prevented, as any leakage due to faulty insulation of the coil table will take place directly through the metallic connection.

The connection from the positive pole to the coil table should be of stout rigid wire, and care should be taken to ensure a sufficient distance between the wire and the core of the coil, at least 12 inches or greater than the alternative spark gap of the hardest tube likely to be employed.

The insulation of the coil table should be as perfect as possible. In damp climates it should be made of unpolished wood and insulated by means of

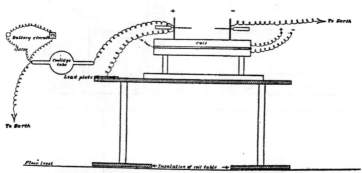

FIG. 2.—Showing connections recommended to prevent surface creeping, etc.

slabs of "ebonite" on "sindanyo," not less than 16 inches square and 1 inch thick. Porcelain and glass insulation is useless in high degrees of humidity owing to deposition of moisture.

Apart from preventing surface creeping over the coil, the arrangement described acts as a "governor" to the whole system, ensuring smooth running, especially at high voltages. This is seen in the steadiness of the needle of the milliamperemeter. This fact has already been mentioned in my former paper (ARCHIVES OF RADIOLOGY AND ELECTROTHERAPY, August, 1917, pp. 7, 8, 9, 10, and 14), from which it will be seen that the use of the "grid," in some instances, at any rate, increases the milliamperage passing through the tube, and ensures steady running. It is difficult to say how this comes about, but it is probable that it acts as a condenser picking up excessive energy (due to irregular action of the inductor unit), storing and discharging it so as to produce a steady flow through the tube. It may be possible to discover some relation between the dimensions of the lead plate and those of the secondary winding, or voltage and milliamperage produced. Such an investigation is outside the scope of the present paper.

In an attempted elucidation of this point the following experiment (Fig. 3) was carried out: An oscilloscope and milliamperemeter were introduced in the positions indicated (Fig. 3), milliampere readings were taken and the oscilloscope photographed, as in my former experiments. To ensure uniform results the same milliamperemeter and oscilloscope were used in the different positions, but the conditions of the experiment as regards amperes in primary circuit and heating current were kept constant.

EXPERIMENT.

Apparatus used :—Coil: Watson's 12-inch, intensified.
Interrupter: Watson's dreadnought, Mark I.
Tube : Coolidge, medium focus.
Amperes in primary circuit, 8.
Amperes in heating circuit, 4·2.
Alternative spark gap, 3½ inches.

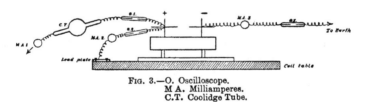

FIG. 3.—O. Oscilloscope.
M A. Milliamperes.
C.T. Coolidge Tube.

RESULTS.

Milliamperes through tube (No. 1 milliamperemeter) - 18
Milliamperes to tube (No. 2 milliamperemeter) - - Slight movement of needle towards table. Not readable.
Milliamperes from earth to coil (No. 3 milliamperemeter) 14

APPEARANCE OF OSCILLOSCOPE.

No. 1 (in tube circuit). No inverse current.
No. 2 (on wire from coil to table). A slight excess of current from coil to table.
No. 3 (on wire from earth to coil). A fair amount of inverse current leaving negative end of the coil.

In the above experiments the camera in each case was placed at exactly the same distance from the oscilloscope, and if we assume that the extent of glow around the negative wire of the oscilloscope is proportional to the current, the length of glow around the positive wire gives us a measure of the inverse current. Photographs (not reproduced here) show that an inverse current represented by a glow 6 mm. long reached the positive end of the coil *viâ* the table; that leaving the negative end of the coil being given by a length of 12 mm. An amount of inverse current represented by 6 mm. of negative glow has, therefore, disappeared in the earth's capacity. This conclusion is supported by a comparison of the milliampere readings.   No. 1 milliamperemeter shows 18 ma. passing through the tube, while No. 3 ma. shows only 14 ma. returning to the coil. The difference in the readings (4 ma.) is due to the passage of inverse current through the milliamperemeter in the second instance.   Furthermore, the oscilloscope shows no inverse current passing through the tube circuit.

From these considerations one may postulate that the inverse potential being unable to force current through the tube is temporarily absorbed by the earth's capacity, the earth's potential being thereby raised momentarily above that of the negative pole of the coil, and that a readjustment between coil and earth takes place during the time the direct potential is effective.   Support is lent to this theory by the fact that a coil can be run below the earth's potential just as well as above (*vide* forthcoming paper).

The experiments, however, throw no light on the action of the "grid" connection beyond showing that a small portion of the direct current leaks to the coil table and a small amount of inverse current returns by this route. Were the table and coil insulation perfect this would not occur.

II. *Danger of Shock from Contact with the Positive Wire.*

This. danger is more imaginary than real.   In my first paper on this subject I explained the general principles of insulation when using this method (ARCHIVES OF RADIOLOGY AND ELECTROTHERAPY, August, 1917). Efficient insulation from coil table, couch, tube box, and earth is therein insisted on.   If, in addition, all metal parts of the couch or neutral stand, including the tube box, are connected up and earthed the patient is effectively screened.   The danger of coming into contact with a charged wire is much diminished when only one pole of the coil is connected to the tube and one end of the apparatus is "dead."   If the apparatus is properly disposed one readily gets into the way of working from the "dead" end.

If necessary, heavily insulated high tension cable might be used for the positive connection, but I think we may brush aside any objections on the score of increased danger to the operator or patient.

In conclusion, I may draw attention to the great advantages this method has over bipolar connections in treatment and dental radiography, owing to the ease with which the tube may be set at any desired angle.

NOTE.

On going to the post I have received the May No. of the ARCHIVES OF RADIOLOGY AND ELECTROTHERAPY, and note an article by Dr. Hernaman-Johnson, in which he goes very fully into the *pros* and *cons* of the "earthed" system.   The present article will, I hope, clear up the situation as regards danger of breakdown in the coil.   The method has now had a very extensive trial at Colaba War Hospital, and since I introduced the "grid" connection "brushing" from the positive high tension lead has been greatly diminished and leakage around the positive end of the coil absolutely stopped. Care must, of course, be taken to prevent the positive lead from being too near any conductor to earth, as pointed out by Dr. Hernaman-Johnson. In treatment, if all the metal parts of the tube box are connected up and earthed, the patient is absolutely screened from risk of shock.

THE EXAMINATION OF THE LIVER, GALL BLADDER, AND BILE DUCTS.

By ROBERT KNOX.

(A portion of this paper was read at a meeting of the Electrotherapeutic Section of the Royal Society of Medicine, held in April, 1919, and formed part of a discussion on the Radiography of Gall Stones.)

(Continued from July issue, p. 52.)

Details of Experiments carried out to ascertain the Absorption Equivalent of Gall Stones.

The experiment detailed in Fig. 17 was carried out to ascertain the degree of penetration obtained through gall stones under the average working conditions employed in ordinary opaque meal examinations.

(a) Exposure of penetration gauge. Gall stones on an X-ray plate without an intensifying screen; exposure 1 second, spark gap 6 in., about 20 millamperes in the secondary circuit. A good picture is obtained showing good detail in the gall stones and the gauge.

(b) Same subjects and conditions, with an intensifying screen. A greatly over-exposed plate was obtained.

(c) Same conditions as (b), but in addition 9 in. of aluminium interposed between the object and the X-ray tube. The plate obtained approximated to that obtained in a subject who had taken a meal. It shows an under-exposure, but good detail in the gall stones and good penetration in the record of the gauge. In all these plates the maximum penetration is about the same; the six spots in the highest scale but one are about equally visible on the plates, some of the detail has been lost in printing.

Gall stones vary greatly in their density, and consequently in their power of absorbing radiations. A small stone which contains a large percentage of calcium salts will be very opaque and will require a larger percentage of tissue to completely block the detail ; as a rule a stone will show through 16 mm. of aluminium, while a very dense stone may be seen through 32 mm. These very dense stones are exceptional ; they approximate in density to the oxalate stones met with in the kidney, and when one is found in the renal area may lead to difficulty in diagnosis.

The statement that an average stone may show through 16 cm. of tissue, when the correct type of plate is obtained, may appear to be contrary to accepted evidence, and possibly to some experimental results which will follow this paper. The statement will be made that liver closely approximates in density to pure cholesterin stones. Pure cholesterin stones are relatively rare, since the accepted description of these allows for 10 per cent. of other substances, and in that percentage is included a small percentage of calcium salt. A cholesterin stone, when radiographed with a " soft tube" and a piece of liver tissue for comparison of density, gives only a faint outline. By increasing the spark length, and necessarily the potential, greater penetration will follow. It should then be possible to differentiate the gall stone from the liver tissue.

The proof that the softer rays are quickly absorbed by the tissues through which the beam passes is readily produced. The following experiment, conducted to ascertain roughly the rate of absorption of the rays, is given in detail.

Filtered and unfiltered rays were used from a Coolidge tube working under the following conditions: heating current, 4 amps.; milliamperes, 4; spark gap, 9 inches.

EXPERIMENT A.—COMPARISON OF THE EFFECT ON UNFILTERED AND FILTERED RAYS THROUGH 4 IN. OF BEEF.

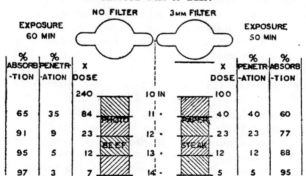

PENETRATION OF UNFILTERED & FILTERED RAYS THROUGH
FOUR INCHES OF BEEF STEAK

FIG. 22.

Twenty 3 min. runs of tube; total
exposure, 60 min.

Ten 5-min. runs ; total
exposure, 50 min.

Four pieces of beef 1 in. thick ; paper on top and between each piece of beef ;
one paper at lowest level, 4 in.

CURVES CHARTED TO SHOW THE PREVIOUS EXPERIMENT.

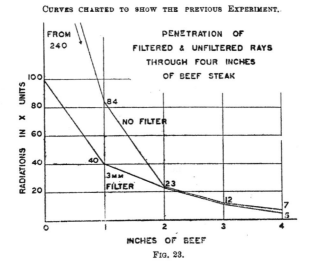

FIG. 23.

The curves representing the filtered and unfiltered rays come to the same value 2 in. from the skin, and follow each other down to the beginning of the fourth inch, where the filtered ray has rather less value than the unfiltered rays. This showing may be the result of a slight experimental error. The unfiltered skin dose is 2·40 X ; focus dose, 7 X in 60 min. The filtered skin dose is 100 X ; focus dose, 5 X in 50 min. The distance from the Coolidge target, 10 in., 11 in., 12 in., 13 in., and 14 in.

The interesting point shown in the experiment is that 65 per cent. of the unfiltered radiation is absorbed by the first inch of tissue, while at a depth of two inches the total absorption is 91 per cent. of the unfiltered rays against 77 per cent. of the filtered rays. At two inches depth the curves practically meet for the two types of rays and proceed onwards together. This clearly demonstrates that the rays from a very soft tube can have very little photographic action when they are passed through the tissues of the body, as they must be when X-raying for gall stones.

With a 6 in. spark gap the following figures were obtained:—

Experiment B.—Comparison of the percentage of rays passing through air and beef with a fixed tube, with filtered and unfiltered rays. The effect of the filter so far as the penetrative power of the ray is concerned was practically negligible. It appears to effect the purpose for which it is used : it cuts down the skin dose. Through 4 in. of beef the time taken to obtain 5 X was 95 min. with the unfiltered ray, while with the filtered ray it took 130 min. to obtain the same value. The dose on the skin paper, however, was 118 as against 161. In the experiments through air with the filtered and unfiltered rays the time taken to produce much more intense effects was much less, but it took twice as long to produce the same result at 4 in. with the filtered rays, the skin dose with the filtered ray being much less.

TABULATED RESULTS OF FILTERED AND UNFILTERED RAYS FROM THE COOLIDGE TUBE THROUGH BEEF AND AIR.

Fixed tube, Beef and Air—no filter; 3 mm. filter; 12 in., 13 in., 14 in., 15 in., 16 in.

			BEEF			AIR	
			No filter	3 mm. filter		No filter	3 mm. filter
Skin	...	...	161	... 118	...	43	... 29
1	...	...	50	... 38	...	29	... 23
2	...	...	22	... 20	...	24	... 20
3	...	...	10	... 8	...	19	... 19
Focus	...	...	5	... 5	...	17	... 18
			95 min.	130 min.		15 min.	30 min.

Amperes, 4·5; milliamperes, 4;   Amperes, 4; milliamperes, 4;
heat, 3·8; spark, 6.   heat, 4; spark, 9.

CHART TO SHOW RESULTS OBTAINED WITH RADIATION THROUGH AIR AND BEEF.

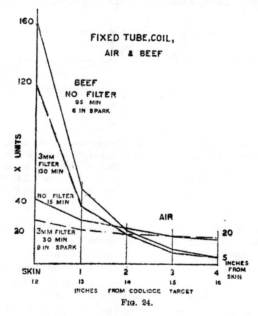

FIG. 24.

The experiments clearly demonstrate that the tissues absorb a large percentage of the " softer rays," and that the rays which give the detail in the organs and even in gall stones are rays of " medium hardness," and that it is a fallacy to depend upon getting detail in substances which are not very opaque with a " soft tube " when these structures are in the interior of the body. A hard tube, if the right exposure is given, will show a shadow of the object; hard rays do not entirely pass through gall stones, as was formerly taught. When so-called soft rays are used the tissues of the body act as a filter and absorb practically all of these soft radiations; the rays which act upon the plate in the radiography of gall stones are the medium and hard rays. Prolongation of the exposure will certainly give denser and more fully exposed radiograms, but that takes place only because a larger percentage of the medium and hard rays get through the tissues and so act on the emulsion on the plate. Prolonged exposure with " soft rays," so long as they do not possess the property of penetrating the tissues, will not give denser plates; the rays will be absorbed by the tissues for an indefinite time. To put the matter into the form of a simple arithmetical problem: If a beam of radiation contains 10 per cent. of rays of a wave length capable of penetrating 6 in. of tissues, and 100 represents the total dose to give a full exposure, then if in an exposure only 10 per cent. gets through, the result will be an under-exposure. Now multiply the exposure by 10 times, then the result will be the correct exposure.

So in radiography, if a full exposure is given with either soft or hard rays the plate when developed will show the effect of full exposure.

Technique for the Examination of the Liver, Gall Bladder, and Bile Ducts.

In addition to the technique employed in the routine examination of the thorax and the abdominal cavity for the investigation of diseases of the thoracic and abdominal organs, there are several special points in technique which should be described in connection particularly with the examination of the region for the determination of the presence of gall stones.

The Special Preparation of the Patient.—This is most important. The bowels should be thoroughly evacuated a day or two before the examination, and on the morning of the examination several enemata may be given in order to ensure that the large bowel is thoroughly emptied. It is of some importance that this should be most thorough, for empty intestines give practically no shadows except when the bowel contains gas; the presence of a gas-distended colon is often very useful, because it gives great contrast in the picture and the presence of adhesions may be suspected from the general contour of the gas-distended colon. No solid food should be allowed on the day of the examination, until the examination has been satisfactorily completed. The patient should be instructed while the exposure is being made to " hold the breath"; difficulty may occur in getting some patients to do this properly. A preliminary drilling of the patient is therefore useful.

The Position of the Patient.—There are several well recognised positions employed in the radiography of the liver and adjoining organs. For fluoroscopy the following are available : (*a*) the upright ; (*b*) the prone or supine upon the couch ; (*c*) the oblique ; (*d*) the lateral. All of these are at times useful in the examination of difficult cases.

Screening is carried out in the general survey of the patient ; the upper surface of the liver is carefully examined along with the diaphragm during respiratory movements. Valuable indications for diagnostic purposes may then be obtained. The lower surface of the liver, the gall bladder, and the duodenum are examined as a routine of the opaque meal technique or independently. The examination of the liver and gall bladder should always form a part of the technique of the opaque meal examination, because it is often possible to get an indication of the condition present, and to confirm it by a later examination, when a more specialised technique is employed.

The positions for radiographing may be similar to those employed for screening. Plates may be exposed in the upright position, but as a rule it is preferable to make the exposure with the patient lying upon the X-ray table, the tube being either above or below the patient. There are three positions which are most valuable for the production of radiograms.

(*a*) Patient prone, with plate placed beneath the anterior abdominal wall. The tube is behind the patient.

(*b*) Patient supine, the plate on the posterior aspect, and the tube in front of the patient.

(*c*) The lateral position.

The several positions are shown in Figs. 29-31. The picture obtained in the Carl Beck position is the most useful in the diagnosis of gall stones, because it favours the production of the picture with the level of the organs well defined, and tends to throw the gall bladder below the lower border of the liver. This is in itself a technical point of prime importance. The chest is raised by placing sand-bags or pillows under it; this tends to throw the gall bladder downwards into the abdominal cavity, and so facilitates the demonstration of the stones. The tube is directed at right angles to the plate placed on the anterior abdominal wall—angling of the tube will aid in obtaining the proper position on the plate.

The Lateral Position.—The lateral position is the most important in all cases, and no examination of the region is complete if this is not employed. It is desirable to call attention to the value of this position in the examination of patients in whom shadows are found in the renal and gall bladder regions. In doubtful cases it provides absolutely positive evidence of the position of the calculus by clearly demonstrating its relationship to the spine. A shadow situated behind the level of the bodies of the vertebræ will, in all probability, be a calculus in the kidney. One found well in front of the anterior border of the spine directs attention to the gall bladder. Fig. 25 is a cross section of the trunk at the level of the second lumbar vertebra. It gives the anatomical relations of the kidney, liver, and gall bladder. The shoulder upon which the patient rests may be raised by placing a sand-bag under it.

For the radiography of kidney and gall bladder cases a special table-top may be used; this consists of a three-ply top which has in the centre a couple of hinges, at each end is a rack arrangement which allows of both ends of the table top being raised if required. For the kidney position both ends are raised so that the region to be examined lies flat upon the table; the plate is placed beneath the region under examination. Relaxation of the abdominal walls is in this way ensured, and when compression is used a very sharp radiogram is obtained. For the anterior position the shoulder end of the table is raised. The table top is shown in Figs. 26-28. These show the construction and the methods of use. It is an extremely useful piece of apparatus, simple in construction, and easily used.

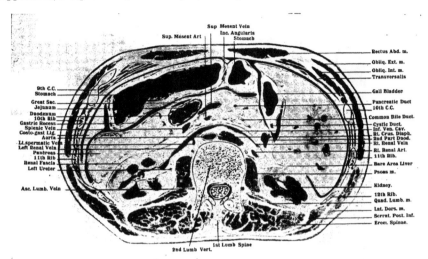

FIG. 25.—Cross section of the Trunk at level of the 2nd Lumbar Vertebra.
(Reproduced, with permission, from Symington's "Sectional Atlas of the Neck, Thorax and Abdomen.")

A compression diaphragm with a small opening should be used ; this aids in the production of very sharp radiograms by fixation of the parts and preventing the secondary radiations from reaching the plate.

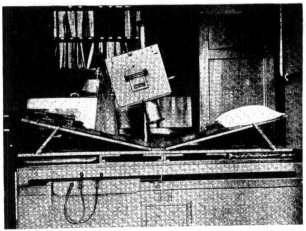

FIG. 26.—Table top employed in kidney and gall bladder radiography, showing method of construction.

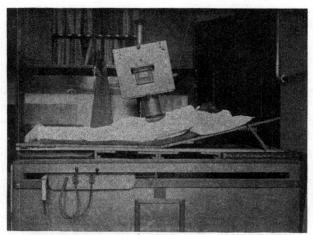

Fig. 27.—Patient in position for anterior view of gall bladder region. The position is the one recommended by Pfahler, in which the body is rotated to throw the right side outwards.

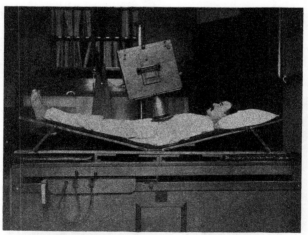

Fig. 28.—Patient in position for kidney radiograph. The shoulder and the lower extremities are raised to obtain a closer approximation of the spine to the plate.

Stereoscopic radiography may be employed in special cases. By its use it may be possible to differentiate calculi and to determine their exact position. The technique is the same as that employed in ordinary routine work; it need not be described further, except to state that accurate depth measurements may be made from the stereoscopic pictures.

FIG 29.—POSITION A.—Postero-anterior.   The usual position for the examination of the kidney.

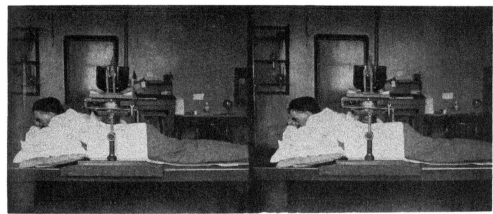

FIG. 30.—POSITION B.—Antero-posterior, with thorax raised.   Carl Beck position.   The angle of the tube may be varied to suit particular cases.

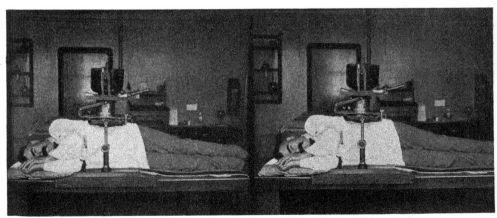

FIG. 31.—POSITION C.—Lateral.   A valuable one for the differentiation of kidney and gall stones.
Stereoscopic photographs of the three positions recommended for the examination of the gall bladder region.

Stereoscopic fluoroscopy may also be found to be useful in the future. It will, before long, be employed in opaque meal examinations.

Little need be said about photographic technique. To enter into it fully would occupy too great space. There are many ways by which photography can help to differentiate shadows which give only very faint outlines, but the employment of these methods necessitates the skill of an expert in photography. The subject may be dealt with fully at a later date.

The exposure should be as rapid as possible. In cases where small gall stones may be present, and the detection of these depends upon absolute sharpness of the radiogram, instantaneous exposures are recommended; if the apparatus is not very powerful intensifying screens should be used. The patient is instructed to hold the breath during the exposure, however short it may be.

The plates should not be over-developed. For the examination of the negatives a strong light should be employed, and it should be possible to vary its intensity so that various types of negative may be scrutinised under conditions which will give the best value for the type.

The important points in the examination of the negatives are fully dealt with in the abstracts from the literature of the subject, which form the conclusion of this paper.

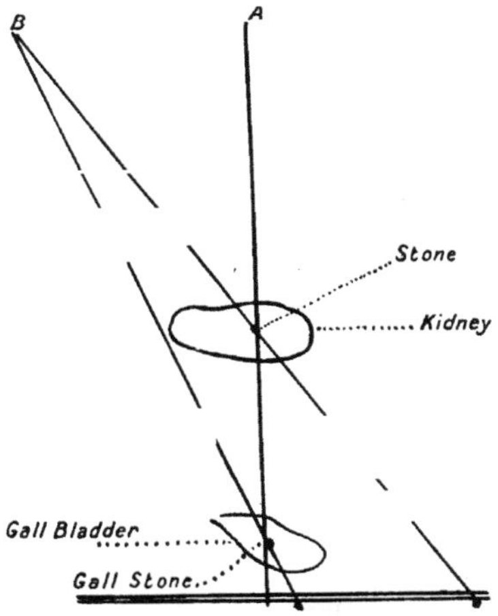

It may be advantageous in a number of cases to distend the colon with air; this, by giving contrast in the bowel shadows, helps in the differentiation of shadows in the region of the gall bladder. The air is introduced slowly through a long rectal tube.

Fig 32.—Diagram to illustrate a simple method for determining the position of a shadow in the renal or gall bladder area, where the shadow in the antero-posterior position might be situated in either the kidney or the gall bladder. A shows the central projection of the rays ; B the oblique. In the latter the shadow nearest to the plate shows the lesser displacement, and so demonstrates that the object casting the shadow is nearer to the plate. The lateral position, however, shows beyond any doubt the true position of the object. This position should always be employed.

The presence of adhesions to the colon and other viscera may be indicated when the colon is considerably dilated with air; palpation may show clearly the area involved if the examination is carried out with the aid of the fluorescent screen.

Situations in which Gall Stones may be found.

These are :—

(*a*) In the gall bladder, at the fundus, the body, or the neck.

(*b*) In the cystic duct.

(*c*) In the hepatic ducts.

(*d*) The common bile ducts.

(*e*) In the liver.

And in the abdominal cavity. A gall stone may cause inflammatory changes which lead to ulceration and the protrusion of the stone into the duodenum or into the colon. It may, if large enough, give rise to symptoms of intestinal obstruction.

It is important to bear these situations in mind when attempting to interpret a radiogram which shows a number of doubtful shadows. The position of the shadow in relation to well known landmarks gives an indication of its location, and in a number of instances this may suffice, but when a shadow appears to be situated in regions other than that recognised as the gall bladder area, then an attempt has to be made to determine its nature and exact position. These points are dealt with under differential diagnosis. A reference to the anatomical figures will facilitate an appreciation of the presence of a gall stone in the normal position of the gall bladder and the ducts ; it must, however, be realised that a pathological gall bladder may not occupy the normal position, it may be found at almost any level in the abdominal cavity.

Differential Diagnosis.

The following are the chief conditions which call for consideration in a differential diagnosis :—

(1) Renal calculi.

(2) Pancreatic calculi.

(3) Calcified mesenteric glands.

(4) Chronic inflammatory lesions of the liver, *i.e.*, liver abscess with calcareous deposits in the abscess cavity; inflammatory conditions of the gall bladder, *i.e*, cholocystitis, with thickening of the wall of the gall bladder, distention of the gall bladder by the products of inflammation, mucus, muco pus, etc.

(5) Fæcal contents.

(6) Adhesions of gall bladder to adjoining structures, *i.e.*, pyloric end of stomach, duodenum, colon, etc.

(7) Foreign bodies.

(8) Calcareous deposits in rib cartilage.

(9) Calcified patches in a tuberculous kidney.

(1) *Kidney Stones.*—The differentiation of gall stone shadows from those given by kidney stones will always be difficult. In a number of cases the distinction is clear and beyond dispute, but there will always be occasions

when it is almost impossible to distinguish between the two on the X-ray plate alone. As a rule kidney stones are larger, denser, and have not the characteristic appearance of particular types of gall stones. A number of writers state that the shadows of kidney stones are clear, sharp, and apparently homogeneous, while gall stones throw a shadow transparent in the centre and having a dense ring-like shadow at the periphery. This is not invariably so, for kidney stones may give detail in the structures in a number of instances, especially if the subject is thin and the quality of the negative is high. Gall stones, if they possess a large percentage of calcium salt, may give a dense round shadow which is indistinguishable from that of a kidney stone. That the mistake may be made is shown by a case recorded by Edling, *Verhandl. der Deutsch. Röntgengs.*, 1912, where a calculus the size of a walnut gave a homogeneous shadow which appeared to be in the hilus of the right kidney. An operation was performed on the kidney with a negative result. At the autopsy a stone was found in the gall bladder, in form and size corresponding to the X-ray picture. A lateral radiogram would have shown at once the position of the stone.

Gall stones vary in shape and size, and the size bears no ratio to the density. A small stone, consisting largely of calcium salt, will give a very dense shadow, while a very large stone, which is chiefly composed of cholesterin, will give only a faint shadow, and this may be lost in the shadows of the parts lying in relationship to it. The position of the shadow may be a guide to its exact nature. This, in the case of gall stones, will vary with the situation in which they are found. If in the gall bladder the shadow will be further from the spine, and may lie at a lower level than a kidney stone if the gall bladder is distended. The stone in the common bile duct will cause more trouble in diagnosis. The most valuable point in diagnosis is to demonstrate clearly by radiography the exact situation of the shadow in relation to other structures, and particularly in relation to well known bony landmarks.

The shadow of a gall stone in the gall bladder will lie in a plane anterior to the kidney shadow, though in the antero-posterior picture it may appear to be directly in front of the kidney. To definitely settle this point plates should be exposed in three positions: (1) dorso-ventral; (2) ventro-dorsal; (3) lateral or lateral oblique. Shadows of stones in the gall bladder will be smaller and sharper when the plate is on the anterior surface of the body, and *vice versa*. The lateral picture will demonstrate almost invariably beyond doubt whether the stone is in the kidney, the gall bladder, or bile ducts. It would appear that in lateral radiography we have the best method of clearly showing the position of a stone whose shadow gives rise to doubt when examined in the first two positions. Lateral pictures should therefore be taken in all kidney and gall bladder examinations. If positive results are obtained a great saving of time results and much anxiety is avoided.

The lateral picture is not easy to obtain, especially in very stout patients. Powerful apparatus is necessary, and the exposure must not be a long one if sharp pictures are required. Intensifying screens on either side of a film coated on both sides will greatly help in the obtaining from thick subjects a lateral picture of value in diagnosis.

In other cases it may be possible in the usual kidney position to show the shadow of the kidney with those of gall stones well outside its shadow. This is beautifully shown in a radiogram by Thurstan Holland, in which the diagnosis is shown at a single glance.

(2) *Pancreatic Calculus.*—These are not frequently met with, or rather, are very rarely diagnosed. The chemical composition of a pancreatic calculus is chiefly calcium carbonate; the shadow will therefore be fairly dense. A calculus situated in the pancreatic duct close to the opening in the duodenum may give all the appearances of a gall stone in the common duct. Only an exploratory operation will demonstrate beyond any doubt its exact location.

(3) Calcified mesenteric glands will be a frequent cause of difficulty. The shadow of such a gland is more irregular in shape and density than either a kidney or a gall stone. The calcification is most irregular, there being hardly any tendency to lamination, and the centre is often more opaque than the periphery. The shadow may be found in different positions in a number of plates. This should be a useful point in distinguishing between all forms of gall stones, except those in a very large gall bladder, where the movement of a stone may be very considerable.

Fig. 33.—Radiogram showing calcareous deposits in mesenteric glands.

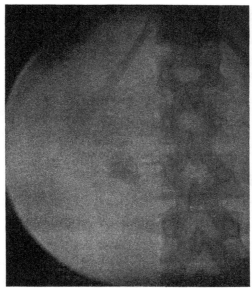

Fig. 34.—Calcified mesenteric glands, situated in the left renal region, in front of the lower pole of the kidney. The outline of the kidney is faintly seen.

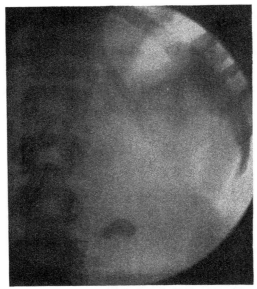

Fig. 35.—From the same patient, radiographed with the plate on the anterior abdominal wall. Note the sharper outline of the group of shadows.

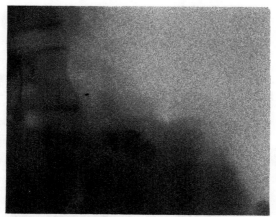

Fig. 36.—Lateral view from same patient, showing group of shadows situated in front of the lumbar vertebræ, at the level of the crest of the ileum.

(4) Fæcal concretions, scybala, etc., may give rise to trouble if the patient is not very thoroughly prepared by a preliminary purgation. All doubtful shadows should be disregarded, an aperient given, and a re-examination made to settle any doubt that may exist.

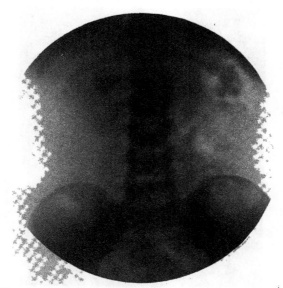

Fig. 37.—Shadows of intestinal contents; these might easily lead to error in diagnosis.

(5) Adhesions of adjoining structures to the gall bladder will give rise to trouble, especially if the inflammatory processes have led to the deposition of calcareous matter in and around the gall bladder. These might show as very indefinite shadows; they should be noted and described for future investigation.

(6) Calcified areas in the liver resulting from old inflammatory processes, such as abscess, etc., may also require consideration.

(7) *Foreign Bodies.*—These are very varied in character, and should always be thought of when examining a plate which presents an unfamiliar shadow in the gall bladder area. Coins, buttons, etc., will be very perplexing if the quality of the radiogram is not very good. A lateral picture will be very helpful in those cases.

(8) The costal cartilages of the lower ribs may show irregular ossification, and when this occurs in a subject suffering from gall stones the shadows thrown by a small area of calcification may give rise to difficulty in diagnosis. A careful examination of the radiogram should be sufficient to distinguish between the two ; the sharpness of the shadow should help to clear up the point ; the position, the direction, and the general appearance of the shadow are distinctive ; a lateral picture will at once dismiss all doubt.

It is only in the very indefinite cases, where the shadows are very indistinct, that difficulty is likely to occur, and such evidence should not be considered seriously; it is obviously imperative that only good plates should be used for diagnosis of this kind ; indistinct shadows do not afford evidence upon which to base a diagnosis of the presence of gall stones.

(9) The kidney area may give indefinite shadows when the organ has been the seat of an earlier tuberculous condition in which degenerative changes have been followed by calcification. There should, however, be no great difficulty with modern technique in obtaining radiograms from which a positive diagnosis of gall stones can be made.

(To be continued.)

A NORMAL OSSICLE IN THE FOOT FREQUENTLY DIAGNOSED AS A FRACTURE.

By A. HOWARD PIRIE, Major, C.A.M.C.

THERE are variations frequently found in the bones of the hand and foot. These have been described from time to time in anatomical papers, principally by Pfitzner and Dwight. In the latest edition of Quain's " Anatomy " these observations have been gathered together, and all the varieties of extra bones in the foot and hand have been figured in diagrams and described. Few of these extra bones can be recognised by X rays, but some can be very definitely demonstrated. In the foot the extra bones one can distinguish by X rays are the os trigonum, os peroneum, os vesalianum, secondary os calcis and the tibiale externum.

In the hand one can recognise the os centrale, the os triangulare, the os vesalianum, and a double scaphoid. I have radiographs of all of these bones, but the object of the present paper is to point out an ossicle which, as far as I am aware, has not had attention drawn to it, and yet it is by no means a rare ossicle. It is seen in a lateral view of the foot, and lies at the upper posterior part of the navicular. Most radiologists have seen it, and many, no doubt, have diagnosed it as a fracture. My attention was drawn to it by the fact that I had to give a diagnosis of fracture of the navicular, when there was no apparent reason why the navicular should have been fractured. After this had happened several times I sent a radiograph of this ossicle to Prof. Arthur

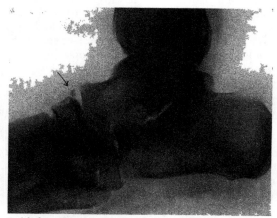

Ossicle found at upper posterior aspect of the navicular bone in eight cases without history of fracture. In one case it was found in right and left foot with no history of accident in its region.

Robinson, of Edinburgh University, asking him if he knew of any extra bone in this region. His reply was that he had never seen one nor heard of one, but that he suspected that it existed because he had occasionally found an articular surface for it on the navicular bone, though the actual bone had always been lost in maceration. My interest in this ossicle was now thoroughly roused, and by watching carefully for it I have during the last two years collected eight cases showing it. The most striking case was that of a man who received a blow on his external maleolus and was radiographed on account of pain over that region. He had no tenderness over the navicular bone, and there was no reason to suspect a fracture of the navicular. The ossicle appeared in the radiograph, and after radiographing the other ankle, which had had no accident to it, an equally developed ossicle was found. This was a clear case of a normal extra ossicle in both feet. The radiographs obtained were very similar in all the other cases in which I had found the ossicle when I had radiographed only one foot.

Occasionally the upper posterior border of the navicular bone, as seen in a lateral radiograph of the foot, presents an extra long lip. This appears as if the ossicle had fused with the navicular. It appears from this to belong to the navicular bone rather than to the astragalus. But I have also found an astragalus with a projection in the corresponding region indicating the probable fusion of the ossicle with the astragalus. One sees a similar condition in regard to the os centrale in the hand. I have radiographs of the os magnum with a small cavity in the border facing the scaphoid. This appears to be the space for the os centrale though the latter may be absent. Other cases show the space with the os centrale lying in it, while others show a projection from the os magnum as if the os centrale had fused with the os magnum. Similarly, the os triangulare may lie free from the styloid process of the ulna, or it may be fused with the styloid process, and the process is then very long.

Variations in the bones of the wrist and ankle are by no means rare. Many extra bones may exist and not be recognisable by X rays owing to superposition, but those mentioned at the beginning of this article can be frequently observed in a large X-ray department.

There is a condition seen in the ankle and wrist which simulates extra bones, viz., a small round or oval body lying apparently over or under a normal bone. These shadows when examined stereoscopically are seen to be inside the bone they appear to cover. They are usually single and resemble the appearance of a sesamoid bone. I have found them in order of frequency as follows: In os calcis, in os magnum, in scaphoid, in semi-lunar, and more rarely in other bones in single instances. Attention has been called to these condensations during the war. It is possible that they are foci of tubercular disease which have caused irritation followed by increased bone formation and extinction of the disease, like calcified spots in the lungs following tubercular disease.

Conclusions.

1. Variations in the bones of the wrist and ankle are not uncommon.

2. There is a normal ossicle not uncommonly found at the upper posterior part of the navicular. It is seen in a lateral view of the foot, and is liable to be diagnosed as a fracture.

3. Fusion of an extra bone to a normal bone of the wrist or ankle causes a projection on the normal bone.

4. Condensations inside normal bones are common and simulate extra bones.

REPORT OF SOCIETY.

SOCIÉTÉ DE RADIOLOGIE MÉDICALE DE FRANCE.

Séance du 13 Avril, 1919.

Une visite à Coolidge à Schenectady.—Le Dr. H. BECLÈRE expose la fabrication des tubes Coolidge et montre les différentes pièces détachee a dont l'assemblage formera le tube définitif. Il signale les nouvelles ampoules en préparation le Baby Coolidge, 30 mill. et l'ampoule spéciale pour la thérapie des cavités (buccale et vaginale).

Nouvel appareillage pour l'utilisation du tube Coolidge à radiateur.--Le Dr. LEDOUX-LEBARD expose les modifications dans l'appareillage radiologique rendues possibles par l'emploi du nouveau modele de tube Coolidge à ailettes et montre les simplifications apportées à toute la technique radioscopique et radiographique, lorsque l'on utilise, en particulier un dispositif à tension constante, supprimant ainsi, quand on dispose du courant alternatif, toutes les parties mécaniques et mobiles, en même temps que les soupapes. Il présente deux appareillages, l'un à tension constante, l'autre à tension variable, réalisés récemment par la maison Gallot-Gaiffe sur les données nouvelles.

La valeur de la teinte dans la radiodiagnostic des affections thoraciques: la densimétrie.—Le Dr. MANOEL de ABREU estime que la teinte est la base même du radiodiagnostic de ces affections. Le poumon normal a ses teintes qu'il faut connaître, les poumons pathologiques aussi. La teinte est un symptôme de la maladie, qu'il faut préciser. La Densimétrie, comme l'auteur propose de l'appeler est son étude et sa mensuration. Deux procédés la réalisent suffisament : 1° une échelle de lames

métalliques de densité semblable à une échelle d'eau de jusqu'à 3 ccm. 2° les repères anatomiques : côtes (équivalentes à 2 à 3 cm. d'eau) ; clavicules (4 à 6 cm.) ; cœur (7 à 8 cm.), etc. Dans le premier procédé on di ra teinte n° 1, 2, 3 . . . (densification) ou moins 1, moins 2, moins 3 . . . (raréfaction) ; dans le second on dira : teinte costale, claviculaire, etc.

Nouvelles acquisitions de la radiothérapie radiculaire.—Les Drs. ZIMMERN et COTTENOT montrent que la radiothérapie radiculaire ne vise pas les radiculites comme on l'on cru par erreur, mais le traitement de toutes les névralgies réputées essentielles et ayant vraisemblablement leur cause anatomique dans une alteration du nerf ou des tissus voisins dans la zone du trou de conjugaison. Indépendamment de la plupart des sciatiques, les névralgies des autres nerfs (intercostaux, occipital, cubital) sont justiciables de l'irradiation roentgenienne exclusive, au point d'émergence du nerf. Les indications de cette méthode semblent devoir aussi s'étendre à certaines dermatoses et certaines névrodermies les A. ayant ou guérir, par ce procédé des prurite rebelles, du psoriasis.

La création des plans en radiographie stéréoscopique. — Le Dr. H. BECLÈRE pour mettre les plans en évidence étend sur la peau examiner de la region à examiner une legère couche de vaseline puis fait un massage avec de la poudre de carbonate de bismuth. Les moindres détails de la peau apparaissent alors nettement. Cette méthode pourra rendre de grands services dans les recherches et données anatomiques.

Le Secrétaire Général : DR. HARET.

REVIEW.

Les Applications de la Physique pendant la guerre. Par H. VIQUERAR. Masson et Cie., Editeurs.

This book of 322 pages is a splendid proof of the part played by the physicist in dealing with a host of problems arising out of the war. While it is doubtless true that practically every one of the many subjects discussed in this book had been under investigation prior to the outbreak of war, the record of achievement since is a very full one.

The book is attractively and very clearly written, mathematical treatment being everywhere avoided; the illustrations are excellent, the one on vision through a submarine periscope being especially good.

Some idea of the range of subjects dealt with will be gleaned from a mention of the main divisions of the book: first come the problems of visibility, range finding, signalling, and the general applications of photography. Then follow sections upon war in the air, conditions of flight of aeroplanes and dirigibles and their range of action.

A comparatively short section on submarines is followed by one on gunnery in all its aspects.

Section V deals with the application of mechanics to the stability of machines of divers kinds. Wireless telegraphy and the part played by the Eiffel Tower form a very interesting section, and the book closes with an account of the localisation of foreign bodies by means of X rays and the electro-vibreur of Bergonié. Altogether a fascinating volume, which should appeal to a very wide circle of readers.

CORRESPONDENCE.

To the Editors of ARCHIVES OF RADIOLOGY AND ELECTROTHERAPY.

SIRS,

I notice in the ARCHIVES OF RADIOLOGY AND ELECTROTHERAPY of March, 1919, a paper by H. C. Orrin, O.B.E., F.R.C.S., on the X-ray demonstration of the vascular system by injections. He calls attention to the fact that only *fifteen* months previously he had discovered that his line of research was not original.

Very many years ago, David Walsh, M.D., published, so far as I know, the first British work on radiography, and in one of the early editions of this work, I think probably the first, he called attention to this subject and published a beautiful illustration showing a human fœtus with all the arteries injected with red lead. In the *fourth* edition of Dr. Walsh's work, dated 1907, the following appears:—

"ANATOMY OF BLOOD VESSELS.

"The injection of blood vessels by some material opaque to the rays, and their subsequent study by the rays, opens up a wide field of anatomical investigation. In this way Dr. F. J. Clendinnen, of Melbourne, demonstrated the arteries of a seven months fœtus, which he had injected with a solution of red lead. His record afforded a sharp and beautiful diagrammatic view of the arteries, even where they passed behind the fœtal bones. A peculiarity, such as that of double high division of the brachial artery, was well shown."

In the latter issue of the same journal (January 20th, 1897), Dr. Clendinnen published some further illustrations obtained in a similiar way. They showed the arteries about the knee and the ankle joint. The small muscular twigs and other minute branches were reproduced with the utmost fidelity.

There can be no doubt that this method may now and then afford a valuable means of showing in a graphic manner the facts of local blood supply, both in normal and in pathological specimens. As an instance of the latter, a perfect picture could be obtained by circulation by anastomoses, say, in a case where during life the femoral artery had been tied for aneurism, or in the stump of an amputated limb.

After Dr. Clendinnen showed me his beautiful results, I then decided to carry out some similiar experiments, and I injected the human lung and published an illustration depicting the vessels injected by this method. Following this work Mr. Fryett, of Melbourne, assistant to Mr. Fred Bird, the eminent surgeon, produced most beautiful stereoscopic pictures showing all the arteries of the body. No more perfect work than this has ever been produced, and several years ago many of these pictures were reproduced in the *British Journal of Radiography.*

I feel it is my duty to call attention to these facts. Mr. Orrin is certainly to be congratulated on his excellent results, but at the same time the pioneers should be remembered in this work, and they should be given the credit due for the work that was carried out in the early days under great difficulties, very different to the easy manner in which such results can be produced now.

HERSCHEL HARRIS, M.B., C.H.M., Sydney.

Honorary Member of the Roentgen Society of America.
Honorary Consulting Radiographer of Sydney Hospital.
Honorary Radiographer of the Royal Prince Alfred Hospital.
Honorary Radiographer of the Royal Alexandra Hospital for Children.
Late Assistant Surgeon of the Sydney Hospital.

THE EFFECTS OF RADIUM BROMIDE IN SMALL DOSES.

To the Editors of ARCHIVES OF RADIOLOGY AND ELECTROTHERAPY.

SIRS,

In his extremely important article * on the possibilities of good effects resulting from the administration of small doses of radium bromide, Dr. Lazarus-Barlow writes thus : " One may fairly argue when a given quantity of radium acting for a given length of time on a given mass of a given variety of cells has been

* W. S. Lazarus-Barlow, " Some Biological Effects of small quantities of radium," ARCHIVES OF RADIOLOGY AND ELECTROTHERAPY, June, 1919.

observed to be followed by degenerative changes, that a sufficient reduction of the quantity of radium, or of the length of time during which it is allowed to act, will induce a stimulative or beneficial effect." Again, he points out that the number of circulating lymphocytes may be increased by small doses of X rays, while massive doses will reduce the number; and he also mentions the mental brilliancy of a patient under minute doses of streptotoxin as compared with the mental hebetude caused by large doses of that toxin.

In view of such remarks it may be of interest to bring forward some facts and experiences, from avowedly heterodox sources, on the basis that it is in the interest of advance to consider anything that may bear on an accumulation of scientific knowledge. In the *Homœopathic World* for Nov., Dec., 1912, and Jan., 1913, there appears a record of a "proving" of radium bromide, that is, the record of the testing of the action of the salt in non-poisonous doses on a series of healthy persons. This was carried out in America by Drs. Dieffenbach, Crump, Sayre, and Stearns, and the results given at the International Homœopathic Congress. The proving "was made from the purest obtainable radium bromide, of an activity estimated at 1,800,000 to 2,000,000, the original trituration being made personally by Mr. E. W. Runyon, of the Boericke and Runyon Homœopathic Pharmacy, of New York, in the presence of Professor Pegram, of Columbia University, who weighed out a definite quantity of radium." The result of the proving is recorded as a series of general systemic effects with their varying symptoms. Amongst these it is interesting to note that the urine of several of the "provers" was radio-active to electroscopic tests, and that there was a marked increase in the proportional number of polymorph neutrophils in their blood.

The complete picture produced by these experiments has given a valuable new remedy to homœopathic practitioners who have studied it. When given in accordance with the correct methods of choice, and the correct rules and principles of the system in question, it has been found to benefit greatly cases showing a similar systemic condition to the recorded "proving." The following two cases will illustrate this. They are recent, and have come under my personal observation, while under the care of Dr. Henderson Patrick at the Glasgow Homœopathic Hospital. I would point out, emphatically, that the action obtained will only take place with the preparation of the drug used when it is given in accordance with the rule that the patient in very many points corresponds with the proving record. This is not meant to indicate that I in any way regard radium bromide as a specific for every case of the diseases mentioned.

Case 1.—S. K., aet. 33, housewife. Subacute rheumatism.

Admitted June 2nd, 1919, suffering from swelling of the right knee, chiefly involving the sub-crureal bursa, but also involving the joint. Onset May 15th, 1919, with sharp shooting pains in the knee followed by swelling, heat, and throbbing. There had been some pain in the left shoulder joint and right mandibular articulation a few days previously. The whole condition seemed to have resulted from a heavy day of washing clothes.

On admission, T. 102°, P. 120. *F*rom date of admission until June 17th, 1919, the T° oscillated between 102° and 99° continuously. On June 17th, 1919, radium bromide was given in minute dose homœopathically prepared. T° immediately subsided, that is, within twenty-four hours, and the swelling began to diminish and the pain to decrease. On July 8th, 1919, she had another dose, and on July 12th, 1919, she was discharged well. The immediate effect of the drug on the T° and swelling was most marked.

Case 2.—E. C., female, aet. 29, Chronic arthritis.

Admitted July 11th, 1919, suffering from aching in wrists, back, and right foot, with swelling of the wrists of two years duration. The condition had become gradually worse, and there was marked tenderness over the wrists, great stiffness and aching of the joints, with pain on movement. The pain in the back was at times very severe, and the navicular of the right foot was distinctly tender.

On July 12th, 1919, radium bromide given at my suggestion. Since that date there has been steady improvement. The tenderness at the foot has disappeared, as has a frequent sharp pain in the back. The aching pain in the back has almost gone, while the wrists have decreased in size and are movable with a very fair range of movement and no pain within that range. She is undoubtedly on the way to very great improvement and probably to recovery.

Only local symptoms have been given. To give the many points which finally determined the use of the drug would be too lengthy.

Wm. E. Boyd, M A., M.D. Glas.

Radiologist to the Glasgow Homœopathic Hospital.

BRITISH ASSOCIATION OF RADIOLOGY AND PHYSIOTHERAPY.

The following member's name should have been included in the List of Donors to the Association published in the July issue:

H. Carew Nott - - - - £1 1 0

ERRATA.

In the List of Donors to the British Association of Radiology and Physiotherapy, on p. 64 of the July issue, "Sir Charles Thurstan Holland" should read "Charles Thurstan Holland," and "Archibald Douglas Reid" should read "Sir Archibald Douglas Reid."

PUBLICATIONS RECEIVED.
Journals.

American Journal of Electrotherapeutics and Radiology, Dec., 1918, Jan., 1919.

Archives d'Electricite Medicale et de Physiotherapie, June, 1919.

British Journal of Dermatology and Syphilis, April-June, 1919.

British Journal of Surgery, July, 1919.

Bulletin et Memoirs de la Société de Radiologie medicale de France, June, 1919.

Bulletin of the Johns Hopkins Hospital, June, July, 1919.

Gaceta Médica Catalana, June 30th, July 15th, 1919.

Good Health, July, 1919.

Hospitalstidende, June 4th, 11th, 18th, 25th, 1919.

Journals—*continued.*

International Journal of Orthodontia and Oral Surgery, June, July, 1919.

Journal of Cutaneous Diseases, May, 1919.

La Radiologia Medica, May-June, 1919.

Le Radium, May, 1919.

Medical Journal of Australia, April 19th, 26th, May 10th, 17th, 24th, 31st, June 14th, 21st, 1919.

Modern Medicine, June, 1919.

New York Medical Journal, June 14th, 21st, 28th, July 5th, 12th, 26th, 1919.

Norsk Mag. for Lægevidenskaben, July, 1919.

Rivista Italiana di Neuropatologia, Psichiatria ed Elettroterapia, May, 1919.

Surgery, Gynæcology, and Obstetrics, July, 1919.

Ugeskrift for Læger, June 26th, 31st, 1919.

NOTICES.

ARCHIVES OF RADIOLOGY AND ELECTROTHERAPY is published monthly.

The index for each volume, which ends with the May number, is supplied with the June number of each year.

Communications to the Editors should be addressed to "ROBERT KNOX, M.D., 38, Harley Street, W. 1."

Communications and illustrations from American contributors may be sent to Messrs. REBMAN COMPANY, 141-145, West Thirty-sixth Street, New York City.

All radiographs and photographs must be originals, and must not have been previously published. Drawings should be supplied on separate paper.

Owing to the scarcity of paper the Publishers are reluctantly compelled—as a temporary war measure—to reduce the number of free reprints of Papers to twenty-five.

Annual Subscriptions, payable in advance, 30/- including postage. Single copies, 3/- (postage 2d.) Single numbers and back numbers can be supplied on application.

Vol. XXIV—No. 4   SEPTEMBER, 1919   No. 230

ARCHIVES OF RADIOLOGY AND ELECTROTHERAPY

THE OFFICIAL ORGAN OF THE

BRITISH ASSOCIATION OF RADIOLOGY AND PHYSIOTHERAPY

Editors.

ROBERT KNOX, M.D., Hon. Radiographer, King's College Hospital.
E. P. CUMBERBATCH, B.M., M.R.C.P., Medical Officer in Charge, Electrical Department, St. Bartholomew's Hospital.
SIDNEY RUSS, D.Sc., Physicist to the Middlesex Hospital.

IN COLLABORATION WITH

A. E. BARCLAY (Manchester); BELOT (Paris); H. MARTIN BERRY (London); W. H. BRAGG (London), N. BURKE (Woodhall Spa); J. BURNET (Edinburgh); W. J. S. BYTHELL (Manchester); J. T. CASE (Battle Creek, U.S.A.); A. ST. GEORGE CAULFEILD (London); H. A. COLWELL (London); FOVEAU DE COURMELLES (Paris); GUNZBURG (Antwerp); HALL-EDWARDS (Birmingham); HARET (Paris); HAUCHAMPS (Brussels); F. HERNAMAN-JOHNSON (London); W. F. HIGGINS (Teddington); THURSTAN HOLLAND (Liverpool); HURST (London); KLYNENS (Antwerp); LAQUERRIERE (Paris); LAZARUS-BARLOW (London); LEDUC (Nantes); ALEXANDER MACKAY (Edinburgh); REGINALD MORTON (London); HARRISON ORTON (London); W. OVEREND (St. Leonards-on-Sea); PFAHLER (Philadelphia); C. E. S. PHILLIPS (London); GEORGE PIRIE (Dundee); HOWARD PIRIE (Montreal); A. W. PORTER (London); R. W. A. SALMOND (London); WERTHEIM SALOMONSON (Amsterdam); S. SLOAN (Glasgow); SOMERVILLE (Glasgow); W. C. STEVENSON (Dublin); W. J. TURRELL (Oxford); HUGH WALSHAM (London); ROBT. WILSON (Montreal).

BINOCULAR VISION AND RADIOGRAPHY.

By R. S. BURDON, M.Sc., Demonstrator in Natural Philosophy, University of Melbourne.

THIS investigation was undertaken in an effort to account for the various difficulties that occur in the use of X rays stereoscopically, and to find a means of overcoming them. The fact that lack of contrast is an inevitable source of trouble makes it the more important to remove all the avoidable causes of error, viz., those connected with the act of vision in the observer and those due to variations in the technique, whether in the use of the stereoscope or in obtaining the plates.

The first portion of the paper deals with the simple theory of stereoscopic vision and illusions that may occur. For this part of the paper most of the available French and English literature on the subject has been consulted, and in particular Quidor's thesis on binocular vision. The application of this theory to radiography is next considered, with particular attention to possible illusions and false reconstructions. The rest of the paper deals with X-ray practice, and is the result of work carried out with University X-ray outfit and the Wheatstone stereoscope (as modified by Professor Laby). The reconstructions resulting from the different methods of inserting the plates, as well as the method of measurement given, were directly verified by radiographs of both simple and complex geometrical objects, the parts of which could be identified without possibility of error, and also by plates of the human body.

The complete lack of perspective in the single radiograph renders precise localization of any point by means of a single plate impossible. All localization reduces to considering every point on the object as the intersection of two straight lines whose positions may be determined. The simplest theory of binocular vision bases our estimation of the distance of a point on the convergence of the two lines joining that point to either eye. The implicit acceptance of this theory as sufficient still stands in the way of a realization of the difficulty of stereoscopic radiography. In reality, whether we view two plates in a stereoscope, or the object direct, *always we see what our experience has trained us to see* and by no means necessarily what the geometric principles of vision would lead us to expect. All visual perceptions are to a large extent subjective in nature.

I.—Factors in Vision, Binocular and Monocular.

1. *Convergence.*—The retinal images of an object, and consequently our perception of it, have maximum definiteness when the images are formed on the fovea centralis for each eye. The effort to bring this about causes the muscular phenomenon of convergence. This is the chief factor in judging the distance of isolated objects which are close to us. The limit of accuracy in so judging a distance will depend on the smallest change in convergence which can be detected. Any process equivalent to increasing the interocular distance will increase the convergence necessary to see a given point clearly, and so far improve the power of judging difference in distance.

2. *Accommodation.*—The effort to focus the image as sharply as possible on the retina brings in the act of accommodation. This enables us to form some idea of the distance of an object seen with one eye only.

3. *Inequality of Retinal Images.*—The visual axis of the eye (line through fovea and optic centre of lens system) does not pass through the axis of rotation of the eye. From this Quidor shows[1] that the retinal images of an object are in general of different size, the larger image being that on the retina which is on the same side of the observer's median plane as the object. Stereoscopic vision is essentially due to the psychic fusion of these two unequal images.

4. *Light and Shade.*—The light and shade over the object or picture are interpreted in terms of distance and relief in a manner determined by our previous experience.

---

[1] *Ann. Chim. e. Phys.*, XIX, 1910, p. 250.

5. *Construction of a Perception of the whole Stage.*—The appearance of other objects, either nearer or more remote, give a framework by reference to which we estimate the distance and dimensions of the particular object of interest. The importance of this factor is evident when we compare our powers of judging the distance and size of (say) a balloon on the ground and the same balloon in the air, when we have round it no familiar stage to assist our judgment by reference to known objects and distances. This perception of the visible region as a whole is built up by extremely rapid movements of the eye, so that each point in turn is imaged on the fovea. To obtain this for objects in the median plane the head too is moved slightly to one side or the other. Stereoscopic plates are taken from two fixed points of view, however, and it is impossible then to get anything equivalent to this sideways movement of the head. In consequence of this two objects in the median plane are not in favourable positions for estimations of their relative distances being made.

6. *Apparent Size of Objects.*—If the object is familiar to us, its apparent size contributes to our estimate of its distance. The fallibility of this is obvious when we consider that there is equally much evidence in support of the converse of this, viz., that if we have a preconceived idea of the distance of an object, the apparent size of the object will be influenced by it in spite of the fixed size of the retinal image.

7. *Diffuseness of Image.*—In vacuo, or in a non-absorbing atmosphere, an object would appear equally bright and sharply defined at all distances. Actually, however, distant objects appear less bright and less sharply defined owing to atmospheric effects. We have learned by experience to interpret this " atmosphere " in a picture in terms of distance, greater diffuseness giving the impression of greater distance.

Of these seven factors the first and third only belong to binocular as distinct from monocular vision. Quidor[2] thus sums up the results of his work on vision : " The perception of relief is due to the inequality of the retinal images and to the system of shades belonging to each. The perception of distance is due to convergence and to variations in apparent size. But there is a synthetic action of all these given factors that produces the actual sensation. Stereoscopic perception is due to the *psychic* fusion of the images perceived by the two eyes." Binocular vision, then, is not amenable to geometric rules but is always largely subjective.

II.—ILLUSIONS IN STEREOSCOPY.

The factors mentioned above may vary independently, and the suppression of one or more of them may permit the remainder to give a totally wrong impression. The following facts of ordinary stereoscopy show the liability to error in interpreting X-ray negatives.

1. *Monocular Vision.*—If, while looking into a Wheatstone stereoscope, a screen be placed over one eye, the observer presently begins to see distance

and relief in the single picture.   This is because the screen prevents the eyes converging and so discovering the distance of the picture.   "Convergence" being eliminated, the light and shade and "atmosphere" of the single picture is then interpreted in terms of distance and relief.   In such a case the perspective is always liable to inversion, unless the observer has a preconceived idea about the picture, in which case he will usually see what he expects to see.

2.   *Inhibition of Retinal Image.*—M. Chauvan[3] gives an account of researches leading to the conclusion that, "if one of two images (of a pair viewed in a stereoscope) contains details rendering it asymmetric with respect to the other, these asymmetric parts may be completely suppressed in the single image seen by the two eyes.   This may occur whenever there is unequal vision in the two eyes, or its equivalent, unequal illumination on the two pictures."   Figures given show that the same pair of plates in a stereoscope may give completely different reconstructions according to the relative intensity of the stimuli received by the eyes.

The reality of this "dominant impression" may be shown as follows. Place two exactly similar coins, one on each illuminator of a stereoscope, in such a way that a single clear image is seen when looking into the mirrors. Now reverse sides of one coin.   On again looking into the mirrors a confusion of the two patterns, or occasionally first one image then the other, is seen by a person of normal vision.   If, however, the illumination on one coin be considerably increased that coin only will be seen and apparently *seen with both eyes.* Its superior visibility has suppressed the sensation from the other eye.   It is only necessary to shut each eye in turn to prove that the retinæ are still receiving different stimuli.

3.   *Reversal of Perspective.*—(a) If the pictures be interchanged, so that the right eye sees the picture intended for the left, the resultant picture has the perspective inverted or is pseudoscopic.

(b) In the use of transparent pictures (as photo plates) the perspective will be inverted if the wrong sides of the plates are turned towards the observer.

III.—STEREOSCOPIC RADIOGRAPHY.

1. It will be supposed that the observer's eyes are situated at the positions of the source of rays, looking through the object towards the plate. Theoretically the plates show geometric projections of the object from these points, and when correctly viewed in the stereoscope should give an impression of the object in relief, as if viewed from the position of the tube.   In practice this simple character of the plates is modified in three ways.

(1) The rays absorbed by the tissues of subject give rise to secondary rays of a softer nature, some of which reach the plate, giving rise to a general fogging which reduces contrast.

(2) A comparatively soft object near the plate, by intercepting this second-

3 C.R. 152, p. 481, and 154, p. 1132.

ary radiation, may give a deeper image than that of a much denser object a short distance from the plate.

(3) Partly owing to the finite size of the source of rays, but mainly owing to secondary radiation, all objects give images less and less sharply defined as they recede from the plate. Thus, contrary to general experience, objects near the observer are less clearly defined than objects further away (nearer the plate).

2. The facts of stereoscopic vision emphasize and explain the following well known rules:—

" The two radiographs should be taken with the plates in the same position with respect to cross wires and to patient, with identically equal exposures and the plates developed to equal density. The plates must be illuminated by diffused light of uniform intensity, and examined by an observer with the power of stereoscopic vision and having approximately equal vision in each eye." Lack of any one of these conditions may so increase the visibility of one plate as to make it give rise to the "dominant image," when the following errors may occur.

(1) *Monocular Vision.*—The "dominant image" alone may be recorded, yet the single eye may give the impression of relief now that the factor of convergence is eliminated. In a radiograph, however, there is no light and shade to give distance and relief, and the "atmosphere" of the picture favours an inversion of perspective since distant objects appear more sharply defined than near ones.

(2) A difference in the two plates may be undetected owing to the asymmetric parts being suppressed (see II, 2, above). Thus, the fact that two plates fuse to give relief is not final evidence that they are correctly inserted in the stereoscope.

An observer having an adjustment by which the illumination on the plates in the stereoscope can be varied continuously and independently can guard against these errors. Looking into the mirrors, and opening and shutting each eye in turn, the illumination is adjusted till the impression received by each eye is of the same intensity. This will correct for inequality of vision of the eyes and also to some extent for unequal exposure or development of the plates.

IV.—TECHNIQUE.

1. *Separation.*—In practice stereoscopic plates are taken for two purposes; firstly for examination in a stereoscope, secondly for localization of objects by measurements on the plate. Unfortunately, the same technique is not best for both of these purposes.

Where the plates are for diagnosis by examination only, experiment shows that Marie and Ribaut's [4] tables give the correct data for obtaining pictures which fuse to give normal relief while placing a minimum of strain on the

4 Marie and Ribaut, C.R. 1897, or Table I at end hereof.

observer's eyes. In practice a wider separation is usually practised in order to accentuate the relief. Now any relief except the normal means that one dimension of the object is seen on a different scale from the others, or the object is distorted. It is doubtful if any advantage gained by wider separation is not counterbalanced by the difficulty in mentally converting depths as seen on one scale in the stereoscope into correct depths in the normal anatomy of the object. *Relative* depths, of course, are not affected by changes in the relief.

Marie and Ribaut's technique, however, does have the disadvantage that where the object is thick (say 25 cms. or over) it must be examined in a stereoscope so as to reconstruct the object at a considerable distance from the eyes. Where the aim is to localize something (*i.e.*, decide the relative position of a number of neighbouring objects), it is an advantage for the eyes to be as nearly as possible at the distance of distinct vision.

Where the plates are intended for measurement, Marie and Ribaut's separations are generally so small as to limit the accuracy with which the depth of any given point can be determined.

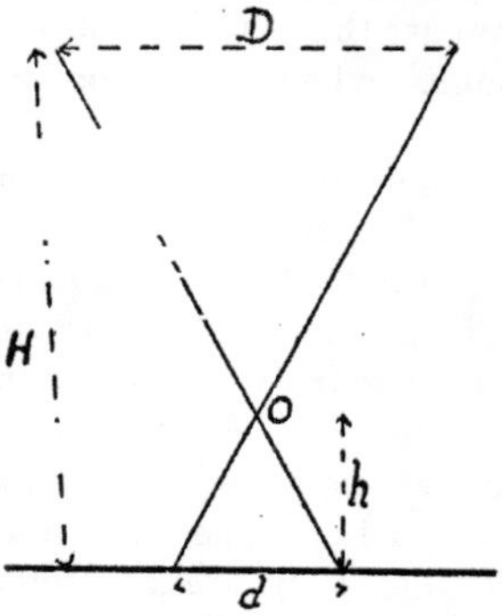

Fig. 1.

The greater the displacement D between the two positions of the focus the greater will be the distance d between the two positions of the image (see Fig. 1), and the more accurately will h be determinable from measurements on the two plates. Further, the position of O may be more accurately determined the greater is the value of h. Increasing the distance of the object from the plate, however, rapidly decreases the definition of the image, and it is in general better to get the point of interest as near the plate as possible. Where plates are to be used for both measurement and examination, it is better to use the widest separation that will give easy reconstruction in the stereoscope.

It is important to realize that no distance can be determined from measurements on the plate with greater accuracy than the following factors permit :—

(1) It must be possible to set the tube so that the focus is accurately situated on the normal to the plate, drawn through the centre of the cross wires (*i.e.* to within 1 mm.).

(2) H should be known with the same accuracy.

(3) The displacement D should be parallel to the X-axis (to within 1°), and should be known to within ·5 mm.

(4) The displacement d is the smallest quantity, and therefore must be known most accurately (within ·2 mm.). This quantity can be rapidly measured by a reseau. This may be prepared by printing on to a photo plate from a sheet of paper ruled with fine lines showing centimetres and millimetres. From this a positive is taken, considerably over-exposed, and development stopped as soon as the lines show up. The rest of the plate will

then be perfectly transparent. The reseau is laid over each plate in turn, and the X and Y co-ordinates of the required points read off. If the Y co-ordinates are not identical, it will show that the tube has not moved parallel to the X-axis in displacement. From these readings the positions of any number of points on the plates may be determined in a few minutes, and hence the position of any object relatively to various bony points or landmarks.

2. *Theory of Measurement.*—Instead of taking the radiographs from two points symmetrically situated with respect to the point of interest and cross wires, the first plate is taken with the focal spot on the normal to the plate through the centre of the cross, and the second from a point distant D to the

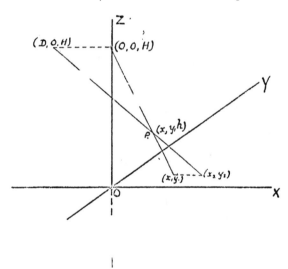

Fig. 2.

left of this point. This simplifies measurements, and it is an advantage (*for examination in a stereoscope*) not to have the object and cross in the observer's median plane (see above I, 5); moreover, the object will always be in the quadrant in which it appears on the first plate.

In Fig. 2 let OX OY represent the cross wires supposed in the plane of the plate.

Let O, O, H, and D, O, H, be the co-ordinates of the two points from which the radiographs are taken.

Let x_1, y_1, and x_2, y_2, be the co-ordinates of the image of the point in question on the two plates.

Let x, y, h, be the co-ordinates of the point P to be localised.

Then $x_2 - x_1 = d$, and $\dfrac{H - h}{h} = \dfrac{D}{d}$, or $h = \dfrac{d H}{d + D}$. . . . (1).

It takes a very short time to prepare a set of tables from this formula, so that the values of h may be read off immediately for all standard values of D and H. (Table II at end.)

Having determined h, the co-ordinate x, y, may be obtained from the *first* plate only, since

$$\frac{H}{h} = \frac{x_1}{x_1 - x} = \frac{y_1}{y_1 - y}. \quad \ldots (2).$$

3. *Examination of Plates in Stereoscope.*—Given a pair of stereoscopic plates, there are sixty-four ways in which they may be inserted in a stereoscope. Of these there are no less than eight ways in which the plates will fuse to give the impression of relief. These eight aspects are all different, and one only will show the object correctly as seen by an observer looking from the position of the tube. These possibilities exist quite apart from any optical defects or illusions, so it is important to eliminate them. This will be accomplished when the observer can at once insert the plates so as to get any desired reconstruction without having to look into the mirrors and " see if they fuse." To insure this each plate must be marked. This marking can be simply accomplished by a device on the plate changer. A small lead letter is fixed over each plate, so that the top left-hand corner of the plate taken with the tube on the left (the west side of a map) has a small W printed on to it, while the other plate (tube to the right) has a small E on the top right-hand corner. If the technique be standardised, so that the plates are always taken in the same order, these letters may be safely made fixtures on the plate holders. These marks in no way interfere with the picture, and they completely obviate the possibility of wrongly inserting the plates, even if a plate has been exposed with the film wrong side up.

Note.—" Left " and " right " are considered to refer to an observer whose eyes occupy the two positions of the focal spot from which the plates are taken, and "top " is the edge of the plate further from the observer, *i.e.*, the terms have the same significance as when applied to a page of print.

The following are the eight methods of insertion, and the resultant re-constructions :—

A. *With plate marked W in left-hand illuminator of a Wheatstone stereoscope, so that left eye sees the plate taken with tube on the left.*

Position 1.—The W mark in the top right-hand corner.
The E mark in the top left-hand corner.

Reconstruction.—Correct, *i.e.*, as seen by an observer whose eyes were at the positions of the focal spot during exposure.

Position 2.—The W mark in the top left-hand corner.
The E mark in the top right-hand corner.

Reconstruction.—Left and right sides of object inverted. Relief inverted. The object appears as if rotated through 180° about the Y-axis.

Position 3.—The *W* mark in the bottom left-hand corner.
The *E* mark in the bottom right-hand corner.

Reconstruction.—Left and right inverted. Top and bottom inverted. Relief inverted. The object appears as if rotated through 180° about the Z-axis, and examined in a mirror at the position of the plate during exposure.

Position 4.—The *W* mark in the bottom right-hand corner.
The *E* mark in the bottom left-hand corner.

Reconstruction.—Left and right correct. Top and bottom inverted. Relief correct. The object appears as if seen in a plane vertical mirror placed on the Y-axis at the edge of the plate.

B *With plate marked E in left-hand illuminator, so that left eye now sees plate taken from right-hand position of tube.*

Position 5.—The *E* mark in the top right-hand corner of left illuminator.
The *W* mark in the top left-hand corner of right illuminator.

Reconstruction.—Left and right inverted. Top and bottom correct. Relief correct. The object appears as seen in a plane mirror on the X-axis at edge of plate.

Position 6.—The *E* mark in the top left-hand corner.
The *W* mark in the top right-hand corner.

Reconstruction.—Left and right correct. Top and bottom correct. Relief inverted. The object appears as if seen in a mirror occupying the position of the plates during exposure.

Position 7.—The *E* mark in the bottom left-hand corner.
The *W* mark in the bottom right-hand corner.

Reconstruction.—Left and right correct. Top and bottom inverted. Relief inverted. The object appears as if rotated through 180° about the X-axis.

Position 8.—The *E* mark in the bottom right-hand corner.
The *W* mark in the bottom left-hand corner.

Reconstruction.—Left and right inverted. Top and bottom inverted. Relief correct. The object appears as if rotated through 180° about the Z-axis.

Conclusion.—In examining stereoscopic plates *Position 1* is the desirable one. If this method is used the plates are film side in, and owing to reflection in the glass surfaces images of one plate will be seen in the other. This can easily be prevented by a black screen mounted on the mirror holder of the stereoscope.

A more serious trouble is that the part of the object near the plate casts a sharper image than the part near the observer. This is contrary to ordinary visual experience, and it favours a psychical inversion of the perspective (see above I, *y*). For this reason *Position 2* is the simplest and safest. In it the object appears as if rotated through 180° about the Y-axis, or as if the observer were looking *through the plate* at it, and the nearest parts are most sharply defined, as is normal. There are thus no factors present which would tend to an incorrect reconstruction, and the simple rotation of the object should not confuse the observer.

The danger of diagnosing from any of the various positions merely because the pictures happen to fuse will be obvious to anyone who knows the difficulties of interpreting from a " mirror image," or who has tried to draw a simple geometrical figure when guided only by the reflection in a mirror.

In practice *Positions 1 and 2* should each be used, and only these two positions, so as not to risk relying on one's memory of all the possible ways of inserting the plates. The change from 1 to 2 is made by merely turning each plate about the Y-axis. If the plates reconstruct unambiguously in each position, it may safely be assumed that no wrong interpretation is occurring. That there is a real danger in using only one position is shown by the following : A good pair of plates showing chest and one arm were obtained. These gave a correct reconstruction for *Position 2*. When the plates were rotated so as to give *Position 1*, the reconstruction showed that the perspective of the arm bones was inverted, as was to be expected, but that the rotation had not affected the appearance of the ribs. The explanation is that the arm bones, being close together, would give images of about the same definition. Consequently, the perspective seen on reconstruction will depend on the geometrical factors. The ribs, however, owing to their widely varying distance from the plate, give images varying from sharpness down to extremely poor definition. The subjective effect of this "atmosphere" in the picture is so great that the clearly defined parts of the ribs appear closer to the observer in spite of the geometrical factors opposing this appearance.

TABLE I.—*Marie and Ribaut's Results.*

P = Thickness of object.

H = Distance from source of rays to nearest part of object.

D = Separation between two positions of tube for normal relief.

x = Distance from eyes to nearest part of object as reconstructed in stereoscope.

	$H = 20$ cm.		$H = 30$ cm.		$H = 35$ cm.	
P	D	x	D	x	D	x
2	4·4	30				
4	2·4	55	5·4	36	6·8	34
6	1·7	77	3·6	55	4·7	46
8	1·4	94	2·8	70	3·7	62
10	1·2	110	2·4	82	3·1	74
12	1·0	130	2·1	94	2·7	85
14	·9	148	1·9	104	2·4	96

TABLE II.—*Showing distance of object above plate for various displacements of the image.*

Symbols have same meaning as in IV, 2, Equation (1).

H = Height of tube above photographic plate.

h = Height of object localised above plate.

D = Displacement of tube.

d = Displacement of image of point localised.

	$H = 50$ cm.			
	$D = 4$	$D = 6$	$D = 8$	$D = 10$
d	h	h	h	h
·2	2·4	1·6	1·2	1·0
·4	4·5	3·1	2·4	1·9
·6	6·5	4·5	3·5	2·8
·8	8·3	5·9	4·5	3·7
1·0	10·0	7·1	5·5	4·5
1·2	11·5	8·3	6·5	5·3
1·4	13·0	9·4	7·4	6·1
1·6	14·3	10·5	8·3	6·9
1·8	15·5	11·5	9·2	7·6
2·0	16·6	12·5	10·0	8·3
2·2	17·7	13·4	10·8	9·0
2·4	18·8	14·3	11·5	9·7
2·6	19·7	15·1	12·2	10.3
2·8	20·6	15·9	12·9	10·9
3·0	21·4	16·7	13·6	11·5
3·2	22·2	17·4	14·3	12·1
3·4	22·9	18·1	14·9	12·7
3·6	23·6	18·7	15·5	13·3
3·8	24·3	19·4	16·1	13·8
4·0	25·0	20·0	16·7	14·3

In conclusion, the writer desires to tender his sincere thanks to Professor T. H. Laby, at whose suggestion this investigation was undertaken. Professor Laby has suggested the scope and method of work throughout, and has made available the whole of the apparatus used, including his improved form of the Wheatstone stereoscope, a description of which is to be published shortly.

ON THE DISTORTION OF STEREOSCOPIC IMAGES.

By Captain E. G. HILL, U.L., B.Sc., and Captain T. W. BARNARD, U.L., Radiographers, War Hospitals, Bombay.

WHILE attempting to devise a method of localisation directly applicable to stereoscopic images, the authors of this paper were struck with the peculiar discrepancies in the proportions of the image when portrayed under ordinary working conditions. They were thereby led to a mathematical investigation of the laws governing stereoscopic effects as applied to radiography. This investigation brought to light the following remarkable facts. Only under specially defined conditions, detailed later, is the stereoscope to be relied upon to portray an accurate representation of reality, and, that if these conditions are not fulfilled, the resulting effects are distorted in a curious manner.

Although the whole of the subject matter is quite elementary, it may be of interest and importance to the radiographer.

As an introduction, a few words may be said about the general principles of localisation. The prolific multiplication, in recent years, of different devices for the localisation of foreign bodies tends to obscure the fact that there is but one principle underlying all methods of localisation, and also of stereoscopy. This is the highly important principle of parallax which is employed, as a powerful method of distance measurement, in many sciences. The distances of the stars are measured in identically the same way, from a mathematical point of view, as we localise the position of a foreign body in the human frame.

The following diagram, with the symbols used in the calculation, are given for reference.

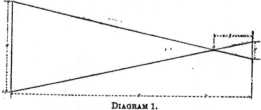

DIAGRAM 1.

d is the distance between the anticathode and the plate.
a is the amount of the shift of the anticathode.
h is the distance between the foreign body O and the plate.
y is the corresponding displacement of the shadow.

By the principles of similar triangles we obtain directly the "localising formula "—

$$h = \frac{d\,y}{a + y}.$$

As before indicated, every method of localisation is a practical application—more or less simple—of this formula, which might well be termed the " Law of Localisation."

Let us consider the application of this formula to the interpretation of stereoscopic effects.

Stereoscopic plates are produced if a lateral displacement of the tube is made while one plate, having been exposed, is replaced by another, and a second radiograph taken in the new position of the tube. This means, mathematically, that every shadow image appearing on the first plate is

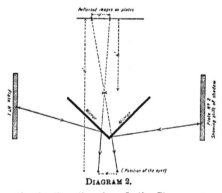

DIAGRAM 2.

Showing the action of a reflecting Stereoscope.

displaced on the second negative by an amount which we have called y^1. By transposing the above formula, we obtain

$$y = \frac{a\,h}{d - h}$$

that is, the displacement varies with the distance of the object from the plate, but is not directly proportional to it.

Let us now consider how stereoscopic images are formed from these two plates. Perhaps the simplest case to consider will be that of the reflecting stereoscope, where reflected images of the two plates are superimposed by a suitable arrangement of mirrors. This superimposition practically reproduces the effect of taking the two radiographs on one plate, thus, the shadow displacements still remain equal to the amount y, this quantity, of course, having the same values and varying as before. On gazing into the mirrors, the eyes immediately attempt to fuse corresponding images into one. The geometrical construction of this " cross fusion " determines the position where any object will be seen in space. A diagram will make this clear.

Suppose now, the distance between the eyes be equal to a distance which we will call a^1, and the distance from the eyes to the image of the plates be d^1, this amount d^1 will be, of course, the sum of the distances of eye to mirror and mirror to plate.

Let any particular image of an object appear to stand out a distance h^1 from the background of the plates, while the real object was a distance h from the plate when the radiograph was taken, what we wish to know is the relation between h and h^1. Since the same principle of parallax applies to this case we may at once deduce the formula—

$$h^1 = \frac{d^1\, y}{a^1 + y}.$$

Eliminating y, we obtain the relation

$$h^1 = \frac{d^1\, a\, h}{d\, a^1 + h\,(a - a^1)},$$

where we see that h^1/h is *not* constant unless $a = a^1$, when

$$\frac{h^1}{h} = \frac{d^1}{d}.$$

Thus, our first inference is, that in order to obtain true proportion in antero-posterior measurements the shift of the tube must exactly equal the distance between the eyes. Also, if this condition is fulfilled, it appears that all antero-posterior dimensions will be proportional in the stereoscope to the original dimensions.

We will go on to consider the effect on lateral dimensions. The shadow images on the plate of an object of lateral size l at the height h from the plate will throw a shadow of size

$$\frac{d\, l}{d - h},$$

where d is the distance of the tube, and a the shift of anticathode as before.

The dimensions of the shadow will be the same on the two plates no matter how much we displace the tube, providing its height remains the same. This, perhaps, would not have been expected.

When viewed stereoscopically, this image will appear to stand out a distance h^1, as before. Suppose that it appears to have, in this position, a lateral size l^1, all viewed under the same conditions as before, then, from the geometrical construction, we may at once write the relation

$$l^1/l = \frac{d}{d^1}\,\frac{d^1 - h^1}{d - h}.$$

So that this proportion is also not constant unless $h = h^1$; but, what is more important, is the fact that—

$$l^1/l \text{ is not, in general, equal to } h^1/h.$$

Thus, our stereoscopic picture is not proportional in the three dimensions of space. The only case in which it is so is when

$$h = h^1 \text{ and so } d = d^1 \text{ and } a = a^1.$$

These results show that, in order to obtain stereoscopic images giving a true representation of reality, the tube shift must always be made equal to the

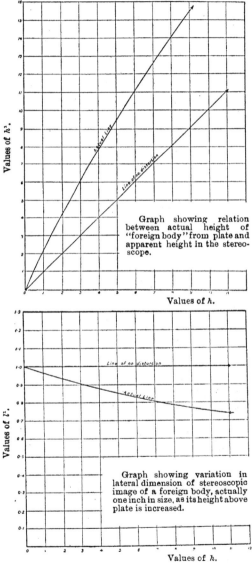

Graph showing relation between actual height of "foreign body" from plate and apparent height in the stereoscope.

Values of h.

Graph showing variation in lateral dimension of stereoscopic image of a foreign body, actually one inch in size, as its height above plate is increased.

Values of h.

distance between the eyes, and also the plates must, in every case, be viewed at a virtual distance equal to that at which the radiographs were taken.

A graphical illustration is appended to this discussion showing the nature of the distortion when the radiographs are made and viewed under other (specified) conditions.

The graphs, made for conditions by no means improbable in actual practice, show that the apparent lateral size diminishes as the depth increases, while the apparent depth increases at a greater rate than the real depth.

All images are, therefore, distorted as though they were stretched in the line of sight and compressed in directions at right angles with this line, and so the apparent position of "foreign bodies" in the stereoscope will appear further from the radiographic plate than they actually are.

FRACTURED SESAMOID BONE OF THE THUMB.

By T. GARFIELD EVANS, M.D. Lond., Capt. R.A.M.C.

Officer in charge, X-ray Department, 34 (The Welsh) General Hospital, Deolali, India.

A FRACTURE of a sesamoid bone in the hand is a rare condition, so I thought it would be interesting to record this case.

History.—Pte. E., A.S.C., M.T.   On January 19th, 1919, patient was playing football, acting as goal keeper.   While saving a shot at goal, the ball landed on the tip of the left thumb, pushing it very forcibly backwards.   The patient definitely felt a "snap" and thought his thumb was broken.   Immediately the thumb became painful, numb, and swollen.

Present Condition.—On January 20th, 1919, patient was sent to the X-ray Department for examination.   The thenar eminence was much swollen, the thumb was kept a little flexed at the metacarpo-phalangeal joint.   Extension, and also active adduction and opposition of the thumb caused a good deal of pain.   A very tender spot was detected on the palmar aspect of the first metacarpo-phalangeal joint towards its ulnar side.

X-ray Report.—There is a traverse fracture of the inner sesamoid on the palmar aspect of the metacarpo-phalangeal joint of the thumb.   This sesamoid bone is developed in the tendon of insertion of the oblique head of the adductor pollicis.   The outer sesamoid bone (developed in the tendon of insertion of the superficial head of the flexor brevis pollicis) is normal, and can be seen on the plate through the head of the first metacarpal.

Diagnosis.—In my opinion the case is one of indirect rupture of the tendon of insertion of the oblique head of the adductor pollicis with the fracture of the sesamoid bone, which is developed in this tendon.

At the time of the accident this muscle was in a state of contraction, at the same instant the thumb was forcibly extended and abducted by the impact of the ball—the tendon of insertion gave way at its weakest point—which in this case was in the region where the sesamoid bone is developed. The history is

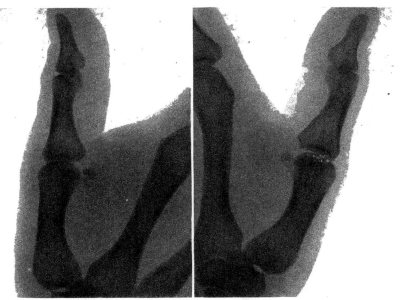

| Fractured Sesamoid. | Normal Sesamoid of Thumb of the other Hand. |

very definite, so that it is fairly certain the fracture was not due to direct violence.

I am greatly indebted to Lieut.-Col. Maturin, Officer Commanding 34 (The Welsh) General Hospital, for kind permission to publish this case.

THE DISTORTION OF THE CARDIAC SHADOWS PRODUCED BY VARYING DISTANCES OF THE ANTICATHODE FROM THE PLATE OR FILM.

By R. W. A. SALMOND, M.D.

IN view of the recent work by the French observers, Vaquez and Bordet, and its elaboration by Morison and White in this country, the following experiments were made to estimate the increase in size of the heart and its great vessels as seen in anterior views of that organ.

A silhouette of the heart and its great vessels was cut in lead, with the maximum transverse diameter of its chambers and the maximum and minimum transverse diameters of the aortic shadow of the same size as seen in a cross-section anatomy, such as Symington's.   The silhouette was then oriented, by means of careful measurements from the cross-section anatomy, in proper relation to the position a plate on the anterior wall of the chest would occupy in an average sized person.   A tube, Macalaster-Wiggin, of medium focus and hardness, was then accurately centred over the middle of the heart, a plate placed in the position of one in the living subject, and radiographs taken at different distances between the anticathode and the plate, the diaphragm for the two feet experiment being three inches diameter, and for the others two inches.

The following table shows the increase in size of shadow of the chambers

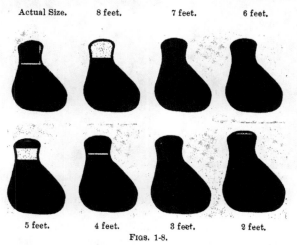

Actual Size.   8 feet.   7 feet.   6 feet.

5 feet.   4 feet.   3 feet.   2 feet.

Figs. 1-8.

of the heart and its great vessels at distances from two to eight feet between the anticathode and the plate.   It will be seen that the vessels show more distortion than the chambers, the reason being that the arch of the aorta, which runs nearly backwards, and the descending aorta are further from the plate than the chambers of the heart at their greatest transverse diameter.

Distance between anticathode and plate.				Percentage increase in transverse diameter of shadow as compared with actual size.	
				(1) Chambers.	(2) Great Vessels.
7 and 8 feet	...	...	...	2·75	3·25
6 ,,	...	...	...	3·25	4·25
5 ,,	...	...	...	3·75	4·75
4 ,,	...	...	...	5·25	6·50
3 ,,	...	...	...	7·00	8·25
2 ,,	...	...	...	11·00	13·00

Figs. 1-8 show the increasing size of shadow as the distance between anticathode and plate decreases.

If the heart is enlarged there will be more distortion than shown on table, as the rays delineating its margin are more divergent, and similarly, if the antero-posterior depth of chest is increased the distortion would be greater.

These experiments clearly show that, to avoid gross distortion of the size of the heart and its great vessels, if an orthodiagraph cannot be used, the distance between the anticathode and the plate should be at least three feet, and more if it can be conveniently arranged.

My thanks are due to Mr. A. O. Forder for his kind help.

THE EXAMINATION OF THE LIVER, GALL BLADDER, AND BILE DUCTS.

By ROBERT KNOX.

(A portion of this paper was read at a meeting of the Electrotherapeutic Section of the Royal Society of Medicine, held in April, 1919, and formed part of a discussion on the Radiography of Gall Stones.)

(Continued from August issue, p. 93.)

The Pathological Gall Bladder.

The demonstration of the presence of gall stones in the gall bladder or ducts is of considerable value in diagnosis. The actual position of a stone or stones may be indicated if the anatomical relations of the gall bladder and the bile ducts are kept in view. It may be possible to indicate that a stone is in the cystic or common bile duct ; in the latter situation jaundice may be a pronounced symptom, while pain on deep pressure may also be a determining factor; stones situated in the ducts will not readily change their position with changes in the posture of the patient. Lateral views will clearly show their position, and should enable a differential diagnosis from kidney stones to be readily made. There are other conditions than gall stones which may be shown by an X-ray examination ; of these the most frequently met with will be adhesions of the gall bladder to surrounding structures, secondary to cholocystitis. The gall bladder may be shown to be distended with mucus or muco-purulent fluid, a faint globular shadow situated beneath the liver is occasionally seen in the examination of cases in which gall bladder trouble is suspected. In exceptional circumstances a normal gall bladder, if distended with bile, may be shown. In good radiograms it may be possible to determine the presence of morbid conditions of the gall bladder without the aid of the opaque meal, though this should always be used as a confirmatory measure in doubtful cases. The colon may be unduly high in position and fixed. A number of cases in which this condition was present have been diagnosed in this way. The pyloric end of the stomach or the duodenal cap may show deformities due to adhesions.

The gall bladder may be shown to be enlarged, its walls thickened, and the presence of adhesions become evident when a radiogram of the correct quality is obtained. Fig. 38 is an example of this kind. A diagnosis of adhesions to

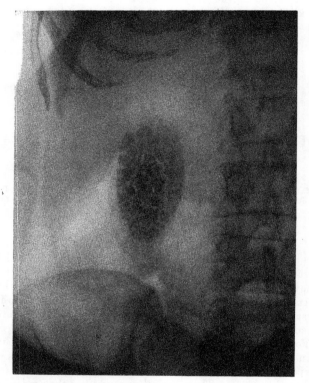

Fig. 38.—CASE 1. Gall bladder containing a large number of gall stones.
Note thickened wall of gall bladder.

the gall bladder was made in this case. The faint outline of a distended gall bladder could also be distinguished. At operation the bladder was found to be distended with muco-purulent material and fairly stout adhesions found bending the colon to the fundus and under aspect of the gall bladder.

The pathological gall bladder has been described by Leonard and George, Ledoux-Lebard, and Macleod, of Shanghai, have also called attention to the possibility of diagnosing other conditions than gall stones by means of X rays. In all work of this kind it is only painstaking attention to detail that will ensure success, and it may be necessary to take a large number of plates before the proper density of negative is obtained. The transformer appears to be more useful than the coil in this relationship; large currents passed through a modern vacuum tube and very short exposures are necessary if success is to be expected.

A tube of 5-6 inch spark gap will allow 50 to 100 milliamperes through the circuit; this should give negatives full of detail in the soft parts. Intensifying screens of very fine grain are also helpful; double coated films with two screens and very short exposures appear to give finer detail. A negative which will show stones with small calcium content should show also detail in

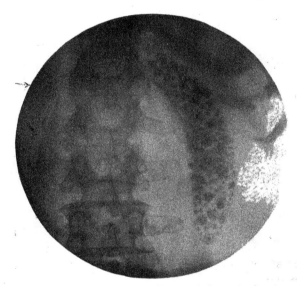

Fig. 39.—Same case as in Fig. 38. Three weeks later, showing change in position of gall bladder. Arrow indicates a fault on the plate.

the bowel, and it should be possible to differentiate bowel contents from a distended gall bladder. A thickened wall of the gall bladder may occasionally be seen. Gall stones in a gall bladder full of bile may show as lighter shadows in a denser mass, if numerous the faceted appearance of the typical distended gall bladder may be seen. (Carmen and Miller.)

The future of the diagnosis of gall stones is full of promise if the investigator realises that it is possible to get very fine detail on the plates, and if he is prepared to devote a great amount of attention to the technique.

The value of recognising pathological conditions of the gall bladder by X rays is further illustrated by the following cases:—

A soldier was sent for X-ray examination with a suggested diagnosis of gall

bladder trouble. No gall stones could be detected, but there was a well
defined shadow below the lower border of the liver. It was fairly dense and
of uniform consistence. A diagnosis of fluid in the gall bladder area was
suggested; the patient had an empyema which was pointing downwards and
had involved the gall bladder. The empyema was drained, and at a later
date bile was found in the discharge. The condition is shown in Fig. 57.

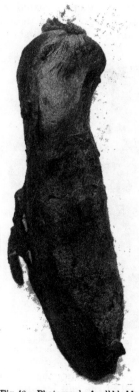

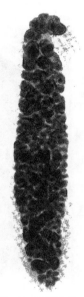

Fig. 41.—Gall bladder
containing stones
radiographed to
show arrangement
of stones *in situ.*

Fig. 40.—Photograph of gall bladder
after removal.

A patient submitted to a barium meal examination showed a well defined
irregular shadow in the gall bladder area. It was obviously connected to the
liver, and from its irregular shape was most likely to be due to the invasion of
the gall bladder by new growth. Post-mortem the bladder was found
invaded by new growth.

The liver is frequently the seat of secondary deposits in cases of cancer ;
these show as general enlargement of the organ, or if localised to a particular
area, bulging of the liver shadow may give a clue to their presence.

Hydatid cyst is also occasionally met with, and should not be overlooked when a perplexing shadow in the liver is shown. Abscesses of the liver are of fairly frequent occurrence, and should be demonstrated by X rays when the proper technique is carried out.

Clinical Details of Cases of Gall Stones in which the Diagnosis was made and confirmed by X-ray Examination.

The value of the diagnosis, or rather the confirmation of a diagnosis, of gall stones is shown in the case next described. A lady, about 55 years of age, was sent for X-ray examination, with the following history : Pain and sense of dragging in the right hypochondria ; pain was spasmodic in character but never approached the degree of colic generally associated with gall stones; it had been present intermittently for several years. There was no jaundice, the urine was clear. On palpation an enlargement could be felt near the inferior border of the liver ; deep palpation gave a sensation of pain ; an elongated irregular mass could be felt between the palpating fingers, it gave a sense of semi-solid material and was irregular to the touch. The diagnosis lay between a distended gall bladder with gall stones and a new growth. The question of malignancy arose, but was dismissed after a careful consideration of the clinical signs, symptoms, and general appearance of the patient. A provisional diagnosis of gall stones in a distended gall bladder was made; the question of the presence of stones in the hepatic ducts or common bile duct was dismissed. A radiogram taken in the kidney position showed a picture seen in Fig. 38. The confused shadow seen in an earlier radiogram was rather disappointing since it gave no very definite evidence of gall stones. So convinced was I that gall stones were present that I determined to examine the case more thoroughly. The patient was placed in the position for the examination of the gall bladder shown in Fig. 30.

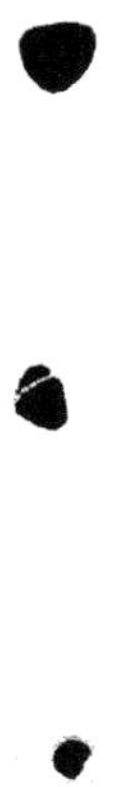

Fig. 42.—Three calculi removed from gall bladder radiographed to show structure.

The picture obtained with a moderately long exposure showed unmistakable evidence of a distended gall bladder, with a large number of gall stones in its interior. The radiogram, however, was far from satisfactory from the technical point of view, accordingly another was taken ; this time an intensifying screen was used, and a short exposure of half a second given. The result is shown in Fig. 38, where a good picture of the typical appearances of numerous gall stones is shown; the outline of the gall bladder is shown at the periphery of the collection of stones.

The diagnosis was now established ; the patient was admitted to hospital a few weeks after and another radiogram taken just before operation. A compression cylinder was used; the picture obtained shows a marked departure in shape from the previous one, the change depicted coincided with a marked change in the shape and size of the tumour when palpation was

made, and, what is perhaps of more significance, a variation in the symptoms
The patient stated definitely that she had lost the sense of distension and the
dragging pain.   This important clinical fact may be explained by the emptying of the liquid contents of the gall bladder in the interval between the
taking of the radiograms.   The importance of realizing that this does occur is
very great ; none of the stones appear to have been evacuated, possibly the
distension at intervals coincided with the blocking of the cystic duct by one

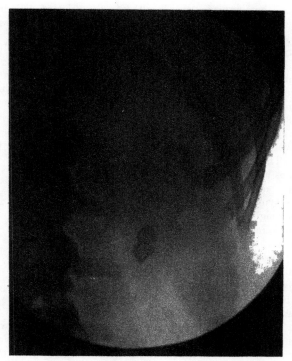

Fig. 43.—Two gall stones in gall bladder. Radiogram by C. Thurstan
Holland. Note well defined shadow of lower pole of kidney. This
offers a very definite diagnostic point.

or more of the stones.   Change of position may have relieved the blocking
and allowed the fluid contents to escape.

The gall bladder with the stones was removed intact.   A radiogram of
the bladder after removal is shown in Fig. 41.

The emptying of the gall bladder is quite a possible occurrence, even when
it contains several hundreds of stones.   One case met with in practice
completely evacuated a greatly distended gall bladder in two or three days.
At least two hundred stones were evacuated in that time.

The next case met with gave a typical history and the clinical signs of a gall stone impacted in the common bile duct. Clinically, a diagnosis was established, the patient was sent for X-ray examination, and a picture obtained; this is shown in Fig. 44. There was a definite round shadow in the right side just below the last rib and close to the spine. There were several irregular shadows in the gall bladder region. The shadow was so definite that some doubt existed as to its exact nature; the possibilities were gall stone, kidney stone, foreign body; the latter was dismissed after a few minutes consideration and an examination of a lateral plate. The suggestion of a foreign body was borne out by the appearance of some irregularity in the centre of the shadow; it gave the appearance of a small button.

A lateral picture of the region was then made and the diagnosis of gall stone

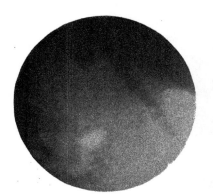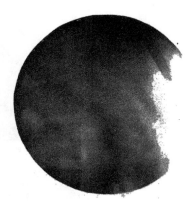

Fig. 44.—Antero-posterior view of a gall stone in the common bile duct, confirmed at operation.

Fig. 45.—Lateral view of gall bladder and stone in common bile duct. The outline of the distended gall bladder is faintly shown.

established (Fig. 45.) The lateral view still showed a round shadow, so a button could be excluded. The shadow lay a little anterior to the anterior edge of the body of the first lumbar vertebra. A kidney stone was accordingly eliminated from the consideration of the nature of the shadow. It remained to determine whether the stone was in the gall bladder or the common duct. Change in position of the patient gave no appreciable change in the position of the shadow, it was apparently firmly fixed. The depth from the anterior surface of the body clearly showed that it was not in the gall bladder, the persistent jaundice indicated obstruction to the flow of bile. A diagnosis of gall stone impacted in the common duct was made; there was obviously also something in the gall bladder. An operation was performed. The stone was found to be situated in the common duct and was removed · The gall bladder contained some debris and a few small stones.

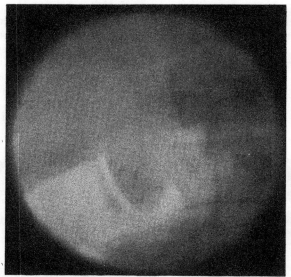

Fig. 46.—Group of shadows on under surface of liver, gall bladder containing stones.

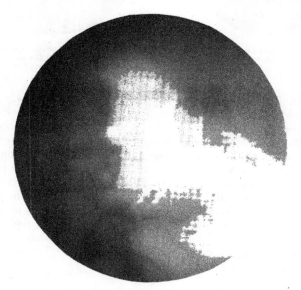

Fig. 47.—Gall bladder area showing inferior border of liver. Two groups of gall stones strapped to anterior abdominal wall. Note, where the gall stones are superimposed on the liver shadow a denser shadow is obtained. These two groups of gall stones are shown radiographed under different conditions of the X-ray tube in Figs. 8, 9, 10, 11, 12, and 17.

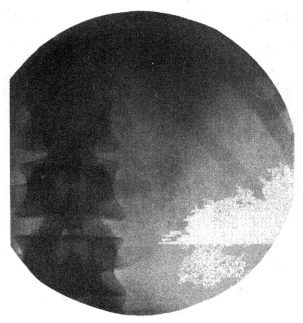

Fig. 48.—Multiple gall stones in gall bladder.   Radiogram by C. Thurstan Holland.

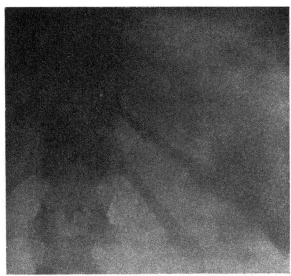

Fig. 49.—Two shadows seen in that of the liver.   ? Gall stones in gall bladder covered
by liver.   Shadows are just above the level of the eleventh rib.

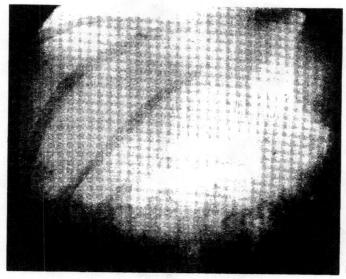

Fig. 51.—Shadow between eleventh and twelfth ribs. Irregular shadows in gall bladder and stone in common bile duct.

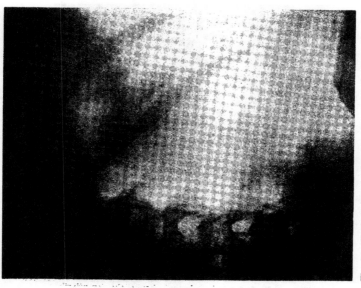

Fig. 50.—Shadow of gall stone between eleventh and twelfth ribs close to spine, debris in gall bladder.

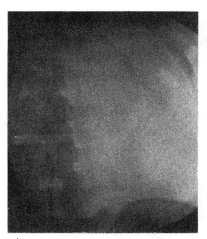

Fig. 52.—Same case as Fig. 51. Gall stone in common bile duct. The plate was taken in the kidney position, and the shadow of the gall stone is nearly lost in that of the first lumbar process.

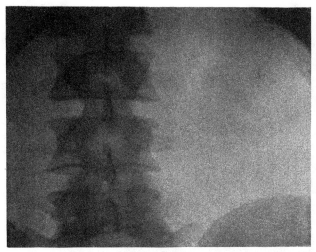

Fig. 53.—Two groups of small shadows in the right renal region. The diagnosis in this case was small calculi in the kidney. The conclusion was arrived at from a consideration of the sharp outline of the shadows, indicating that they were close to the plate, and most probably on the posterior aspect of the kidney.

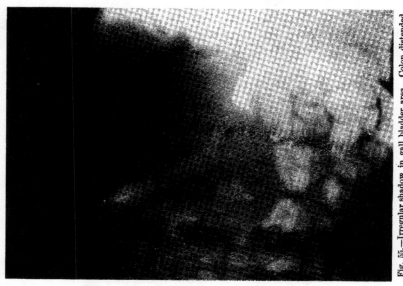

Fig. 55.—Irregular shadow in gall bladder area. Colon distended with gas. ?Enlarged thickened gall bladder with adhesions to colon.

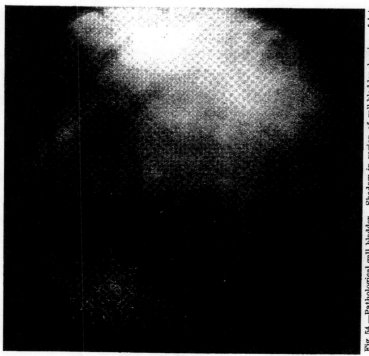

Fig. 54.—Pathological gall bladder. Shadow in region of gall bladder showing a faint outline above and below the twelfth rib. The case was sent for examination for gall stones; none were demonstrated, but the suggestion was made that the shadow described might be that of a distended gall bladder. Mr. G. B. Mower White has kindly supplied the following notes of the condition found at the operation: "The gall bladder was greatly distended with clear mucus, two small gall stones were found blocking the cystic duct. The under surface of the gall bladder was attached to the colon by firm adhesions."

Fig. 57.—Large shadow on under surface of liver. This was found to be an abscess passing down from the pleural cavity and involving the gall bladder.

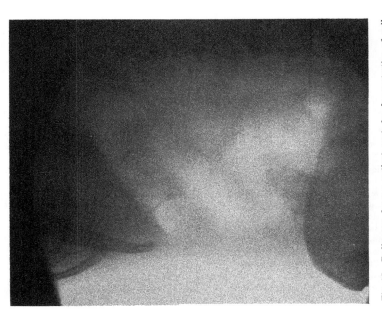

Fig. 56.—Radiogram from a patient sent for demonstration of gall stones. None were found, but on several plates a fairly definite shadow was obtained. A diagnosis of enlarged gall bladder with adhesions was suggested. Mr. Mower White kindly supplied the following notes: "Gall bladder distended, adherent to the stomach, under surface of the liver. There were no gall stones present." The interesting features in this radiogram are: (1) the fairly definite shadow of the distended gall bladder; (2) the gas distended colon; (3) the angle at which the gall bladder lies pointed inwards towards the middle line.

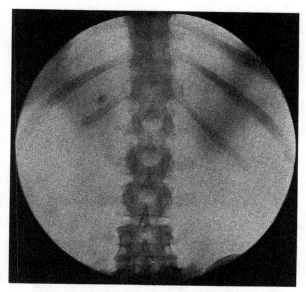

Fig. 58.—Small dense shadow close to twelfth rib, probably calcareous deposit. A shadow of this kind in the gall bladder region might easily be mistaken for a gall stone. The diagnosis was clearly established after thorough purgation, all the shadows had disappeared.

(To be continued.)

REPORT OF SOCIETY.

SOCIÉTE DE RADIOLOGIE MÉDI-CALE DE FRANCE.

Séance, du 13 Mai, 1919.

Présentation de radiographies d'un calcul de la vésicule biliaire.—Le Dr. RONNEAUX montre la radiographie d'un Malade présentant un état douloureux ancien de la fosse iliaque droite à propos duquel on avait fait les diagnostics d'appendicite, syphilis, ulcère du duodénum, du pylore, etc. L'examen rad. montra qu'aucun de ces organes n'étaient en jeu. Une radiographie, fait sans technique spéciale, dans le but d'avoir une image gastro-intestinale révéla la présence d'un volumineux calcul de la vésicule biliaire dans une région très différente du siège habituel à la vésicule. Le diagnostic fut confirmé opératoirement.

Trois préparations pour l'examen des voies digestives : lait, repas, lavement. — Le Dr. HARET présente trois préparations au sulfate de baryte gélatineux, les deux premières sont édulcorées, aromatisées, et toutes prêtes à être employées, pour la dernière il suffit d'ajouter 500 gr. d'eau chaude. A part le coté pratique permettant au radiologiste d'avoir à tout moment les émulsions préparées, l'A. rappelle les voeux émis en 1913 et 14 pour l'unification du repas opaque et montre les avantages qu'on aurait à y souscrire ; le repas qu'il présente est conforme aux désirs des Radiologistes.

Tumeur de l'apophyse coracoide.—Le Dr. VIGNAL rapporte une obs. intéréssante de tumeur assez volumineuse, régulière, englobant l'apophyse coracoïde et déterminant des phénomenes de compression vasculaire.

Nouvel appareillage pour l'utilisation des tubes Coolidge.—Le Dr. BECLÈRE présente et fait fontionner cet appareil construit par la maison Drault et Raulot-Lapointe. Tres puissant et enfermé dans un meuble à roulettes il se relie directement a une prise de courant comme les lampes électriques usuelles et, par la facilité de sa manœuvre, met, sans apprentisage, l'exploration radiologique à la portée de tous les Médicins. Il suffit pour provoquer ou pour suspendre l'émission du rayonnement de Röntgen, d'abais ser ou de relever la clef d'un interrupteur usuel, tandisque, pour augmenter ou pour diminuer l'intensité de ce rayonnement, pour augmenter ou pour diminuer son pouvoir de pénétration, il suffit de tourner dans le sens des aiguilles d'une montre ou en

sens inverse, la poignée circulaire d'un régulateur d'intensité ou celle d'un régulateur de pénétration; le fonctionnement de chacun de ces deux régulateurs demeure d'ailleurs tout à fait indépendant de celui de l'autre.

Un cas de ptose hépatique.—Le Dr. HADENGUE relate un cas d'hepatoptose observé auvcours d'une grossese. La foie occupant sa situation normale dans le decubitus horizontal pouvait facilement ètre attiré en bas par le palper profond, et s'abaisser spontanément d'environ un travers de main dans la situation verticale. Cette ptose provoquait l'apparition d'une plage lumineuse en forme de croissant entre la coupole diaphragmatique et le dôme hepatique.

Le Sécrétaire Général: Dr. HARET.

NOTES AND ABSTRACTS.

Stereoscopic Radiography.—The late SIR J. MACKENZIE DAVIDSON (*Proc. Roy. Soc. of Med.*, April-May, 1919, Sect. of Elect. Therap., pp. 1-8).—The author predicts that the day will soon come when all important X-ray examinations will be conducted by stereoscopic fluoroscopy. He points out one factor of great importance in producing correct stereoscopic photographs, and that is, upon the displacement of the tube to produce the second image, the most complete immobility possible in the part being photographed must be maintained. If this is not observed, an erroneous stereoscopic picture is produced, for example, a piece of metal on the outside of the chest may appear as if inside.

R. W. A. S.

The Sharpness of Radiographic Images.—A. LUMIÈRE (*Jour. de Radiol. et d'Elect.*, Dec., 1918, pp. 97-102, with 20 Figs.)—Experimenting with gas tubes, such as Pilon and Muller, Lumière found as follows:—

The surface of impact on the anticathode is slightly modified whilst a tube is running. The modification consists of a slight increase.

Differences of the intensity of current do not appear to have any appreciable influence on the sharpness of the image.

The focus of the cathodal stream appears to

undergo modifications according to the degree of hardness or softness of the tube, but these modifications are not of much importance.

From the point of view of sharpness of image, each tube has its own characteristics, which are relatively slightly modified by the conditions under which the tube is running.

Lumière confirmed the fact, already well known, that the sharpness increases with increasing distance between the anticathode and the plate.

The want of sharpness, then, seems to be due to the fact that the source of origin of the rays is not punctiform, but formed by a surface from whose different points the rays are emitted.

R. W. A. S.

The Necessity of Using a Special Radiographic Technique for Certain Parts of the Skeleton.—LAQUERRIERE AND PIERQUIN (*Jour. de Radiol. et d'Electrol.*, March, 1919, pp. 145-148, with eight radiograms and two figures.)—The authors show that in certain cases it is necessary to make use of special techniques in addition to the usual positions.

Techniques for demonstrating the posterior aspect of the lower end of the humerus, the internal condyle and the superio-inferior projection of the olecranon, the superio-inferior view of the spine of the scapula, the posterior halves of the condyles of the femur and the intercondyloid notch, the longitudinal view of the patella, etc., are described.

R. W. A. S.

Fistula of the Parotid.—P. P. COLE and R. KNOX (*Lancet*, June 7th, 1919, pp. 971, 972).—In cases of incomplete fistula of the duct or fistula of the gland, these observers record good results with treatment by radium or radium and X rays combined.

R. W. A. S.

Some Points about Bone Grafts.—W. I. de C. WHEELER (*Brit. Med. Jour.*, Feb. 1st, 1919, pp. 119-120, with 7 radiograms).— From a study of thirty cases the author has formed the following conclusions :—

Whatever the histological *rôle*, the clinical usefulness of a bone graft is not affected.

The final success of bone grafting in cases in which a gap is bridged depends upon the operation of Wolff's law, *i.e.*, the graft, stimulated by strains and stresses, changes its internal architecture and external conformation until the required strength is attained.

The periosteum should be left on the graft, because, although not essential, it is the medium through which new blood vessels enter the graft and the surrounding structures. Furthermore, in removing the periosteum superficial layers of osteoblasts may be sacrificed. A periostium covered graft is less likely to become rapidly absorbed.

To provide the necessary strains and stresses it is advisable to allow the graft to functionate as early as possible, but in most cases preliminary fixation for three months is essential.

In old ununited fractures with false joints, the bone in the critical area (near the site of fracture) is sclerosed and avascular, and makes an unsuitable soil for that portion of the graft in contact with this area. Growth in the graft is impeded by the surrounding sclerosis. Dense sclerotic bone has no osteogenetic power.

In such cases, a periosteal covered graft may become attenuated and absorbed, or break in the critical area five or six months after operation.

In the same class of case very prolonged fixation is particularly unfavourable to osteogenesis, to the establishment of blood supply,

and bony union. Early movements and the bearing of mechanical stress and strain, on the other hand, may lead to yielding of the graft and failure.

But for slightly slower osteogenetic powers and a real tendency to fracture, the intramedullary peg is effective. This method is satisfactory in the case of the radius and ulna.

In the case of the humerus and femur, long, stout inlay grafts give the best results. Sliding grafts should only be used in simple and fresh cases.

The bone graft has inherent bacteria resisting properties.

Absolute fixation of the graft in its bed, either as part of the operation, or afterwards, by splints or plaster, is essential to success..

As in the operation of tendon transplantation and nerve suture, the operation of bone grafting should be preceded by correction of any deformity, and by the freeing of adhesions in neighbouring tendons and joints.

R. W. A. S.

Effect of Stimuli from the Lower Bowel on the Rate of Emptying the Stomach.—F. W. WHITE (*Amer. Jour. of the Med. Sciences,* Aug., 1918, p. 184-189).—The X-ray method was used to study the effect of stimuli from the lower bowel on the rate of emptying of the stomach ; the effect of mechanical filling and distention of the colon by enemata in men and cats ; the effect of chemical irritation of the cæcum in cats ; the effect of diseases of the lower bowel in 120 cases of chronic colitis, tubercular ulceration and cancer of the colon, chronic and acute appendicitis, and adhesions of the lower ileum and colon.

The results all point the same way ; (1) delay in emptying the stomach is the exception in lesions of the lower bowel ; (2) a strong stimulus is needed from the lower bowel to slow the stomach, for it was found that the stomach emptied a barium meal within the normal time in some cases of ileal stasis of two or more days duration, and in most cases with good-sized 12-hour residue in the ileum, also when the colon was distended with a large enema, also in most cases of chronic appendicitis and chronic inflammations and tumours of the colon.

Clinical and experimental observation in lesions and irritation of the upper bowel (duodenum and jejunum) have shown that they often delay emptying of the stomach.

Experiments on animals showed that when the colon was irritated by injections into the cæcum, variable results were obtained; intense irritation caused vomiting; less marked irritation caused either delay in emptying the stomach up to about twice the normal time or rapid emptying of the stomach and whole digestive tract; moderate or slight irritation had no effect. These experiments would suggest that different degrees of inflammation of the appendix may affect the stomach in a corresponding way.

Marked delay in emptying the stomach is far more often the result of actual lesions about the pylorus than of reflexes from the bowel. "Stomach symptoms" in intestinal cases are not, as a rule, the result of slow emptying of the stomach but are largely toxic on the result of referred pain or distress.

R. W. A. S.

Hilus Tuberculosis in the Adult.—C. RIVIERE (*Lancet*, Feb. 8th, 1919, pp. 213-216). —The term hilus tuberculosis of adults is not here used to include those evidences of obsolete tubercle which are to be found in every X ray plate, and which are apt to bulk large in the radiological report on a suspicious chest, but refers to a fresh and active process involving the deep areas of the lungs where remain the old foci of childhood infection, and thence spreading outwards towards the surface. It thus stands in close relationship to the common form of tuberculosis in childhood, though with less tendency to glandular involvement.

The clinical and physical signs, symptoms, and differential diagnosis are discussed by the writer.

The radiographic appearances, he says, may be divided into three types, according to the activity of the process, as follows :—

1. Chronic and quiet disease with little or no evidence of activity. This represents perhaps the commonest type of case, the evidences of activity being entirely dependent on other factors than the X-ray picture. The main point about the radiogram is the abnormal visibility of the whole lung reticulum, which appears thick and strongly shadowed in all its "twigs" right out to the

periphery. The main branches appear thickened, often wide and tape-like, or may appear as rings or figures of eight, with or without some dilatation of their lumen. The whole picture has a general "fibrous appearance," nodules may be absent and yet the case tuberculous, or there may be a nodular appearance throughout. In many of these chronic cases the radiogram may present so "fibrous" a picture that it is hard to believe any activity can be present. Yet the patient may present symptoms and develop a fresh pleurisy as evidence that the process is not obsolete.

In hilus tuberculosis, of whatever form, it often appears that the diseased area is, roughly, equal on the two sides and often reaches nearly to the periphery; it may present a sharply-marked outer margin, giving a butterfly appearance, and strongly suggesting a simultaneous spread out to this point rather than a slow creeping outwards. From X-ray and post-mortem experience, the writer is convinced that a simultaneous "sowing" of disease over a wide area occurs not infrequently, though the gradual outward spread presumed in the general description of the disease is perhaps the rule.

2. More active disease.—This may show itself in a more woolly and less sharp-cut appearance of disease, which yet remains to X-ray examination purely "peribronchial." The thickening of the bronchi is more marked both round the root and farther out in the lung, and a nodular or even "budding" appearance may be seen. The finer net-work of the lung is thickened irregularly or nodular shadows of various size and not very sharp outline may be linked up in it.

3. Active and acute disease.—The strands of the lung net-work vanish and the pulmonary fields become filled with woolly bronchopneumonic shadows of smaller or larger size with eventual coalescence and cavity formation.

R. W. A. S.

Two rare Cases of Ossification of the Ligaments Diagnosed by X rays.—C. GUARINI (*La Riforma Medica*, March 16th, 1918, p. 208).—This observer records two cases of what he interprets as the above following injury. The first, apparently an ossification of the spheno-mandibular ligament, and forming a solid bridge between the cranium and the mandible, interfering greatly with the movements of the lower jaw.

The second, seen as an ossification extending from the fractured margin of the acetabulum

towards the greater and lesser trochanters. This followed the line of the capsular ligament and was thought to be an ossification of that ligament.   R. W. A. S.

PUBLICATIONS RECEIVED.
Books.
Constipation and Allied Intestinal Disorders. By Arthur F. Hurst, M.A., M.D. Oxon, F.R.C.P. London: Hy. Frowde, Hodder & Stoughton. 16s. net.

Journals.
American Journal of Electrotherapeutics and Radiology, Mar., 1919.

American Journal of Roentgenology, July, Aug., 1919.

Archives d'Electricite Medicale et de Physiotherapie, July, 1919.

Bulletin of the Johns Hopkins Hospital, Aug., 1919.

Gaceta Médica Catalana, Aug., 1919.

Good Health, Aug., 1919.

Hospitalstidende, July 2nd, 8th, 16th, 23rd, 30th; Aug. 6th, 13th, 20th, 1919.

Il Policlinico, July, 1919.

Journals—*continued.*
Journal de Radiologie et d'Electrologie, Vol. III., No. 6, June, 1919; Vol. IV., No. 7, Aug., 1919.

Le Radium, June, 1919.

Medical Journal of Australia, June 7th, 28th; July 5th, 12th, 19th, 1919.

Modern Medicine, July-Aug., 1919.

New York Medical Journal, Aug. 2nd, 9th, 16th, 23rd, 1919.

New York State Journal of Medicine, Aug. 1919.

Proceedings of the Royal Society of Medicine, July, 1919.

Rivista Italiana di Neuropatologia, Psichiatria ed Elettroterapia, June, 1919.

Sunic Record, No. 8.

Ugeskrift for Læger, July 24th, 1919; Aug. 7th, 14th, 1919.

"Yadil" Clinical Notes, Aug.-Sept., 1919.

NOTICES.

ARCHIVES OF RADIOLOGY AND ELECTROTHERAPY is published monthly.

The index for each volume, which ends with the May number, is supplied with the June number of each year.

Communications to the Editors should be addressed to "ROBERT KNOX, M.D., 38, Harley Street, W. 1."

Communications and illustrations from American contributors may be sent to Messrs. REBMAN COMPANY, 141-145, West Thirty-sixth Street, New York City.

All radiographs and photographs must be originals, and must not have been previously published. Drawings should be supplied on separate paper.

Owing to the scarcity of paper the Publishers are reluctantly compelled—as a temporary war measure—to reduce the number of free reprints of Papers to twenty-five.

Annual Subscriptions, payable in advance, 30/- including postage. Single copies, 3/- (postage 2d.) Single numbers and back numbers can be supplied on application.

Vol. XXIV—No. 5   OCTOBER, 1919   No. 231

ARCHIVES OF RADIOLOGY AND ELECTROTHERAPY

THE OFFICIAL ORGAN OF THE
BRITISH ASSOCIATION OF RADIOLOGY AND PHYSIOTHERAPY

Editors.

ROBERT KNOX, M.D., Hon. Radiographer, King's College Hospital.

E. P. CUMBERBATCH, B.M., M.R.C.P., Medical Officer in Charge. Electrical Department, St. Bartholomew's Hospital.

SIDNEY RUSS, D.Sc., Physicist to the Middlesex Hospital.

IN COLLABORATION WITH

A. E. BARCLAY (Manchester); BELOT (Paris); H. MARTIN BERRY (London); W. H. BRAGG (London), N. BURKE (Woodhall Spa); J. BURNET (Edinburgh); W. J. S. BYTHELL (Manchester); J. T. CASE (Battle Creek, U.S.A.): A. ST. GEORGE CAULFEILD (London); H. A. COLWELL (London); FOVEAU DE COURMELLES (Paris); GUNZBURG (Antwerp); HALL-EDWARDS (Birmingham): HARET (Paris); HAUCHAMPS (Brussels); F. HERNAMAN-JOHNSON (London); W. F. HIGGINS (Teddington); THURSTAN HOLLAND (Liverpool); HURST (London); KLYNENS (Antwerp): LAQUERRIERE (Paris), LAZARUS-BARLOW (London); LEDUC (Nantes); ALEXANDER MACKAY (Edinburgh); REGINALD MORTON (London); HARRISON ORTON (London); W. OVEREND (St. Leonards-on-Sea); PFAHLER (Philadelphia); C. E. S. PHILLIPS (London); GEORGE PIRIE (Dundee); HOWARD PIRIE (Montreal): A. W. PORTER (London); R. W. A. SALMOND (London); WERTHEIM SALOMONSON (Amsterdam): S. SLOAN (Glasgow); SOMERVILLE (Glasgow); W. C. STEVENSON (Dublin): W. J. TURRELL (Oxford): HUGH WALSHAM (London); ROBT. WILSON (Montreal).

ON THE MODE OF SPREAD OF CANCER IN RELATION TO ITS TREATMENT BY RADIATION.

By W. Sampson Handley, M.S.

Surgeon to the Middlesex Hospital and its Cancer Charity.

[Reprinted from the Proceedings of the Royal Society of Medicine, 1919, Vol. XII. (Section of Electrotherapeutics), pp. 41-49.]

THE rôle played by radiation in the treatment of malignant disease is one of increasing importance, both on the preventive and curative sides. In a number of cases of cancer the efforts of the surgeon, if unsupported by those of the radiologist, would be unavailing, and of course the converse proposition is equally true. Now, I have found, as a surgeon, that a detailed study of the mode of dissemination of cancer has been of the greatest use to me in my operative work. It has enabled me to substitute carefully planned rational operation for empirical and haphazard procedure. In the belief that a knowledge of the process of dissemination must form a necessary foundation in planning the radiological, just as much as the operative, treatment of cancer, I venture to-night to ask your attention to some facts and observations about the spread of cancer. I ask you also to consider my paper as a tribute of gratitude from a surgeon to his radiological colleagues for help received.

As might be expected, the mode of dissemination of cancer was first worked out in the commonest form of external cancer—namely, breast cancer. Internal cancers are not accessible to observation until after death, and the picture then presented is so complicated and confused that it may defy analysis. Moreover, such cases are at present largely beyond the domain of radiological and still more of surgical treatment. My remarks to-night will refer chiefly to breast cancer.

A rare form of external cancer—namely, melanotic sarcoma—has also been accurately studied as regards its method of dissemination. Here research has been simplified by the fact that the dark colouration of the growth is practically the equivalent of a specific stain for cancer tissue, a desideratum at present lacking for other growths. The mode of dissemination in melanotic sarcoma has proved to be very similar to that found in breast cancer, and it can easily be demonstrated to the naked eye. (Figs. 30 to 38.)

The spread of cancers of the mucous glands, and especially of cancer of the stomach, can sometimes be demonstrated by the use of the stain mucicarmine, which stains mucus red while leaving other tissues unstained. Wherever a degenerate cancer cell is present and mucus is formed, a pink stain is produced. Thus, in situations where mucus is normally absent the track of a cancer can be followed with certainty. When a gastric cancer reaches the parietes at the umbilicus, an event which is not very rare, it is found to spread in the abdominal wall in exactly the same fashion as a breast cancer spreads from its point of origin. (Figs. 39 and 40.)

There is thus a strong presumption that all carcinomata and sarcomata which cause infection of lymphatic glands spread after the same fashion, and mainly by a process which I have termed permeation of the lymphatic vessels.

Definition of Permeation.—Permeation is the continuous tendril-like growth of lines of cancer cells, by their own proliferative power, along the smaller lymphatic vessels. It is to be sharply distinguished from infiltration, which is the growth of cancer cells through the intercellular spaces. (Figs. 1 and 2.)

Lymphatic Anatomy.—For the proper understanding of the process we must consider some of the facts of lymphatic anatomy. What immediately concerns us is the arrangement of the lymphatics of the body-wall, of the skin, subcutaneous tissue, fascia and the superficial muscles. Here the leading fact is the existence, just superficial to the deep fascia, of a plexus of vessels of microscopic size forming an investment for the body as complete as the skin itself. This plexus, the fascial lymphatic plexus, is the main highway for the spread of cancer in the superficial tissues. When invaded by cancer it becomes a kind of shirt of Nessus, in which the victim perishes. (Fig. 3.)

It is important to insist on the unity of this plexus, and on the fact that it offers no barrier anywhere to the spread of cancer through its meshes. It is drained by certain lymphatic trunks, which convey its lymph to the cervical, axillary, and inguinal glands. The imaginary lines separating the tributary areas of these three sets of glands run at the level of the clavicle and of the umbilicus. These lines, together with the middle line, divide the plexus into six areas, each of which has its own set of trunk lymphatics. No trunk lymphatics cross these lines, but the continuity of the plexus itself is not interrupted by them.

The fascial plexus is fed by little vertical tributaries which reach it on both aspects, from the skin above and from the muscles beneath. The lymphatics of origin of the skin are little blind huger-like processes, one in each papilla of the skin. A number of these unite to form one of the little vertical tributaries which run down to empty themselves in the fascial plexus.

Summary of Conclusions on Dissemination.

Dissemination is usually accomplished by the actual growth of cancer cells along the finer vessels of the lymphatic plexuses—" permeation." Embolic invasion of the regional lymphatic glands, though it almost invariably occurs, only leads to invasion of the blood stream after long delay ; and the work of M. B. Schmidt shows that cancer cells which reach the blood usually disappear without giving rise to metastases.

Permeation takes place almost as readily against the lymph stream as with it. It spreads through the lymphatic vessels around the primary neoplasm in much the same way as would a thick injection fluid introduced into the tissues by a syringe. If in a late case of breast cancer one examines the region immediately around the macroscopic primary growth, no permeated lymphatics can be detected. Here and there are secondary nodules of growth entirely isolated from one another and from the primary neoplasm.

If, however, the investigation is pushed still further from the primary growth, by the examination of long radial sections of the skin and underlying tissues, we arrive at a region beyond the remotest visible naked eye metastasis and often lying far from the primary growth. In this region the microscopic growing edge of the carcinoma will usually be detected by careful microscopic search. The microscopic growing edge is to be sharply distinguished from the infiltrating edge of the primary neoplasm where interstitial invasion of the surrounding tissues is occurring. At the peripheral microscopic growing edge there is no interstitial invasion of the tissues, but the principal lymphatic plexus of the part—the plexus which lies upon the deep fascia—is found permeated throughout—that is to say, its vessels are obstructed by the growth of lines of cancer cells along them. (Figs. 7, 8 and 9.)

The disappearance of permeated lymphatics in the area which intervenes between the annular " microscopic growing edge " and the primary neoplasm is due to the destruction, after a time, of the cancerous permeated lymphatics by the defensive process of " perilymphatic fibrosis." The recognition of this process at once removes the difficulty that permeated lymphatics are absent in the region immediately surrounding the naked eye primary growth. (Figs. 21 to 29.)

The process of permeation follows the line of least resistance, and extends, at first exclusively, in the plane of the principal lymphatic plexus into which the lymph drainage of the cancerous organ passes. The annular microscopic growing edge of a breast cancer is therefore found in the plane of the fascial lymphatic plexus, upon, or just superficial to, the deep fascia. It is covered over by normal skin and has normal muscles lying beneath it.

If, however, the tissues are examined at points successively intermediate between the microscopic growing edge and the apparent edge of the primary growth, the cancer will be found penetrating the adjoining layers, the super-jacent skin and the subjacent muscle, to a greater and greater depth, and forming nodular deposits therein, which may, however, be sporadic and few in number, and in some cases may be altogether absent. (Figs. 13 to 17.)

Cancer thus spreads in the parietal tissues by permeating the lymphatic system like an invisible annular ringworm. The growing edge extends like a ripple, in a wider and wider circle, within the circumference of which healing processes take place, so that the area of permeation at any one time is not a disc but a ring. The spread of cancer in the parietal tissues is, in fact, as truly a serpiginous process as the most typical tertiary syphilide. But in the case of cancer the spreading edge is invisible ; and, moreover, the advancing microscopic growing edge of a cancer, owing to the failure at isolated points of the defensive process of perilymphatic fibrosis, may leave in its track, here and there, isolated secondary foci, which give rise to macroscopic metastases. Such nodules, in spite of their apparent isolation, arise in continuity with the primary growth, but perilymphatic fibrosis has destroyed the permeated lymphatics which formed the lines of communication.

We must now turn to the question of treatment.

TREATMENT OF BREAST CANCER BY RADIATION WITHOUT OPERATION.

In a number of cases, either because the disease is too advanced, or on account of some constitutional disease, surgical operation is excluded, and the treatment of breast cancer must be conducted solely by radiation.

Hitherto, in many cases, the only idea which has governed the exact site of application of X rays to growths of the breast has been that the breast itself should be irradiated, with the additional proviso that attention should be devoted to the axillary glands. Such an idea belongs to the same stage of development as the surgical idea that the operation required for breast cancer is an amputation of the breast, combined with removal of the axillary glands. In radiography, as in surgery, it is necessary that advances in pathological knowledge should be reflected in practice. Now that the idea of cancer of the breast as a local disease of an organ has to be replaced by the conception of it as a centrifugal invasion by permeation of the lymphatic system of the body, starting at the point of origin of the primary growth and spreading in a constantly enlarging circle which has no respect for anatomical boundaries, it is obvious that blindfold methods of applying X rays require revision. It is especially necessary that the radiographer should know the exact site of origin of the primary growth in the breast, for otherwise he can only vaguely locate the area of his work. On the first occasion he sees the patient he should insist on making a complete inspection of the chest with the clothes removed. A chart should be made out on which the point of origin of the growth, as ascertained from the patient or the surgeon, should be marked, and a rough outline of the presumed circle of infected tissues should be traced with a flesh pencil upon the skin, and drawn upon the chart as a guide to future work.

Omission of the simple precaution of fixing the site of the primary growth may lead to an error of as much as 5 in. or 6 in. in the location of the circle of tissues to be radiated. In a case I saw a day or two ago a small carcinoma was situated in the fold below a voluminous breast. The 12 in. circle of presumed infection would extend at least down to the umbilicus. Yet if this case had been treated on general lines simply as a cancer of the breast without removal of the clothes and inspection of the growth, it is almost certain that the abdomen would have escaped radiation altogether. In view of the known facts as to invasion of the abdomen directly through the linea alba in the epigastric angle the whole treatment might have been vitiated by the omission.

Position of the Patient during Radiation.—This same case raises another point. The small growth, lying in the fold below the breast, was protected in front from radiation by the whole thickness of the voluminous and pendulous mamma. It is therefore a question to be considered by the Section whether in certain cases of breast cancer the X-ray treatment should be conducted in the recumbent position and with other precautions, such as the use of a sling or bandage to the breast for exposing the growth to the full force of the radiation. Growths of the outer edge of the breast are similarly protected against radiation by the whole thickness of the breast, if the organ is well developed, unless the radiologist has previously secured himself, by inspection of the growth and suitable placing of his tube, against this unnecessary addition to his difficulties. Here, if the case is treated on stereotyped lines, simply as one of cancer of the breast, the whole axillary region, or at least the scapular region, will probably escape radiation, and thus again the treatment may be vitiated. These points are obvious, but they are of fundamental importance, and I believe they are sometimes ignored by radiologists. Undue restriction, and perhaps still more often, bad centring of the area of irradiation are, in my opinion, frequent causes of failure. The second error is inevitable unless pains are taken to investigate the peculiarities of the individual case by questioning and inspecting the patient.

Undue Restriction of the Field of Radiation.—It is not sufficient to apply radiation to the primary growth alone, nor even to apply it to the whole of the breast. We have seen that the most active portion of the growth is an invisible circle of permeation spreading through the lymphatics, quite inappreciable by clinical methods, and often reaching a diameter of 10 in. or 12 in.

in moderately advanced cases. The most important service to be hoped for from radiation is not the destruction of massive deposits of already more or less degenerate cancer cells, but the arrest of the spread of this growing edge of active cells. The achievement is unlikely to be attained unless it is deliberately aimed at. It involves the radiation of an area of the parietal tissues centred upon the primary growth and rather larger than the presumed area of the extension of permeation. The diameter of the radiation circle should, I estimate, lie between 12 in. and 16 in. It is not for me to suggest how this large area should be dealt with, but its periphery is perhaps even more important than its centre, because the cells at the periphery are all young and active, while the massive primary growth resembles a half extinct volcano. On the other hand, a microscopic filament like a permeated lymphatic, is more easily penetrable than a naked eye mass of cancer cells.

The Section should consider whether, and to what extent, the use of diaphragms is advisable in the X-ray treatment of breast cancer. In view of the large area to be covered it seems unadvisable to stop-down the tube. And in view of the facts I have adduced it is a question whether the area submitted to radiation is not frequently too small. A few days ago a case of breast-cancer came under my notice, where a well marked circular area of skin pigmentation, not more than five inches in diameter, mapped out the region to which X rays had been restricted.

Prophylactic Radiation.—During the last fourteen years every case of breast cancer upon which I have operated has received, usually at the hands of your President, a prophylactic course of X rays. I have not adopted the practice of irradiating the wound before closing it, believing that it is unnecessary and that it involves risk of sepsis, and of impairing the vitality of the flaps by chilling them. In my series of cases recurrence in the skin has been almost absent. Three of the five cases in which it took place occurred among the small percentage of cases which had escaped the usual prophylactic course of X rays. This striking fact establishes, to my mind, the great prophylactic value of irradiation. In undertaking prophylactic irradiation the operator should bear in mind before beginning the irradiation : —

(*a*) *That the operation may have failed to extirpate a portion of the microscopic growing edge,* and for the reasons already stated the area submitted to radiation should be a circle of 12 in. or 14 in. in diameter, centred upon the primary growth. It should not be forgotten that the periphery of this circle may be its most dangerous part, and that in fixing it regard should be had to the site of the growth in the breast. Neither the radiologist nor the surgeon can afford to ignore the law of centrifugal spread from the primary growth. The isolated nodules left in the track of the process of permeation, after its spread like a smouldering fire through the lymphatics, are often very amenable to radiation. But unless the spread of permeation at the microscopic growing edge be arrested no permanent good will result. It is to the peripheral region, just beyond the remotest visible deposits, that the special attention of the radiologist should be given. Here he may hope to arrest the process of dissemination by killing the microscopic growing edge. If his radiation is confined to the region of visible deposits he can only hope for palliation. He must remember that in the long run the naked eye manifestations of the disease are less important than its invisible microscopic extensions by which it ultimately reaches the vital organs.

(*b*) *That microscopic foci may lurk in the supraclavicular or the anterior mediastinal glands of the same side.* Of course, the whole region of the growth must be irradiated, but if a method of operation has been employed aiming at extirpation of the microscopic growing edge, recurrence, if it takes place, will usually be late, and will be found at the inner edge of the second, third, or fourth intercostal spaces or in the supraclavicular triangle of the same side. It is a question, therefore, whether the dangerous regions thus indicated should not receive an extra dose of radiation.

(*c*) *In late cases where the surgeon has found advanced infection of the axilla the lateral chest wall must receive special attention.* Modern methods of operating have almost abolished axillary recurrence, but in advanced cases radiation of the axilla with the arm abducted is advisable.

It is not within the scope of this paper to consider the methods and dosage of radiation. But pathology and lymphatic anatomy must be as fundamental for the radiological as for the surgical treatment of cancer. In that belief I offer no apology for the claim upon your attention which I have made to-night.

NATURAL CURE OF CANCER.

It is not possible to form a correct estimate of the value of radiation in cancer without taking into account the natural tendency of the disease to undergo local repair. In a lecture on this subject I came to the conclusion that, "Every aggregation of cancer cells, after increasing in size for a varying period and for a varying rate, tends spontaneously to undergo certain degenerative or regressive changes. These changes begin at the centre of the mass, spread centrifugally to its circumference, and may terminate in the replacement of the mass of cancer cells by a fibrous scar." (Figs. 18 to 20.)

These changes, which are exemplified in the ulceration of a primary growth, and in the umbilication of secondary deposits in the liver, appear to depend upon a breakdown of the improvised vascular commissariat of the growth, and upon the harmful internal pressure produced by the active proliferation of the cancer cells. These degenerative changes can be seen beginning even when the collection of cancer cells is still of microscopic size, as is a permeated lymphatic. Their onset is invariably accompanied by the advent to the neighbourhood of collections of lymphocytes. It is thus possible that in every carcinoma we have to deal with a comparatively small number of perfectly healthy and active cancer cells, and with a large mass of more or less degenerate or dying cells. The former class of cell is to be found in the permeated lymphatics of the microscopic growing edge, and at the edge of macroscopic nodules of growth which are still in the actively infiltrating stage.

It seems likely that these two classes of cell differ widely in their reaction to radiation. It is probable that the crowds of degenerate cells which constitute the mass of a carcinoma may fall a ready prey to the reaction of radiation. Even the earliest attempts at the destruction of secondary nodules by X rays were often locally successful. The shrinkage and disappearance of local masses of cancer may possibly indicate nothing more than the acceleration and completion of this natural process of destruction.

The real problem is not to dispatch the wounded but to attack the cancer cell in full vital activity, and to determine how it responds to radiation as compared with the degenerate cancer cell, and what is the amount and character of the radiation necessary to destroy it. Such a research is quite practicable but necessarily laborious. It would require the co-operation of a radiologist and a histologist. Cases of breast cancer showing a moderate and regular dissemination of subcutaneous nodules round the growth should be selected, and a sector of the microscopic growing edge just beyond the region of visible nodules should be submitted to radiation, and compared post-mortem with untreated sectors of the microscopic growing edge.

So long as investigation is directed to macroscopic masses of mostly degenerate or dying cells its results must remain indeterminate and confused. Definite results can only be obtained by experiments upon the standard healthy cancer cell of the microscopic growing edge, not the edge of the primary growth or of any of the visible secondary deposits, but that of the ripple of permeation which is extending from the primary growth, through the patient's lymphatic system. The detection of the microscopic growing edge of permeated lymphatics provided the key to the understanding of the process of dissemination. It is quite possible that a careful study of its behaviour under radiation may supply a master-key to the therapy of cancer.

DESCRIPTION OF FIGURES.

SLIDE 1.—Active infiltration at the edge of a primary carcinoma of the breast.

SLIDE 2.—Permeation of a lymphatic vessel seen in longitudinal section. From the true microscopic growing edge of a breast cancer at a point 10 inches distant from the point of origin of the primary growth. Note the endothelium of the lymphatic. Normal blood vessels are seen above and below.

Slides 1 and 2 contrast the two main processes concerned in dissemination, namely, permeation and infiltration. Infiltration is the growth of cancer cells along the intercellular spaces. Permeation is the tendril-like growth of cancer cells along lymphatic *vessels*. It ultimately assumes much greater importance than infiltration.

SLIDE 3.—A plate from Sappey's " Vaisseaux Lymphatiques," showing the fascial lymphatic plexus, and the trunks which drain it into the cervical, the axillary, and the inguinal glands. This plexus lies upon the deep fascia and forms a complete investment for the body. It is the main highway of permeation for cancers originating in the parietes, and the process spreads indefinitely in it like a ripple. The plexus receives tributaries from the skin above and the muscles beneath, hence after a time the skin and muscles are invaded by the up-stream extension of permeation along these tributaries. The lymph stream plays no part in permeation, either as an obstacle or an adjuvant.

SLIDE 4.—The mucous lymphatic plexus of the intestine (Sappey). Inserted to show the general characters of a lymphatic plexus.

SLIDE 5.—Schematic representation of the pectoral portion of the fascial plexus, along with the axillary glands. A circular area of permeated lymphatics (coloured black) is present in the fascial plexus as the result of a cancer in the overlying breast. The arrows indicate the future centrifugal spread of this area. Lymphatic embolism along the trunks (a process of minor importance) has led to the infection of the axillary glands. These glands act as a barrier for a long time to the spread of the growth beyond them to the supraclavicular glands, but there is no obstacle to the indefinite extension of permeation in the fascial plexus.

SLIDE 6.—Up-stream invasion of the skin lymphatics by permeation often leads to the appearance of secondary subcutaneous nodules. These nodules begin *close to the growth*, and spread from it *centrifugally*, occupying a circular area around it. The slide represents this process moderately advanced. (From Sheild's "Diseases of the Breast.")

SLIDE 7.—The *microscopic growing edge* of a breast cancer, situated in the abdominal wall about five inches above the umbilicus, forming Plate I. in Handley's "Cancer of the Breast," *q.v.* There is here no interstitial invasion of the tissues, all the cancer cells are confined within lymphatic vessels, and are restricted to the plane of the deep fascial lymphatic plexus. The section is taken radially away from the primary growth. Other radial sections showed similar appearances at about the same distance away from the primary growth.

SLIDE 8.—The microscopic growing edge of a breast cancer, taken post-mortem from the deltoid region of the arm (Plate II. in Handley's "Cancer of the Breast"). The disease is spreading like an invisible ringworm in the fascial lymphatic plexus.

SLIDE 9.—A high-power photograph of the permeated lymphatics of the extreme growing edge. Same case as Slide 8.

SLIDE 10.—Frontispiece, *loc. cit.* A sagittal median section in the intermammary region of the parietes in a case of breast cancer. The section shows skin, subcu'aneous tissue, and a layer of muscle (pectoralis major and rectus abdominis). Numerous naked eye nodules of cancer are seen upon the anterior layer of the rectus sheath, while the skin over them is quite normal. To emphasise the fact that the primary plane of spread of breast cancer is that of the deep fascial lymphatic plexus.

SLIDE 11.—Diagrammatic vertical section through skin, subcutaneous tissue and deep fascia, taken radially through the edge of a breast cancer, P. Though subcutaneous nodules may appear at N N and N successively, this does not mean that the cancer is spreading *along the skin*. The plane of spread is along the deep fascia, and only secondarily up to the skin at isolated points. The microscopic growing edge will be found in the deep fascia well beyond the furthest skin nodule. It is indicated by a heavy dotted line.

SLIDE 12.—A fascial nodule upon the linea alba in the epigastric angle in a case of breast cancer. Infiltration of the linea alba is proceeding, and thus the cancer cells will soon reach the subperitoneal fat and the peritoneal cavity (epigastric invasion of the abdomen).

THE FORMATION OF SUBCUTANEOUS NODULES.

SLIDE 13.—The up-stream extension of permeation along one of the cutaneous tributaries of the fascial plexus. This process leads to the formation of nodules in the subcutaneous tissue and the dermis.

SLIDE 14.—Above is seen the deep aspect of the true skin riddled with cancer cells. Beneath this is the subcutaneous fat with fan-shaped lines and groups of cancer cells running along the fibrous septa.

Below is seen the deep fascia, and upon it a permeated lymphatic, almost destroyed by the fibrotic process later to be described. A late stage of the process seen in Fig. 13.

THE INVASION OF THE MUSCLES BY PERMEATION.

SLIDE 15.—A section through a fibrous septum of the rectus abdominis muscle in the epigastric angle, showing infiltration by cancer. Naked eye nodules, the result of permeation of the fascial plexus, were present upon the anterior layer of the rectus sheath.

SLIDE 16.—A permeated lymphatic in the pectoralis major muscle, ruptured by the pressure of the growth within it.

SLIDE 17.—A permeated lymphatic from the rectus abdominis muscle, seen under a high power.

NATURAL REPAIR IN CARCINOMA.

Every aggregation of cancer cells, after increasing in size, for a time tends spontaneously to undergo degenerative and reparative changes. These changes begin at the centre of the mass, spread to its circumference, and may terminate in the replacement of the mass of cancer cells by a fibrous scar. The three succeeding slides illustrate this process.

SLIDES 18 and 19.—From a case of breast cancer in which nearly every secondary nodule showed a central area of liquefaction. Sometimes, as in Slide 19, the central degenerate area was occupied by inflammatory round cells.

SLIDE 20.—From the central portion of an old secondary deposit of carcinoma in the liver. Nothing is seen but fibrous tissue ; all the cancer cells have been destroyed.

REPARATIVE PROCESS FOLLOWING PERMEATION.

The succeeding nine slides show the successive stages of the process of *perilymphatic fibrosis*, which normally succeeds the permeation of a lymphatic. This process destroys the lymphatic, replaces it by a fibrous cord, and is the main cause of the lymphatic oedema so often seen in cancer.

SLIDE 21.—Permeation of two small lymphatic earliest stage, from the extreme microscopic growing edge. There is no distension of the lymphatic, and no surrounding round-celled infiltration. Between the lymphatics is a normal blood vessel.

The section is taken from the anterior surface of the rectus sheath in a case of breast cancer.

SLIDE 22.—Permeation, earliest stage. A small branch lymphatic, itself intact, is seen entering the permeated lymphatic, which is cut transversely. Same case as Fig. 21.

SLIDE 23.—From the same case as Slides 21 and 22, but taken at a point *nearer the primary growth.* *Distension* of the permeated lymphatic is beginning, but there is still no inflammatory reaction.

SLIDE 24.—A permeated lymphatic, greatly distended by the growth of the cancer cells within it. Degeneration of the cancer cells from mutual pressure and malnutrition. Round cells of inflammatory origin are now collecting round the permeated lymphatic.

SLIDE 25.—Rupture of the permeated lymphatic, like a water pipe in a frost, by the continued growth of the cancer cells within it. The high pressure has led to permeation of the small branch lymphatics seen in the neigbourhood.

The trauma of the rupture has led to local extravasation of blood and to a dense collection of inflammatory round cells in the neighbourhood.

SLIDE 26.—A further stage. The inflammatory round cells have organized into young fibrous tissue, which is contracting upon and destroying the already degenerate cancer cells.

SLIDE 27.—Same stage as Slide 26, but with a less definite fibrous capsule around the cancer cells.

SLIDE 28.—Fibrosis of a permeated lymphatic nearly completed. A few cancer cells remain in a solid thread of adventitious fibrous tissue.

SLIDE 29.—From the same lymphatic as Slide 28, but at a different point. Higher magnification. The cross section of the lymphatic occupies the whole field. It contains only a few ghosts of cancer cells. In the last stage of all, found in the regions between the primary growth and the microscopic growing edge, the permeated lymphatics have been entirely destroyed by the completion of this process of perilymphatic fibrosis.

DISSEMINATION IN MELANOTIC SARCOMA.

(Slides 30 to 40). See Appendix, Handley's "Cancer of Breast," slide 30. The distribution of the secondary nodules in a case of melanotic sarcoma of the right heel. Note especially the centrifugal spread of the nodules round a mass of right inguinal glands.

(For full descriptions of slide 30 and most of the Slides which follow, see Handley's "Cancer of the Breast" (John Murray, 1906, p. 203, *et seq.*).

SLIDE 30.—Fig. 46, Handley's "Cancer of Breast."

From a case of melanotic sarcoma of the right heel, showing the distribution of the secondary nodules visible on the skin. To demonstrate the mode of spread around the infected right inguinal glands a strip of tissues was taken in the situation marked A B.

SLIDE 31.—Strip A B rendered translucent (Fig. 47, *op cit.*).

SLIDE 32.—From a strip cut parallel to the strip A B and examined microscopically.

A permeated lymphatic cut transversely, showing branch lymphatics cut longitudinally, also permeated. From the strip near its distal end, and beyond the region of visible nodules. The lymphatics lie in the substance of the fascia lata.

SLIDE 33.—Taken through muscle, fascia lata, and subcutaneous fat, also near the distal end of the strip shows permeation of the fascial lymphatic plexus upon the fascia lata.

In the subcutaneous fat are seen (*a*) at two points, a small artery and vein, with comitant permeated lymphatics; (*b*) a small infiltrating nodule of growth, no doubt formed by the rupture of a permeated lymphatic.

SLIDE 34.—A drawing, showing two permeated lymphatics comitant to a small artery and vein—a frequent and typical appearance, showing that the spread is primarily by the lymphatics and not by the blood stream.

SLIDE 35.—A section across an artery and vein, which are accompanied by a diffuse cord of melanotic growth, produced by the rupture of a comitant permeated lymphatic.

SLIDE 36.—A drawing, showing the rupture of a permeated lymphatic and subsequent perivascular infiltration. *Cf.* Slide 35.

SLIDE 37.—The wall of the vein has been infiltrated by growth which has reached its lumen. The artery is still intact. Figs. 35, 36, and 37, taken from the proximal end of the strip, show a late stage of dissemination with invasion of the blood stream, an event which appears to occur a short time before death.

SLIDE 38.—(Fig. 48, *op. cit.*) The latest stage in which the artery is invaded and its lumen occupied by a mass of melanotic growth.

PERMEATION IN STOMACH CANCER.

SLIDE 39.—A gastric carcinoma beginning to invade the abdominal parietes at the umbilicus. Three small subcutaneous nodules, indicated by dotted lines, were palpable at the umbilicus.

SLIDE 40.—In cases such as Slide 39 a centrifugal spread of subcutaneous nodules from the umbilicus begins, just as it occurs in breast cancer from the focus in the breast. Slide 40 shows a case in which this process had extended very widely. The case is recorded in the "Pathological Transactions," I think by Rolleston.

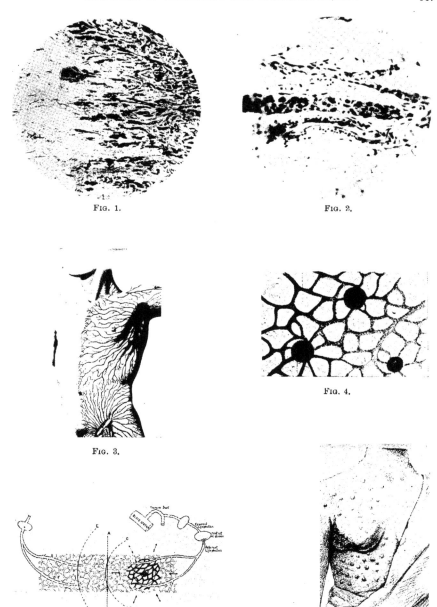

Fig. 1.

Fig. 2.

Fig. 3.

Fig. 4.

Fig. 5.

Fig. 6.

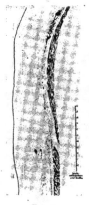

FIG. 7.

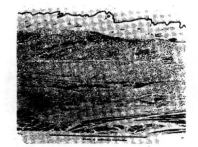

FIG. 8.

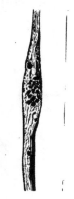

FIG. 10.

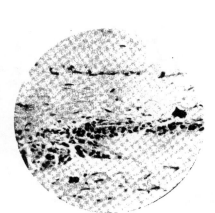

FIG. 9.

| Subserous fat. | Linea alba. | Cancer nodule. | Subcutaneous fat. |

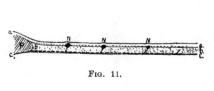

FIG. 11.

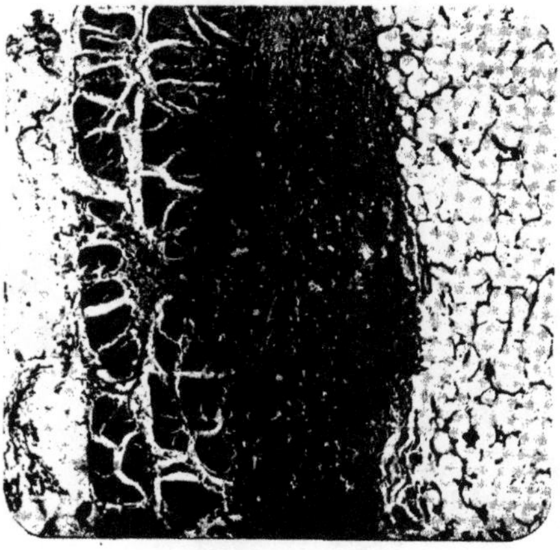

FIG. 12.

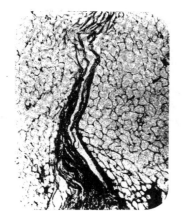

Fig. 13.

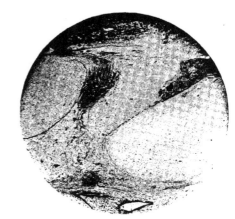

Fig. 14.

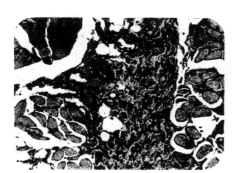

Fig. 15.

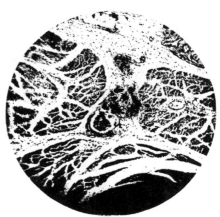

Fig. 16.

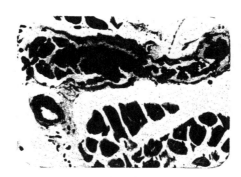

Fig. 17.

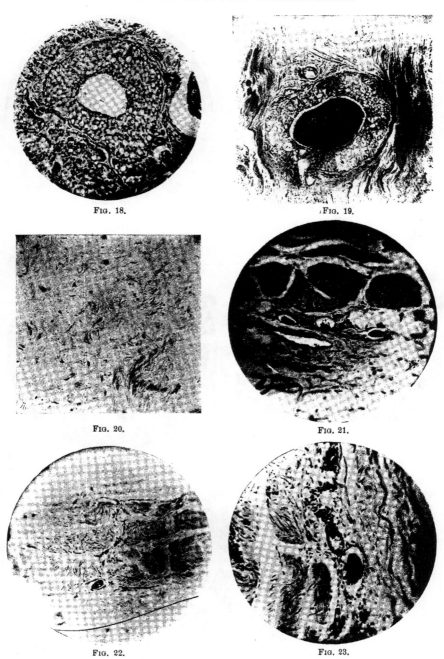

FIG. 18.   FIG. 19.

FIG. 20.   FIG. 21.

FIG. 22.   FIG. 23.

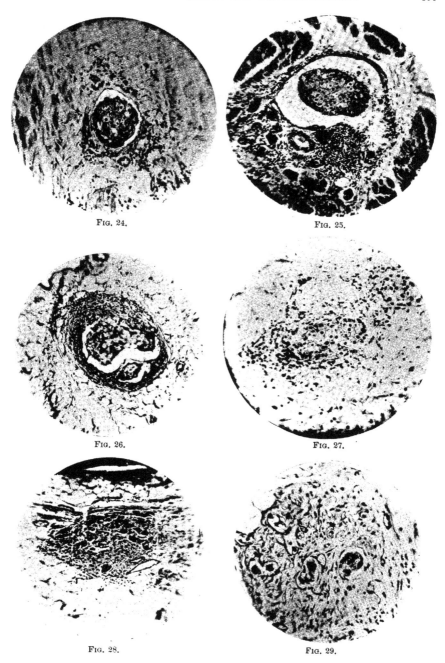

FIG. 24.

FIG. 25.

FIG. 26.

FIG. 27.

FIG. 28.

FIG. 29.

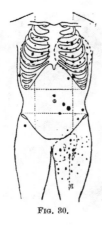

FIG. 30.

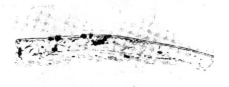

FIG. 31.

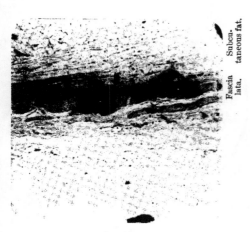

FIG. 32.

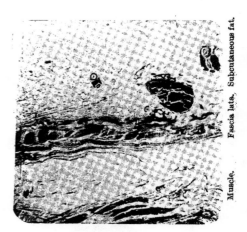

FIG. 33.

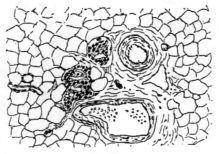

FIG. 34.

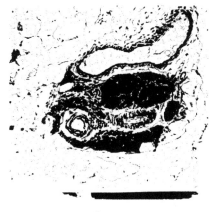

FIG. 35.

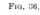

FIG. 36.

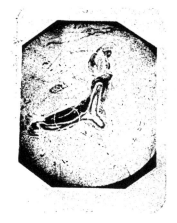

FIG. 37.

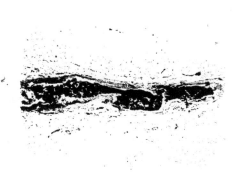

FIG. 38.

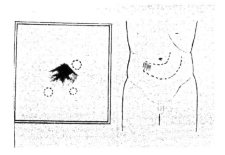

FIG. 39.

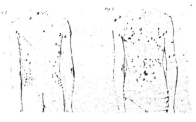

FIG. 40.

LYMPHO-SARCOMA TREATED BY RADIUM.

By DAWSON TURNER, M.D., F.R.S.E.

In charge of the Radium Treatment at the Royal Infirmary, Edinburgh.

A MALE patient, aged 38, a coal miner, was recommended by Mr. Hodsdon, on December 19th, 1918, for radium treatment.

The patient was suffering from a very large lympho-sarcoma on the left side of the neck, which interfered with the movements of the head. The growth was hard and quite inoperable. The patient had first noticed the swelling twelve months previously. The circumference of the neck over the growth

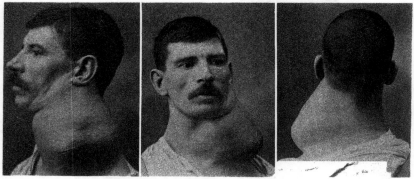

December 27, 1918. Before Radium Treatment.

was $23\frac{1}{4}$ inches (3 photographs). When the writer first saw the patient he was of opinion that the tumour was too extensive for successful treatment with the amount of radium at his disposal, but after consultation with Mr. Hodsdon he decided to do what he could to benefit the patient. Radium treatment was begun on December 27th, 1918, by the insertion of radium tubes into the growth, by Mr. Struthers, while, at the same time, external applications were made. A section taken for microscopical examination confirmed the clinical diagnosis. The position of the internal tubes was changed three times, and the external applications were continually shifted, so as to subject, as far as was possible, the whole of the tumour to sufficient radiation. In nine days time Mr. Struthers observed that the growth was generally much smaller, and was movable, and one or two enlarged glands above had markedly diminished. On January 8th the neck measured 19 inches. The treatment was finished on January 9th, the total dose being 18,080 mg. hours, a screen of $1\frac{1}{2}$ mm. of silver being used. On January 30th, 1919, the growth was much smaller, the neck circumference was 17 inches, and the patient was permitted to go home.

A lump of the size of a small egg had, however, appeared in the left axilla. On February 13th, 1919, a little over six weeks since the treatment was begun, the second series of photographs was taken, which show that the original tumour had almost disappeared (3 photographs). On March 11th there was only a fibrous thickening over the left side of the neck, but the growth in the axilla had increased to the size of a fist, and a new swelling had appeared on the right side of the neck, with enlargement of the supraclavicular glands on that side.

On March 21st, 1919, the fresh swellings were treated by radium, tubes being inserted by Mr. Struthers into the axillary growth and the swelling on the right side of the neck, while external applications were also made. A tube for precaution's sake was also put into the small fibroid mass which represented all that was left of the original tumour. The treatment was stopped

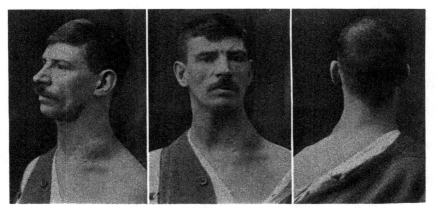

February 13, 1919. After Radium Treatment.

on March 26th, 1919. The right hand growth had received 3,000 mg. hours, the axillary 3,540 mg. hours, the supraclavicular glands 1,500 mg. hours, and the fibroid lump on the left side 750 mg. hours. Almost by the time the treatment was interrupted the axillary growth and the supraclavicular glands had disappeared, the right hand swelling followed suit, and by the middle of April the parts treated by radium were found by Mr. Hodsdon to be practically free from disease.

Lympho-sarcomas of all malignant growths appear to be the most susceptible to radium rays, insomuch that Dr. Howard Kelly, of Baltimore, is of opinion they should not be operated on, but should, in all cases, be subjected to radiation treatment. Whether this view be generally accepted or not, the effects of the radium treatment in this case were truly wonderful.

THE EXAMINATION OF THE LIVER, GALL BLADDER, AND BILE DUCTS.

By ROBERT KNOX.

(A portion of this paper was read at a meeting of the Electrotherapeutic Section of the Royal Society of Medicine, held in April, 1919, and formed part of a discussion on the Radiography of Gall Stones.)

(Continued from September issue, p. 132.)

Historical Notes and Abstracts from the Literature of the Radiography of the Liver, Gall Bladder, and Bile Ducts.

Carl Beck, of New York, showed the first X-ray plates of gall stones, in 1899. From that date on the references to X-ray diagnosis of gall stones becomes increasingly frequent as time lapses. Holland showed the first X-ray plates of gall stones in this country.

Dr. Macleod, of Shanghai, has published two papers in the ARCHIVES OF RADIOLOGY AND ELECTROTHERAPY which clearly prove the value of radiography in the investigation of the liver, gall bladder, and bile ducts. His results are very convincing, and a great deal of credit is due to this worker, who must carry out his investigations under great disadvantages.

Carl Beck, of New York, in 1899, detected two large stones in the gall bladder, three similar ones in the liver, and one in the cystic duct. In 1904, Kohler demonstrated a large gall stone, the character of which he substantiated by repeated examinations. Mikuliez, writing in 1905, believed a positive result seldom attainable. In the same year Holland (ARCHIVES OF THE ROENTGEN RAY, 1905) published his first gall stone case. He found a ring-like shadow in the right upper hypochondrium, but did not interpret it as gall stone since he had never before seen anything similar. At operation two large gall stones were found. Matthias and Fett reported from Konigsberg two cases in 1906. Before the American Roentgen Ray Society, in 1910, Pfahler reported three positive diagnoses of gall stones, and Hænisch, of Hamburg, and Cole, each reported three positive diagnoses on the same occasion. After this date the references in literature become much more frequent.

THURSTAN HOLLAND, in a paper before the Liverpool Medical Institution, December 19th, 1912, stated that until recently it had been considered impossible to obtain a sufficiently distinctive shadow to differentiate gall stones from stones in the kidney or calcareous glands. But in three recent cases he had been able to recognise shadows as those of gall stones. It was found that owing to the composition of the stones the greater part was transparent, but they had a crust of lime salts which gave a marked shadow with a transparent centre. He showed, on the screen, photographs of the cases and of the stones after removal, and demonstrated how the ring of shadow differed from the shadow of a calcareous gland, which resembled a blackberry, and from that of a renal calculus, which was clear, sharp, and homogeneous.

EDLING (*Verhandl. der deutsch. Röntgengs.*, 1912) reported two positive cases of his own, and one from the Kommunehospitalet investigated by Fischer. In this last the patient gave a history of colic in the right side, with hæmaturia, and was referred for examination for kidney stone. In the location of the hilus of the right kidney was seen a homogeneous shadow about the size of a walnut. It was diagnosed as a renal calculus, but none was found on operation.

At autopsy a stone was found in the gall bladder in form and size corresponding with the X-ray picture.

CASE (ARCH. ROENT. RAY, Vol. XVIII, 1913, p. 135) states that it is rare to find a stone composed of pure cholesterin. The cholesterin stones nearly always contain some pigment, generally a calcium salt. In a series of one thousand cases submitted for bismuth meal examination he had found gall stones in forty individuals. In eight other cases gall stones were found. Hence, in approximately a thousand individuals gall stones were found in nearly five per cent. of the cases. He believed that, with proper technique, gall stones might be shown radiographically in 40 or 50 per cent. of cases in which they were present. A negative opinion as to the presence of gall stones based on an X-ray examination did not rule them out, but they were demonstrated with such frequency that it was distinctly worth while to make search for them in every case in which they were suspected. Suspicious shadows in the right upper quadrant of the abdomen, which were most likely to be confused with gall stone shadows, were those due to calcareous deposits in the costal cartilages, renal calculi, calcareous deposits in a tuberculous kidney, and calcified mesenteric glands. Stereoscopic radiograms and pyelography were occasionally required definitely to identify the right upper quadrant shadow. Stereo-roentgenograms following the ingestion of a bismuth meal would often show the relation of the suspected shadow to the pyloro-duodenal shadow in a manner further serving to identify it. *Points of special technique for studying the gall bladder are : Carl Beck's position may be employed*, the patient lying on the abdomen with three pillows beneath the clavicles, the elevation thus produced permitting the extrusion of the gall bladder. *The approximation increased by turning the patient slightly to the right and raising the left side.* Pfahler *had recommended that the patient lie prone upon the abdomen, with the trunk as sharply bent to the left as possible.* Béla Alexander's method of plastic roentgenography ought to be of special value here. *The author himself preferred the stereoscopic method. Moderately soft, comparatively new tubes, penetration 5 or 6 Benoist, instantaneous exposures, and the use of an appropriate compression diaphragm, all important factors. The patient should hold the breath absolutely. Careful bowel cleansing an additional precaution which should not be overlooked. In studying roentgenograms of the gall bladder region for suspicious shadows, it is important that the illumination should be the most favourable. The intensity of the light should be easily regulated, and oblique illumination has sometimes permitted the detection of shadows which would otherwise have been overlooked.*

The same article by CASE also appears in *Journal American Medical Association*, September 20th, 1912.

THURSTAN HOLLAND (ARCHIVES OF THE ROENTGEN RAY, Vol. XVII, 1913, p. 374) states that when stones contain or have on their surface lime pigment salts—the carbonate of phosphate—in sufficient quantity, it is quite possible to obtain plates showing their shadows; this, however, is not sufficient for diagnostic purposes, as it will be necessary to differentiate these shadows from kidney stones and other things, such as calcareous glands. He suggests certain differentiations between kidney stones and gall stones, and says that gall stone shadows have marked characteristics which, when found, should put the radiographer on the right track. The calcareous salts are deposited especially on the exterior of the calculi. This construction is clearly defined radiographically. The centre of the stone is less opaque, whereas the lime salts deposited on the exterior wall give a shadowgraph which is denser at the circumference. This stone will, therefore, have a definite circumference, denser than the central portion. If the calculi are in the gall bladder they will probably be movable; and if more than one is present, different radiograms will show them in different positions as regards one another. Further, it may be possible to show the shadows outside the lower margin of the kidney shadow, which in these cases would probably be in its normal position. He gives particulars of three successful cases, his first successful radiogram of gall stone having been taken as long previously as 1905.

RUBASCHOW (*Zentralbl. f. Chirurgie*, May 16th, 1914) summarizes the main points in the diagnosis of gall stones by X rays. *From the radiographer's point of view there are two forms* of gall stones ; some are of uniform density, and cast an oval or round shadow; others have a clear centre and appear as rings on an X-ray plate. The density of either type is much less than that of renal calculi. The size of the shadow cast by stones in the living patient may vary from a pin-head upwards. A single stone is rare ; when it occurs it is usually in one of the ducts. A group of shadows resembling a bunch of grapes is characteristic of biliary calculi, and the stones are then certainly in the gall bladder. The shadow on the plate lies between the eleventh and twelfth ribs, and is further from the vertebral column than the shadow of a kidney stone. As a rule, the shadow falls outside that cast by the liver. A differential diagnosis must be made from (1) renal calculi. Renal stones cast a denser shadow, often have a characteristic form, and generally lie nearer the vertebral column. Béclère's method may be used ; it consists in taking two photographs, one dorso-ventral and the other ventro-dorsal; in the first, gall stones are smaller and sharper in outline ; renal shadows stand out more distinctly in the latter. (2) Intestinal contents, which should be eliminated by adequate purging. (3) Chalk deposits in the costal cartilages are distinguished by their sharp outlines, elongated form, and (usually) symmetrical arrangement. (4) Calcified lymph glands, which occasionally have a clear centre, and may cast a ring shadow; they are nearer the mid-line, and never show the bunch-of-grapes formation.

GEORGE AND GERBER (*Boston Medical and Surgical Journal*, April 30th, 1914; see also *Lancet*, May 23rd, 1914) began to find the shadows of gall stones by accident during the course of bismuth examinations of the alimentary tract. Gradually the accidental findings became so frequent that they found it advisable to look for gall stones in every case. *They have now adopted the routine of examining the gall bladder in every patient before giving the bismuth meal.* Pure cholesterin stones do not interrupt the X rays to any appreciable extent, so that shadows of them cannot be distinguished. Fortunately, such stones are not common, or at least do not cause many chronic disturbances. When the gall bladder is chronically inflamed by repeated infection, the stones deposited have the characteristic lamellae of calcium and bile salts encrusted on the cholesterin core. It is only the calcium ingredient that is shown by the X rays, and the clearness of the demonstration on the plate depends on the amount of calcium present. As a rule, in nearly every case in which symptoms referable to gall stones are present there is some calcium present. The authors think it will soon be possible to study whether gall stones containing calcium are present or not. *Their technique for demonstrating gall stones is very simple. The patient lies upon the table with his face down. The plate is placed under the right hypochondriac region. The maximum of definition is obtained with a very small diaphragm, 1½ in. in diameter, and a very small cylinder placed close to the back. It is preferable to use a fairly soft tube with a rapid exposure. It is better not to use intensifying screens, but the small plates as in kidney work.* The gall stone shadows will vary according to their calcium content. Often there will be a central light area with a peripheral calcium shadow. Occasionally, irregular deposits of calcium corresponding to the lamellated structure may be made out. As a rule, the faceted outlines are clear, but a shadow suggesting a single mass may be due to closely packed gall stones. Evidences of gall bladder disease are usually shown at the subsequent bismuth examination in the form of signs of pericholecystitis. The commonest sources of error in the diagnosis of gall stones are due to the presence of renal calculi, calcified mesenteric glands, and costo-chondral ossification. Gall stones may be distinguished from renal calculi by taking plates with the patient lying first on the abdomen and then on the back. Gall stones are nearer to the anterior abdominal wall. Therefore the anterior plate will show the shadows small and sharp, whereas the posterior will show them large and blurred. The reverse holds in renal calculi. Calcified mesenteric glands will be found to occupy different positions in different plates on manipulating the abdomen between the exposures. A calcified costal cartilage will be continuous with the rib.

THURSTAN HOLLAND (*Liverpool Med.-Chir. Jnl.*, 1914, p. 308) reports further successful cases, is in agreement with Cole as to the unreliability of the negative evidence, and suggests that gall stones cannot be shown in more than about 30 per cent. of the cases in which they are actually present. In this paper the differential diagnosis from other shadows (kidney stones, calcareous glands) is again discussed, and the more characteristic features of the gall stone shadow pointed out.

PFAHLER (*Journal American Medical Association*, 1914, LXII, p. 1304) believes that *50 per cent. of gall stones can be demonstrated, but that negative findings never can be interpreted as indicating the absence of gall stones. The patient should be thoroughly purged, and the stomach if possible emptied. The patient is placed on the abdomen, with the plate under the gall bladder region, the arms extended toward the head, and the upper part of the body then bent strongly to the left (not rotated). This opens the space between the lower ribs and the crest of the ilium, through which the rays can best reach the gall bladder. He generally does a second examination by passing the rays directly through the liver, between the eleventh and twelfth ribs, which serves to differentiate foreign substances or concretions in the bowel. The tube is set so that the rays will pass obliquely through the steps between the last rib and the crest of the ilium towards the gall bladder. A diaphragm cylinder eliminates many of the secondary rays. Exposure is made while patient holds the breath. The vacuum of the tube should be the same as that used in making kidney examinations—from 6 to 7 on the Benoist scale.* Stones containing a very minute quantity of calcium salts will sometimes be demonstrated by inflating the colon with air. He does not expect to find the gall stones during the bismuth study of the gastro-intestinal tract, but makes a direct preliminary study for gall stones, and follows this up with the bismuth study. In only one of thirty-four cases of gall stones did he find the stones during the bismuth study of the gastro-intestinal tract, and in that case the stones were so dense that no one could overlook them. His conclusions are :—

1. Gall stones can be shown only when they are composed of a substance of greater or less density than the surrounding tissues. This will usually mean that they must contain lime salts, though this quantity may be small.

2. As regards showing positive findings, one can generally count on more than 50 per cent. being demonstrable. At present a negative diagnosis has no value.

3. It is possible that with improved technique, when the gall bladder is found small, and still no stone is found, it may become of more value in negative diagnosis.

4. The estimation of the value of this method of diagnosis must be based only on the work of roentgenologists who have mastered a good technique and who are thorough in their work.

5. Definite information will be obtained only by continued co-operation between surgeon and roentgenologist.

In most of his cases the stones contained only a little lime salts, and could be seen only by a very clear plate and by careful oblique illumination. For the demonstration of these light stones screens are unreliable. He has rarely been able to recognise the stone on plates used with intensifying screens.

COLE (*Surgery, Gynecology, and Obstetrics*, Vol. XVIII, 1914, p. 218) had been led to the routine examination for gall stones in all cases presenting symptoms referable to the right hypochondrium. The number of positive diagnoses he has been able to make proves that the examination was justified, but he states that a negative diagnosis should never be made where there is no X-ray evidence of calculus. Roentgenographic indications of gall stones are direct and indirect. Direct evidence consists of a characteristic localised area of increased density corresponding in size and shape with the calculus. Indirect evidence is afforded by the distortion of the adjacent hollow viscera by adhesions from an accompanying cholecystitis. And if it be true, as Moynihan states, that it is now a matter of general acceptance that gall stones are caused by infection, the *indirect evidence is more valuable than the direct.* He believes that the deformity of the cap and pars pylorica, or the kinking and constriction of the hepatic flexure, are stronger roentgenological indications for surgical procedure than the presence of a calculus in the gall bladder, without evidence of adhesions involving the hollow viscera. The important point to determine in cases of unimpacted calculi is whether the stones are associated with cholecystitis extensive enough to cause symptoms. The accompanying adhesions manifest themselves in the alteration of the lumen of the stomach, cap, or hepatic flexure of the colon. As to direct evidence, the possibility of detection depends upon the percentage of mineral salts in the stone, or surrounding a cholesterin nucleus, upon the thickness and density of the surrounding tissue, and the penetration of the tube. *A soft tube, a very short exposure, and the use of an intensified screen will give a wealth of detail impossible to obtain by ordinary methods.* Intestinal content is often thus accentuated, and must not be mistaken for gall stones. In some cases the calculus is so indistinct that it can be discovered only by making several roentgenograms, superimposing two or three of them, and examining them carefully against the sky. Occasionally an accumulation of gas or air artificially injected into the colon will accentuate the stone in a remarkable manner. He gives some aids to differentiation between biliary and renal calculi. Biliary calculi show more distinctly and appear smaller when the plate is placed on the abdomen than when the plate is placed on the back; the opposite is true of renal calculi. A ring-like shadow is cast by a biliary calculus when there is a calcareous coating to the cholesterin nucleus. Renal calculi seldom, if ever, have this appearance. When three or more biliary calculi are present they are likely to have faceted surfaces which are readily recognised roentgenographically. If more than one renal calculus is present, one is usually larger than the others, and the group frequently has the appearance of a large branching phosphatic calculus. Moving the tube from side to side alters the relation of a biliary calculus to the kidney, but it does not alter the relation of a renal calculus to the kidney. To differentiate from duodenal ulcer, gall bladder infection is usually more extensive; it involves the greater curvature, and draws the stomach to the right, causing an angulation of the cap. The cap may be involved in the adhesions, but not more so than the pyloric end of the stomach.

PFAHLER (*American Journal of Radiology*, 1915, I, p. 774) *suggests a new position for the demonstration of the stone, one which he claims to be of importance, inasmuch as it throws the shadow of any gall stone outside that of the kidney. For this the patient is placed obliquely upon his right side, whilst the compressor is directed into the epigastric region and tilted so that the centre of the cylinder is resting posterior to the right costal border; the angle must be varied according to the thickness of the patient.* This is only one of a series of plates taken in different directions. The author lays great stress upon the examination of the plates and the lighting to be used.

CALDWELL (*American Journal of Roentgenology*, 1915, II, p. 816) protests against the making of positive diagnoses on the insufficient evidence of very indefinite shadows, and says that if *only enough plates are taken it is possible to obtain these suspicious shadows in the gall bladder region of any normal individual.* He believes that the personal equation of the individual observer is more important in this field of X-ray work than in any other, and that this accounts for some reporting 85 per cent. of results and others only 5 per cent. "It is very easy to make a roentgen diagnosis of gall stones. The difficult thing at present is to avoid making such a diagnosis occasionally when no stones are present."

HUBBARD (*Boston Medical and Surgical Journal*, September 23rd, 1915) puts in a strong plea for operation as soon as the diagnosis of gall stones is made. He brings forward statistics from the Boston City Hospital, which show that stones in the gall bladder killed 11 per cent. of those who had them, while stones in the ducts killed 43 per cent.—an argument for operating while the stones are in the gall bladder.

CARMAN (*Journal of the American Medical Association*, LXV, 1915, p. 1812) gives an account of the radiological demonstration of a barium-filled gall bladder in a living patient. The patient had had a cholecystostomy for gall stones. In the scar of the operation wound were two sinuses, discharging pus, and surrounded by a movable nodular mass. On roentgen examination, far up in the right abdominal quadrant, was a dense collection of barium with streak-like branches, and from its situation it was believed to be the gall bladder indicating a communication between it and the upper intestinal tract. The tendril-like branches were deemed to be due to the extension of barium into the hepatic ducts. At operation the external sinuses were found to lead into a dense carcinomatous mass surrounding the gall bladder and involving the stomach. The gall bladder itself, which was excised, simply showed a chronic cholecystitis, with particles of barium adherent to the mucosa. The fundus of the gall bladder communicated with the duodenum through the perforation.

PANNER (*Hospitalstidende*, Denmark, February, 1915) reports eight positive diagnoses of his own, and dwells at length on the ring-like shadow as being the characteristic roentgen picture of gall stones. He says that if it can be regarded as settled that in a number of cases we can detect the presence of gall stones by the roentgen examination, it is just as certain that we shall most frequently get negative results of a sort to which there can be given no significance whatever. Only a very small proportion of gall stones offer favourable conditions for reproduction on the photographic plate, for they usually consist, to a great extent, of so considerable a quantity of organic substance that they cannot be differentiated from the surrounding tissues. Pigment, lime, and other inorganic ingredients are, as a rule, diffused through the whole stone, so that their proximity is not capable of altering the conditions.

COLE (*Journal American Roentgen Ray Society*, February, 1915) sought to determine how a variety of gall stones, *extra corpus*, would appear on the photographic plate when suspended in air, water, and bile, as compared with a selected "keystone" fairly rich in calcium content. About 20 per cent. of the gall stones showed more calcium deposited than the keystone. About 26 per cent. showed a trace of calcium less than the keystone. About 54 per cent. showed practically no calcareous deposit, in other words, they were practically pure cholesterin. Eighty per cent. of the stones submerged in bile cast a shadow less dense than the bile surrounding them. This observation would seem to preclude the hope of a positive diagnosis of gall stones in more than 20 or 25 per cent. of the cases. But the cholesterin stones are so much less dense than the bile surrounding them that they appear like bubbles of air, and when many stones are present the bile surrounding them appears more dense than the stones and gives the area of the gall bladder a honeycomb appearance or the ring-like shadow typical of gall stones. He has made a definite or probable diagnosis of gall stones in thirty cases. In only one case was there the amount of calcareous deposit which six months previously he had deemed necessary to justify one in making a safe diagnosis of gall stones. Sixteen out of the thirty cases have been operated on. Of these sixteen cases twelve were correctly diagnosed roentgenographically; three incorrectly diagnosed, and one very provisional diagnosis was incorrect.

COLE AND GEORGE (*Boston Medical and Surgical Journal*, Vol.CLXXII, p. 326, 1915) claim that "it would now appear that we can show gall stones in all cases where they are really present," and that the positive diagnosis can be made in such a large percentage of cases where gall stones are present that the negative diagnosis has become far more important than it was previously considered to be. Until within three or four years ago gall stones were rarely detected by X rays. During the last few years several roentgenologists, including ourselves, consider that they have detected gall stones in about 50 per cent. of the cases examined. This was estimated in different ways by different men. Experience has shown that gall stones may be detected about twice as frequently as formerly by: (*a*) a *special* technique for making the roentgen plates; (*b*) a *thorough* intimacy with the roentgenographic appearance of gall stones. By applying the new method of interpretation gall stones have been detected on many roentgen plates made by the old technique, and formerly diagnosed as negative. By means of the special technique for making and interpreting roentgen plates, a positive diagnosis may be made in so many cases that the negative diagnosis has become of considerable significance. Much care and study will be necessary properly to interpret the additional detail which can be obtained by the special technique, and undoubtedly some erroneous diagnoses will be made. If there is no direct roentgen evidence of gall stones, the stomach, cap, duodenum, and colon should be examined for adhesions from an accompanying cholecystitis. If there is no *direct* or *indirect* roentgen evidence of gall stones, the clinical history should be more characteristic than usual before one resorts to surgical procedure.

ORAM (Paper read at British Medical Association Annual Meeting, 1914, and reported in ARCHIVES OF THE ROENTGEN RAY, XIX, p. 438, 1915) says that the chief constituents of gall stones are three in number : cholesterin, bile pigment, and calcium carbonate. Cholesterin and bile pigment cast practically no X-ray shadow. Calcium alone gives evidence of its presence. One large class of gall stones containing over 90 per cent. cholesterin, therefore, cannot be demonstrated. Laminated cholesterin stones, containing 75 to 90 per cent. cholesterin with layers of calcium between, give a radiographic shadow of a characteristic annular appearance. A third class, usually found in the gall bladder, with a soft nucleus and hard laminated crust containing calcium, will be annular when visible. A fourth type, the mixed bilerubin calcium stone, usually large and with 25 per cent. cholesterin, casts an annular shadow. Pure bilerubin calcium stones, rarely larger than a pea, and containing but little cholesterin, are demonstrated by X rays with a fair amount of ease. The first step in the diagnosis of gall stones is the demonstration of their shadow; the next, the differentiation of that shadow from other shadows in the same region representing stones in the right kidney and calcified abdominal glands. Calcareous glands are usually multiple and freely movable by pressure ; gland shadows also are usually characteristic in appearance, having ill-defined and blurred edges and showing within their area regular mottling of light or dark spots. The differential diagnosis from kidney stones is more difficult. The situation of the shadow does not give material assistance, but the annular outline which is more or less characteristic of gall stones is seldom seen in kidney stones, which are usually of uniform density ; where the lower pole of the kidney can be shown on the plate, assistance in diagnosis may be obtained, first, from the fact that it is seen to lie below or outside the kidney shadow, and secondly, even though the shadow may lie within the renal area, a series of negatives may demonstrate that its relation to the lower pole of the kidney is so variable that even a calculus in a disorganised kidney may be ruled out of court, and the diagnosis of gall stones established. When the shadows are multiple and bear different relative positions to each other in the series of plates, their location in the gall bladder rather than in the kidney becomes probable, for gall stones lying in the gall bladder would be permitted a considerable degree of relative motion, while kidney stones, unless the kidney be very much disorganised, are fixed relatively to each other. Stereoscopic negatives also will demonstrate gall stones as lying near the anterior wall of the abdomen, and kidney stones near the posterior. Again, if two exposures are made, one with the patient's abdomen applied to the plate, gall stones will be smaller and sharper on the abdominal plate because they are nearer to it, while kidney stones will show smaller and sharper on the posterior plate for the same reason. The shadows cast by calcified cartilages often show very clearly in the gall bladder area. The cartilage shadows are, as a rule, linear and are not likely to cause confusion with other shadows, but more or less circular patches of calcification, should they occur, might cause difficulties in diagnosis. The author adds particulars of eight cases.

CASE (*American Journal of Roentgenology*, III, 1916, p. 246) publishes some very interesting statistics as to gall stones, based on a series of three hundred operation cases in which X-ray examination was made, and the results confirmed or otherwise by operation. His results appear to justify the conclusion that it is possible to show gall stones definitely in 50 per cent. of positive cases. He considers that the time has arrived when, admitting that the negative diagnosis is of no value, X-ray examination should be made in every suspected case.

O'BRIEN (*Boston Medical and Surgical Journal*, CLXXIV, 1916, p. 309) believes that for preparation catharsis is valuable, and prefers an effervescing saline. Catharsis by the mouth may be aided by an enema. Screen examination has absolutely no place in the direct diagnosis of gall stones, though it may be of value for studying the indirect manifestations. Serial plates alone should be employed. The patient should first be examined prone, then the movements of Pfahler and Cole employed, such as bending the body sharply to the left, and directing the rays obliquely through the liver, using if one wishes an 8×10 piece of board, as described by Pfahler, to bring the gall bladder closer to the plate, or the circular plate-holder of Cole, which can be pushed up under the gall bladder for the same purpose. He uses a fast, finely-grained intensifying screen in all gall bladder work. Soft tubes are essential; has used two Coolidge tubes now for eight months with the utmost satisfaction. The plates should be read only when thoroughly dry. Direct illumination by the northern sky is often particularly helpful. The roentgenographic appearance of gall stones will differ according to the amount of lime salts present. The more lime salts present in the calculus the more readily it shows up on the roentgenogram. A simple method of differentiation between biliary and renal calculi is to make plates with the patient prone and supine. If the shadow is more distinct with the patient supine the shadow may be considered a kidney stone, and *vice versa*, a gall stone if the shadow is more distinct with the patient prone. This method, however, is far from exact. A lateral view may save the necessity of catheterisation of the ureter. If one sees the shadow lying against the vertebræ one can be reasonably certain that one is dealing with a kidney stone.

MACLEOD (ARCHIVES OF RADIOLOGY AND ELECTROTHERAPY, XXI, 1916, p. 117) gives an account of several cases of suspected gall bladder disease, in which radiographic examination was successful. The notes are concerned, not with the definitely margined shadows indicating biliary calculi, but the more frequently occurring ones where shadows are not definitely margined, but which nevertheless indicate not only calculi but other gall bladder abnormality. Of 29 cases examined, 17 were reported as presenting abnormal shadows; of these, 9 were operated on and the interpretation confirmed, the other 8 being without features regarded as justifying operation so far. He has applied compression in every case with a rubber cushion, used perpendicularly to the plate by an apparatus consisting of a vulcanite ring fastened to two uprights.

Abstract from the " Journal de Radiologie et d'Electrologie."

SOME EXAMPLES OF THE IMPORTANCE OF THE RADIOLOGICAL EXAMINATION OF THE INFERIOR SURFACE OF THE LIVER.

By Dr. R. LEDOUX-LEBARD.

While the examination of all parts of the digestive tract proper has benefited greatly by the extension and perfecting of radiodiagnostic procedures, the adjacent organs have remained rather outside the influence of this wave of progress. There would even seem to be indicated a slight movement of recoil as far as the inferior surface of the liver and the bile ducts are concerned.

Those physicians who expected to see radiography supply them with positive information as to the presence of gall stones, or as to the hepatic origin of a malady, deceived by constant negative reports, came to the conclusion that the radiological examination could throw no light on such cases, and was therefore useless. Nevertheless, leaving entirely on one side the superior surface of the liver, so well defined by the transparency of the lung substance, and adhering strictly to the lower surface and the bile ducts, one is soon convinced by an impartial study of published facts and a systematic examination of liver diseases, of the importance of radio-diagnosis, and of the very precise information which radioscopy and radiography, carried out perseveringly and in accordance with a well thought out technique, can supply.

It is necessary to insist on the point of technique, for it plays a very important part. It is well, in the first place, to try to establish clearly the hepatic margin by gas differentiation, which insufflation of the colon, carried out under control by radioscopy, renders possible in an ideal manner, with no danger, and with much less discomfort to the patient than is caused by the similar distension of the stomach.

It is then necessary to take plates in at least three positions:—

1. In the ventral decubitus, a plate of the entire region.

2. In the dorsal decubitus, a plate of the gall bladder region, taken in accordance with the technique for kidney examination.

3. In the vertical position, the examination being completed by a screen and plate examination of the stomach region after the ingestion of a bismuth meal.

It is surprising what definite information such an examination will yield, and enables us to understand how the American investigators who follow this procedure, such as Case, can present a series of radiographs of gall stones which seems at first sight surprising, and boldly proclaim the necessity of hepatic radiographs. It must be admitted that these examinations are long and tedious, but it is better, in our opinion, not to undertake the radiological examination of the liver at all than to carry it out in a perfunctory manner and without a good technique.

It is hardly necessary to add that it is best to use an installation powerful enough to permit always of instantaneous radiographs. Like Case, we recommend the use of soft rays of about 5B. From the clinical point of view, there are three questions which the radiologist is most frequently asked :—

(I) He is asked to diagnose if there is hepatic disease, and especially if, in the case of a palpable tumour in the abdomen, this is of hepatic origin. The following case, taken from

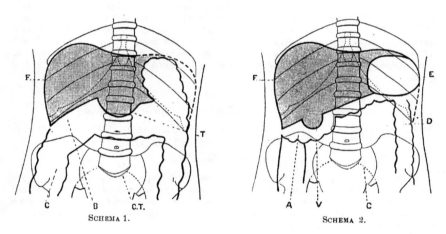

SCHEMA 1.   SCHEMA 2.

among three similar ones, is an example of this, and shows that it is often possible to give a categorical answer to this question.

(a) Madame V., aged 47 years, a highly nervous woman, with no special antecedent history, thought she had a small swelling in the epigastric region, which several surgeons whom she consulted declared to be imaginary. Her doctor, however, thinking he did not feel a tumour, took her to M. A. Gosset, who asked us to make a radiological examination of the liver and stomach. After insufflation of the colon, radioscopy showed a rounded tumour, the size of an apple, on the anterior margin of the liver in a line with the vertebral column.

Schema (1) was drawn from a radiograph taken in the course of the examination. Our diagnosis was, "a tumour on the lower surface of the liver, having the characteristics of a cyst." Operation (Dr. Gosset) showed a hydatid cyst, corresponding in size, shape, and situation to the shadow observed.

(II) The radiologist is often asked to determine whether there is any disease of the gall bladder or not. The positive verification of the shadow of the gall bladder, if it is possible to obtain it, will enable him to give an affirmative answer. In the interpretation of the shadows it must not be forgotten that the right kidney sometimes shows up with great clearness, even in radiographs taken in the ventral decubitus with the plate under the abdomen.

(b) Madame N., aged 39 years, had attacks of pain closely simulating those of gall bladder origin. Nevertheless, before operating, Dr. Reymond wished to be satisfied that the condition was one of the gall bladder and not of the kidney. On radioscopy a shadow could clearly be perceived, which seemed to correspond to the gall bladder, and in concurrence with Dr. Enriquez, who was present at the examination, we had no hesitation in interpreting it as such.

The radiograph gave the shadow reproduced in Schema (2). The stomach examination indicated a condition of adhesive pericholecystitis. Operation demonstrated a gall bladder filled with pus, with very thickened and sclerosed walls. The bladder contained a stone and was everywhere adherent.

(c) A lady of about 50 years had suffered for a long time from pain in the right side. An indefinite mass could be felt which might be either gall bladder or kidney. The radiograph reproduced in Fig. 61 showed the liver, the kidney prolapsed and increased in size, and a mass which could only be the gall bladder, a hypothesis which operation confirmed, demonstrating to M. Gosset a hydro-cholecystitis with a degenerated stone, the presence of which was suspected rather than seen on the plate.

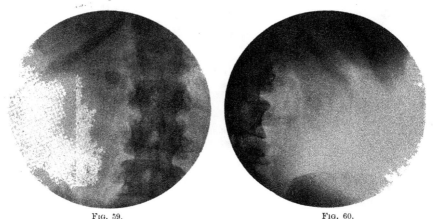

FIG. 59.　　　　　　　　　　　　　　　　FIG. 60.

(III) Are there any gall stones? This is certainly the question most frequently put to the radiologist in regard to the liver.

The report of Messieurs Desternes and Baudin on this subject, published in the Journal, gives all the indications of general use, and we will not dwell further on it. We will merely recall the fact that Case showed, at the Congress in London, in 1913, a series of forty radiographs of gall stones collected in the course of 1,000 hepatic examinations.

Now, since October, 1914, we have ourselves met in forty-seven patients, radiographed from this point of view, four cases where gall stones were diagnosed with certainty and one doubtful case. Our statistics, therefore, would seem to be not inferior to those of Case, which demonstrates clearly that the question is one *of technique alone*, and not of a chemical composition peculiar to transatlantic gall stones.

(d) Madame S., 44 years of age, had many hepatic crises--jaundice present. A radiograph, in the abdominal decubitus, showed a shadow resembling a stone situated between the two first right transverse processes. This shadow is clearly shown in Fig. 59. Another, Fig. 60, showed a radiograph of the same patient taken with the usual kidney technique. In it is seen much more clearly the liver, shown at the level of the top of the right kidney, small and atrophied, and the characteristic quadrilateral shadow less dense in the centre, which evidently corresponded to a gall stone with a calcareous coating.

Operation enabled M. Gosset to remove a single gall stone, which was very fragile, and which broke under examination. This was put together and radiographed, Fig. 64.

(e) Another case, Fig. 62, shows a gall bladder full of stones. The plate was taken

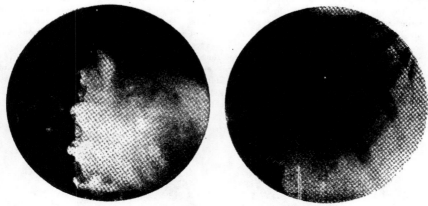

FIG. 61.   FIG. 62

with the usual kidney technique. The patient was a lady who had had repeated attacks of gall stone colic extending over many years. We believe, therefore, that it is necessary to carry out more often than is usually done the radiological investigation for gall stones, which, with a good technique will give us, a little oftener perhaps than is thought, proof of their presence, and in many other cases will enable us to make interesting verifications.

We reproduce here, Fig. 63, the radiograph of a giant stone, a true cast of a large gall stone, removed by M. Gosset. It would have been interesting to radiograph the patient before operation.

In cases which occur fairly often, where there is clinically some doubt between the gastric and the gall bladder origin of the symptoms observed, the doctor can ask the radiologist to examine and determine a doubtful diagnosis. Sometimes this will reveal a lithiasis which had been very doubtful, as happened to us recently in the case of a young girl who presented very grave symptoms,

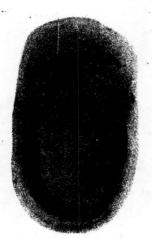

FIG. 63.

FIG 64.

which might have been either gastric or duodenal in origin, and in which we verified numerous stones in the gall bladder.

In other cases, on the contrary, the examination may show a gastric or intestinal origin for the observed symptoms, while it must not be forgotten how difficult interpretation may be in the absence of characteristic shadows.

These few illustrations, taken from among our cases of radiological examinations of the inferior surface of the liver, seem to us, in spite of their small number, sufficient to prove the usefulness of the examination, and compel us to urge that it should be carried out more systematically and in accordance with a suitable technique.

GEORGE AND LEONARD (*American Journal of Roentgenology*, IV, 1917, p. 322) put forward the working hypothesis that only when some pathological change has taken place in the walls of the gall bladder or its contents can the shadow be demonstrated on the X-ray plate. They do not question the possibility that the time may come, with improved technique, when the normal gall bladder will be demonstrated. It may even be true that in a large series of cases one individual, by reason of a freak plate, or possibly by an unusually favourable condition, may show the outline of a normal gall bladder.

SHOUP (*American Journal of Roentgenology*, IV, 1917. p. 580) reports an unusual case of abdominal pain involving the gall bladder, in which the clinical signs were insufficient to make a reliable diagnosis, and where, with the aid of the roentgen interpretation, the nature of the condition was sufficiently revealed to warrant an operation, which verified the suspicions of the roentgenologist. The shadows in the region of the duodenum suggested a diverticulum of the duodenum, a perforating ulcer, or even barium in the gall bladder. On operation dense adhesions were found between duodenum and liver, hiding the gall bladder from view. The fundus of the gall bladder was found to be connected with the duodenum by means of a tube half an inch in length and as thick as a normal appendix. No bile was present in the gall bladder, but on further exploration it was found to harbour a soft cholesterin stone, which completely filled its neck and blocked the entrance to the cystic duct.

CASE (*Annals of Surgery*, July 1917 ; also *Lancet*, December 8th, 1917) divides gall stones into three groups : (1) Composed of pure cholesterin, and quite invisible to X rays ; (2) containing a relatively large quantity of lime salts, and easy to detect ; (3) the largest class, made up of stones in which the amount of lime is relatively low. It is the detection of these last cases which determines the success or failure of the method. A chemical analysis was made for Dr. Case of the lime content of a number of gall stones. Where the X rays were negative, and yet gall stones were found at operation, the percentage of calcium oxide in relation to the total weight of the stone was 0·30. Among the positive cases the lowest proportion of calcium oxide was 0·425 per cent. Dr. Case finds that in a series of 1,000 consecutive bismuth meal examinations there were 40 instances of gall stones ; in Cole's series of 500 similar cases gall stones were found in 20 cases—the same percentage. The figure 4 per cent. represents roughly the number of positive findings ; in autopsy statistics from 19 American and European authors the average frequency of gall stones was given as 5·9 in 18,892 autopsies. Hesse summarises 17,402 autopsies done in 10 years in Petrograd, and finds gall stones in less than 3 per cent. Dr. Case, however, accepts a generous 10 per cent. of probable gall stones in his gastro-intestinal and genito-urinary cases combined, and thus finds that positive X-ray examination has been made in roughly 50 per cent. of cases. Similarly, in a series of 5,000 consecutive patients examined for suspected disease of the gastro-intestinal tract, lumbar spine, or right kidney (instances in which the region of the gall bladder would be automatically included), positive findings were made in 4·5 per cent. of the cases. Again, accepting 10 per cent. as possible gall stones, 45 per cent. of these were demonstrated by X rays. These are, of course, only estimated figures. Accordingly, Dr. Case took a series of 300 consecutive abdominal cases operated upon, in which the gall bladder was examined at the time of operation as well as by X rays beforehand. Gall stones were found on operation in 41 cases, and of these 20 had been reported positive by X rays; here, again, roughly, half of the gall stones can be detected in this way. X rays are claimed as of value also in gall bladder disease, in many cases showing right upper quadrant adhesions with fixation, and even sometimes the thickened gall bladder. Finally, the author says, "We can therefore conclude that it is definitely possible to show gall stones in approximately 50 per cent. of the positive cases, and to show a gall bladder lesion in 85 per cent. of cases of gall bladder disease. . . . Gall stones are demonstrable with much greater frequency than has until lately been conceded. The frequency with which stones may be shown is so great that I believe the time has arrived when the X-ray examination should be required in every suspected case."

OTHER REFERENCES.

ASCHOFF AND BACKMEISTER : *Die Cholelithiasis*, Jena, 1909.

BECK. Chapter on gall bladder. Groedel's *Atlas der Rontgendiagnostic in der inneren Medizin.* Munchen, 1909.

LENNE. *Experimentale Untersuchungen bezenglich der Darstellung von Gallensteinen durch Röntgenstrahlen*, Erfurt, 1912. G. Richters

RUBASCHOFF (S. M.) *Rontgenodiagnosis of biliary calculi.* 1913, *Kharkov, M. J.*, 1913, XVI, 102.

BYTHELL AND BARCLAY : *X-ray diagnosis and treatment*, 1913, London : Hodder and Stoughton. (Merely a reference that " gall stones are so transparent to the X rays that, unless they happen to be encrusted with lime salts—an exceedingly rare occurrence—they throw no shadow distinguishable in even the most perfect radiograms.")

CHAUFFARD. *Leçons sur la Lithiase Biliare.* Paris: Masson et Cie. 1914.

SZERB. *Cholelithiases Rontgendiagnosia. Budapesti orr. ujság*, 1914, XII, 531.

COSSET. Presentation de radiographies d'un calcul de la vésicule biliare. *Bull. et mém. Soc. de chir. de Paris*, 1914, n.s., XL, 206.

WITTE. Ein Fall von besonders deutlichem Gallensteinnachweis durch Röntgenlicht. *Fortschr. a. d. Geb. d. Rontgenstrahlen.* Hamburg, 1914, XXII, 217.

TANDOJA. L'indagine Röntgen nella calcolosi biliare. *Atti d. Cong. ital. di radiol. med.*, 1913, Pavia, 1914, I, 172.

NILES. Detection and diagnosis of gall stones by the Roentgen ray. *Southern Medical Journal*, U.S.A., Vol. VIII, 1915.

CASE. The value of the Roentgen examination of gall stones. *Internat. Clin.*, Philadelphia, 25. S. 1915, IV, 145.

LIPPMANN. Routine radiological demonstration of gall stones *Calif. State J. M.*, San Francisco, 1915, XIII, 475.

PESCI. Sulla visibilità ai raggi Röntgen dei calcoli biliari. *Radiol. med.*, Torino, 1915, II, 228.

GEORGE, A. W. Further notes on the Roentgen diagnosis of gall stones. *Interstate M. J.*, St. Louis, 1916, Suppl. Roent., II, 13.

SCHUTZE. Die Rontgenologische Darstellbarkeit der Gallensteine. *Med. Klin.*, 1916, Berlin, 1916, XII, 429

OSMOND. The importance of X-ray examination in clinical diagnosis with report of a case showing gall stones, symptoms of which suggested duodenal ulcer. *Cleveland M. J.*, 1916, XV, 256.

The short clinical histories attached to a number of the cases illustrated should suffice to show the importance of always considering the case from all points of view. It is important that wherever possible an examination of the patient should be made at the time of the X-ray examination; inspection of the abdomen may reveal an alteration in the contour of the abdominal wall, and on deep inspiration changes may be detected which will aid in the diagnosis. Palpation of the abdomen, with the patient in several positions, will also be helpful. The dorsal decubitus, with the anterior abdominal wall relaxed, is the best for deep palpation of the kidney and gall bladder area. By its aid the gall bladder may be satisfactorily palpated. Though it is not essential for the radiologist to perform this clinical examination, it will often be a valuable aid when an obscure case is sent for investigation.

The illustrations have been selected from a number of plates of cases in which doubtful shadows have been shown. These by their presence stimulated a desire to investigate the case more thoroughly, and after repeated examinations some more definite evidence has been obtained. The establishment of a diagnosis of a provisional nature has been followed by an exploratory examination by the surgeon; the collaboration of the radiologist with the surgeon has been of the greatest possible value. In a number of the cases the explanation of the doubtful shadow has been obtained in this way, and experience gained which is of value in the interpretation of these very difficult cases. It is obvious that if systematic work is undertaken in this way the diagnostic value of radiography will be greatly increased. The object of entering into the many interesting points in the paper as thoroughly as possible is to stimulate other observers to carry on the work, and there is no doubt that if an observer is prepared to devote time and skill to the investigation of conditions of the gall bladder and bile ducts he will find that the percentage of accurate diagnoses will increase proportionately with the care devoted to the work.

The short historical notes and abstracts from a large number of important papers on the subject should be useful in giving an account of the technique employed, the success attained by various workers, and some indication of the accuracy of the examination in diagnosis.

The investigation of the region of the liver and gall bladder should always be employed when symptoms point to a lesion in that region. The examination must be very complete, and no detail should be omitted which is likely to ensure success. It has been shown that it is possible to demonstrate in a number of cases the presence of gall stones, and from a consideration of the experimental evidence it is clear that all gall stones will give a shadow on the photographic plate. The probability of demonstrating the presence of gall stones will be dependent upon one factor only, the density of the stone and that of the surrounding tissues; when these are equal the chance of showing the gall stone when it is overlaid by the tissues is very slight, unless it is possible by posture and angling of the X-ray tube to get the gall stone out of the line of the tissue. In a number of cases the difference between the gall stone density and that of the tissues may be very small, then it will be necessary to obtain plates which will show these small variations; it is in these cases that the greatest difficulty will arise, and in which only very high class technique will be likely to succeed. Experience in examining the plates and the use of suitable illumination will greatly add to the percentage of accurate diagnoses. All doubtful shadows should receive very careful consideration.

With increasing experience in technique, and particularly in the radiographic details, the individual value of the observer will increase.

In conclusion, the writer would like to acknowledge the valuable help received from his colleagues on the staff of King's College Hospital, the Cancer Hospital and the Great Northern Central Hospital. Without this help the value of the observations would have been much less.

THE END.

ERRATA.

Page 92, Fig. 36, "ileum" should read "ilium."
Page 120, sixth line from top, should read, " Fig. 54 is an example," etc.
Page 132, last sentence of inscription under Fig. 58 refers to Fig. 37, not Fig. 58.

NOTES AND ABSTRACTS.

Syphilitic Aortitis and its Early Recognition.—G. E. BROWN (*Amer. Jour. of the Med. Sciences*, Jan., 1919, pp. 41-54, with 6 radiograms).—The physical signs in aortitis are of considerable value, and upon them the diagnosis is made with certainty. The normal aorta of a young adult man should measure 5 to 7 cm. in the transverse diameter. At the age of fifty, 8 cm. It is somewhat less in women. In aortitis, the aorta is enlarged in both diameters, and it is upon alterations in width and contour that the diagnosis is made. This change may be detected by percussion from without inward in the second and third interspaces. There is a group of cases, however, in which no percussion changes will be noted.

The X-ray diagnosis is by far the most satisfactory method for demonstrating changes in the aortic arch. X rays show that specific aortitis may show one or more of the following changes in the normal aortic curve:—

1. Enlargement of the aortic shadow to the right. This is usually the earliest demonstrable change, as this is the portion of the aorta first involved in the syphilitic process.

2. Enlargement to the left, with obliteration of the normal aortic knob.

3. Enlargement both to right and left. Increased density of the aortic shadow is suggestive, as is also reduction of the aortic pulsation.

The aorta should be examined both fluoroscopically and with plates. The latter should be taken in the upright position and at a distance of from 6 to 7 feet. These seven-foot plates give, it is stated, an accurate size of the heart and aortic shadow.

R. W. A. S.

Some Observations of Mastoid Structure as Revealed by Roentgen-Ray Examination.—I. GERBER (*Amer. Jour. of Roent.*, Jan., 1919, pp. 1-11, with 13 radiographs and 5 photographs).—This observer describes and illustrates the various types of mastoid structure according to Cheatle's classification. He considers it absolutely essential, for the proper differentiation of these types in the living, to make a stereoscopic view of each mastoid. It is pointed out that while bilateral symmetry is usual, it is by no means a fixed rule.

The X-ray examination of the mastoid, with due regard to the structural type, helps one to predict with much greater exactness the clinical course and prognosis of a middle-ear infection.

In the infantile types, by recognising their presence, a chronic infection of the mastoid can be prevented by early drainage of the antrum, regardless of the absence of the classical mastoid signs. If there is merely a middle-ear suppuration, with definite drooping of the postero-superior canal wall, and an infantile type of mastoid seen by X-ray examination, the patient should be given the benefit of the doubt by early antral exploration.

With the pneumatic type of mastoid, however, even in the presence of acute symptoms, operation should not be hastened at the outset. The re-establishment of positive mastoid pressure by means of proper punctures of the drum-membrane may be sufficient to produce prompt cure. Of course, if actual destruction of the cell walls, or the presence of a perisinus or epidural abscess, can be made out, then the indication for operative interference is definite.

Gerber takes exception to the frequently reported "sclerotic" condition of the mastoid by radiologists when very little cellular structure is visible. The term "sclerosis," when properly used, can be applied only to conditions where there has been actual inflammation, with subsequent repair and new bone production. The majority of so-called sclerotic mastoids, he points out, are really those in which no cellular structure was ever present, and are cases of the infantile type of mastoid. R. W. A. S.

A Case of Hydro-pneumo-cranium with Air in the Ventricles.—H. E. POTTER (*Amer. Jour. of Roent.*, Jan., 1919, pp. 12-16, with 4 radiograms). — A number of days after a fracture of the frontal bone, air entered the cranial cavity. Two weeks later, this air cavity had extended and become partially fluid filled. With the entrance of fluid, the cavity did not shrink, but the air was gradually displaced by the fluid, and at this stage there existed a fluid filled cavity very like a cyst. Coincident with the increase of gas in the cavity, there was a partial filling of the lateral ventricle with gas. From the completeness with which all the gas disappeared, it seemed as if it had been expelled as well as absorbed, since a nitrogen residue is said to persist for some time after the oxygen content of air has been absorbed.

Potter thinks from the above events that air insufflated into the cranial cavity, following fracture through pneumatic sinuses, could easily play an important *rôle* in the formation of certain traumatic cysts filled either with cerebro-spinal fluid alone or this fluid mixed with hæmatogenous elements.

In the above case, it is a reasonable question whether the air in the sub-dural cavity did not gain entrance to the ventricle by the roundabout passage formed by the foramina of Magendie and Luscka, the fourth and third ventricles and the foramina of Munro.

Potter believes that many cases of intra-cranial air are overlooked because of the infrequency of X-ray examination two or three weeks after the injury, when pneumatic sinuses are fractured into. If this examination became routine, he has no doubt that in a short time we should have a complete knowledge of the hydrostatics involved.

R. W. A. S.

The Recognition and Significance of Fractures of the Patellar Border.— R. W. A. SALMOND (*Brit. Jour. of Surg.*, Jan., 1919, pp. 463-465, with 5 radiograms).—Attention is drawn in this article to the recognition of fissure fractures of the border of the patella. These are caused by *indirect* injury or strain, which may be so slight that the patient does not realise at the time that anything unusual has happened, and they are generally not diagnosed as fractures. The line of fissure, or fracture, is either longitudinal or obliquely downwards and outwards. Recurrent syno-

vitis, with effusion into the joint, is a frequent accompaniment, though in reality it is secondary to the condition of the patella.

In a series of cases observed by the writer, all degrees have been found, from a fine fissure without any displacement to a condition approaching in character the well known fracture of the patella by muscular action. This observation suggests that the finer injuries are either a minor degree of the latter, with the line of force acting in a slightly different direction, or that they are due to an overpull of the ligaments, as in the so-called sprain fracture.

The Roentgen Rays in the Diagnosis of Appendicitis.—G. E. PFAHLER (*Amer. Jour. of Roent.*, Feb., 1919, pp. 78-82).—After describing his technique, the author gives the diagnostic points in chronic appendicitis obtained by radiology. Of these, localized tenderness is the most valuable sign, and is elicited either by direct palpation under the screen by the gloved hand or better by means of the wooden spoon. It is pointed out that physicians and surgeons are apt to look for tenderness over McBurney's point, but, from his experience in radioscopic examinations, Pfahler says that we would be much in error if we depended upon this point for the localized tenderness.

If no tenderness is present over a visualised appendix, and if at the same time the cæcum is freely movable, Pfahler thinks that one can say that no appendicitis exists.

The differential diagnosis from other conditions in the right lower quadrant of the abdomen is given.

R. W. A. S.

The Unsuspected Foreign Body as a Frequent Cause of Chronic Bronchitis.— D. R. BOWEN (*Amer. Jour. of Roent.*, March, 1919, pp. 111-119, with 9 radiograms).—This writer believes that unsuspected foreign bodies in the lung are much more frequent than previous experience has indicated. The usual diagnosis has been chronic bronchitis or, less frequently, slowly advancing tuberculosis. Eleven cases from the clinic of Chevalier Jackson are described.

R. W. A. S.

The Effect of the X-ray upon the Response of Tadpoles to Thyroid Stimulation.—C. P. McCORD and C. J. MARINUS (*Endocrinology* Vol. II., No. 3, pp. 289-300).—Selected tadpoles were subjected to the action of X ray, in small amounts. Certain of them were then treated with preparations of thyroid glands, and the rate of their metamorphosis compared with that of (1) normal tadpoles, (2) thyroid-fed tadpoles which had not been irradiated, and (3) irradiated but not thyroid-fed tadpoles. The results of these experiments indicate that irradiation is without apparent effect upon normal tadpoles, but determines a slight but distinct increase in the susceptibility of young tadpoles to thyroid stimulation.

If further experiments show that large doses of X rays produce an effect opposite to the above results, these observers think it may be inferred that the thyroid hormone normally acts in conjunction with the intracellular enzymes to produce the phenomena commonly associated with thyroid activity.

R. W. A. S.

PUBLICATIONS RECEIVED.
Journals.

American Journal of Electrotherapeutics and Radiology, June, 1919.

American Journal of Roentgenology, Sept., 1919.

Gaceta Médica Catalana, Aug 31st, 1919.

Hospitalstidende, Aug. 27th; Sept. 10th; Oct. 3rd, 1919.

International Journal of Orthodontia and Oral Surgery, Aug., 1919.

Journal of Cutaneous Diseases, July, 1919.

Journal de Radiologie et d'Electricite, Sept., 1919.

Journals—*continued.*

La Radiologia Medica, July-Aug., 1919.

New York Medical Journal, Aug. 30th; Sept. 6th, 13th, 20th, 1919.

New York State Journal of Medicine, Sept., 1919.

Norsk Mag. for Lægevidenskaben, Sept., 1919.

Surgery, Gynæcology, and Obstetrics, Sept. 1919.

Ugeskrift for Læger, Aug. 28th; Sept. 4th, 11th, 18th, 25th, 1919.

NOTICES.

ARCHIVES OF RADIOLOGY AND ELECTROTHERAPY is published monthly.

The index for each volume, which ends with the May number, is supplied with the June number of each year.

Communications to the Editors should be addressed to "ROBERT KNOX, M.D., 38, Harley Street, W. 1."

Communications and illustrations from American contributors may be sent to Messrs. REBMAN COMPANY, 141-145, West Thirty-sixth Street, New York City.

All radiographs and photographs must be originals, and must not have been previously published. Drawings should be supplied on separate paper.

Owing to the scarcity of paper the Publishers are reluctantly compelled—as a temporary war measure—to reduce the number of free reprints of Papers to twenty-five.

Annual Subscriptions, payable in advance, 30/- including postage. Single copies, 3/- (postage 2d.) Single numbers and back numbers can be supplied on application.

Vol. XXIV—No. 6   NOVEMBER, 1919   No. 232

ARCHIVES OF RADIOLOGY AND ELECTROTHERAPY

THE OFFICIAL ORGAN OF THE

BRITISH ASSOCIATION OF RADIOLOGY AND PHYSIOTHERAPY

Editors.

ROBERT KNOX, M.D., Hon. Radiographer, King's College Hospital.
E. P. CUMBERBATCH, B.M., M.R.C.P., Medical Officer in Charge. Electrical Department, St. Bartholomew's Hospital.
SIDNEY RUSS, D.Sc., Physicist to the Middlesex Hospital.

IN COLLABORATION WITH

A. E. BARCLAY (Manchester); BELOT (Paris); H. MARTIN BERRY (London); W. H. BRAGG (London), N. BURKE (Woodhall Spa); J. BURNET (Edinburgh); W. J. S. BYTHELL (Manchester); J. T. CASE (Battle Creek, U.S.A.); A. ST. GEORGE CAULFEILD (London); H. A. COLWELL (London); FOVEAU DE COURMELLES (Paris); GUNZBURG (Antwerp); HALL-EDWARDS (Birmingham); HARET (Paris); HAUCHAMPS (Brussels); F. HERNAMAN-JOHNSON (London); W. F. HIGGINS (Teddington); THURSTAN HOLLAND (Liverpool); HURST (London); KLYNENS (Antwerp); LAQUERRIERE (Paris); LAZARUS-BARLOW (London); LEDUC (Nantes); ALEXANDER MACKAY (Edinburgh); REGINALD MORTON (London); HARRISON ORTON (London); W. OVEREND (St. Leonards-on-Sea); PFAHLER (Philadelphia); C. E. S. PHILLIPS (London); GEORGE PIRIE (Dundee); HOWARD PIRIE (Montreal); A. W. PORTER (London); R. W. A. SALMOND (London); WERTHEIM SALOMONSON (Amsterdam); S. SLOAN (Glasgow); SOMERVILLE (Glasgow); W. C. STEVENSON (Dublin); W. J. TURRELL (Oxford); HUGH WALSHAM (London); ROBT. WILSON (Montreal).

ELEVATION OF THE BODY TEMPERATURE BY THE DIATHERMY CURRENT. PATH OF THE CURRENT IN THE BODY.

By E. P. CUMBERBATCH, M.A., B.M. (Oxon), M.R.C.P.

WHEN the current generated by the diathermy machine is passed through the body no sensation other than heat is perceived.* The readiest way of demonstrating this is to grasp a cylindrical electrode in each hand and set the machine in operation. Nothing whatever is felt at first, but as the strength of the current is increased warmth is perceived in the wrists. As the current continues to flow the wrists are felt to become hotter, and, at the same time, warmth is perceived in the narrower parts of the forearms. Gradually the whole of the forearm and upper arm perceives the warmth, while the wrists and lower parts of the forearms become still hotter. Heat is now perceived in the rest of the body, particularly the face and chest. When the wrists

---

* Occasionally a sensation resembling that caused by the faradic current is felt, and slight contraction of the muscles noted. This is usually due to dryness of the skin in contact with the electrodes, and can be abolished by slight damping of the skin.

become very hot a curious and unbearable sensation is felt in them, and the hands seem to lose their grip of the electrodes.   Further heating cannot be tolerated and the current must be interrupted.

The following experiments were made to ascertain the degree to which various parts of the body could be heated by the diathermy current:—

EXPERIMENT 1.—A current of 0·4 amp. was passed for twenty minutes.   A cylindrical metal electrode was grasped in each hand.   The subject of this experiment was seated, and the elbows and knees were semi-flexed.

The following rises of temperature were noted in different regions:—

Front of wrist 6° (from 94 to 100).
Front of elbow 4° (from 95 to 99).
Axilla   -   2·4° (from 98·8 to 101·2).
Mouth   -   2·6° (from 97·6 to 100·2).
Groin   -   1·2° (from 98·8 to 100).
Popliteal space 3° (from 98 to 101).
Between first and second toes no rise noted.

This experiment shows that the passage of the diathermy current from hand to hand along the upper extremities caused a rise of temperature, not only of the upper limbs, but also of other parts of the body.   The amount of the rise varied in different regions, but was higher in the upper limbs than in more remote parts such as the groin and knee.   The temperatures recorded were, strictly speaking, skin temperatures, except that noted in the mouth, which may be regarded as the temperature of the interior of the body.

The difference in the amount of the rise in different parts can be explained in the following way:—

The arms and forearms form a narrow path for the current and so offer a high resistance.   The wrist, being the narrowest part, offers the highest resistance, and so feels the heat first and attains the highest temperature.

The rise of temperature in other parts, such as the mouth, groin, etc., is not due to the passage of the current along them.   The exact path which the current takes in the tissues is not accurately known, but if we assume that when it passes across the trunk its lines of flow diverge, its density must, in consequence, fall considerably, while in distant parts, such as the mouth and lower limbs, the density must be infinitesimally low, and its heating power nil. If, on the other hand, the current flows direct, by the shortest path, across the trunk, from shoulder to shoulder, without any deviation, it will not reach the lower part of the trunk or lower limbs or head.   Another reason must, therefore, be sought for the rise of temperature in these parts.

The rise is due, doubtless, to the circulation through them of blood heated in its passage along the hot arms and forearms.   The current, in its passage along the upper limbs, heats not only the fixed tissues but also the circulating fluids.   The heated blood passes to other parts of the body and a rise of temperature can be recorded where the heat is not too rapidly lost.

The distribution of the heat in the upper extremities is not uniform.   The maximum degree of heat is felt and recorded in the narrowest parts, viz. the wrists. The front of the wrist reaches a higher temperature than the back, and the anterior part of the elbow becomes hotter than the posterior. If the operator holds the electrodes and passes the current along his arms he will note these differences. The front of the forearm will also feel hotter than the back.

EXPERIMENT 2.—A current of 0·5 amp. was passed from hand to hand. The following rises of temperature were recorded in the elbow after the current had passed for ten minutes. The elbow was maintained in a position of full extension :—

Front of elbow   ·   -   -   6·5° (from 93·5 to 100).
Back of elbow (by side of olecranon) 5° (from 90 to 95).

In this experiment the current had to be interrupted after ten minutes, because the heat became intolerable in the wrists and the hold on the electrode could not be maintained. In the next experiment a current of 0·65 amp. was passed from hand to hand. After four minutes it had to be switched off. The following rises of temperature were recorded :—

EXPERIMENT 3.   *Front of wrist.*   *Back of wrist.*
After 2 minutes   -   12° (from 91 to 103).   -   9° (from 86 to 95).
After 3 minutes   -   16° (from 91 to 107).   -   13° (from 86 to 99).
After 4 minutes   -   20° (from 91 to 111).   -   16° (from 86 to 102).

The last two experiments show that the temperature rose higher on the flexor aspect of the wrist and elbow than on the extensor aspect. This is probably due to the fact that the posterior (extensor) region of the wrist and elbow is occupied mainly by cartilage and bone. These tissues offer a higher resistance to the current than the vessels, tendons, etc., which occupy the anterior (flexor) region. The major portion of the current, therefore, travels along the latter region.

If the current is passed along the limb *when the joint is flexed*, a still greater difference is seen in the rise of the temperature on the flexor and extensor region.

EXPERIMENT 4.—Current of 0.5 amp. passed for ten minutes from hand to hand, elbows flexed to a right angle. The following rises of temperature were noted :—

Front of elbow   -   -   -   9·2° (from 93 to 102·2).
Back of elbow (by side of olecranon) 3·4° (from 88 to 91·4).

This considerably greater rise of temperature on the front of the elbow when flexed is probably due to the fact that the path for the current is shorter along the flexor region, and so has a lower resistance. Also, as pointed out above, less resistant tissues lie on the flexor region.

When an electrode is placed on the palm and the wrist flexed to a right angle, the major portion of the current will flow along the anterior region of the wrist, which, consequently, will be heated to a higher temperature than the posterior region. Along the anterior region is the shorter path and the less resistant tissues. If, on the contrary, the electrode is placed on the back of the hand and the wrist dorsi-flexed as far as possible, the shorter path for the current will be along more resistant tissues, and there will be less difference between the temperatures attained on the posterior and anterior surfaces of the wrist.

> EXPERIMENT 5.—Electrode on *palm*. *Palmar-flexion* of wrist. Current passed for ten minutes. The following rises of temperature were noted :—
>> Anterior aspect of wrist 16° (from 89 to 105).
>> Posterior aspect of wrist 6° (from 89 to 95).

> EXPERIMENT 6.—Electrode on *back* of hand. *Dorsi-flexion* of wrist. Current passed for ten minutes. The following rises were noted :—
>> Anterior aspect of wrist 12° (from 93 to 105).
>> Posterior aspect of wrist 12° (from 92 to 104).

When the current is directed along the lower extremities, by way of metal plate electrodes placed in contact with the soles, the ankles feel the heat first and attain the highest temperature ; the thighs feel the heat last, and their temperature rises only slightly. The trunk, head, neck, and upper limbs are heated *indirectly* by means of the circulating blood.

> EXPERIMENT 7.—Same subject as in Experiment 1. Sitting position with knees semi-flexed. A current of 0·7 amp. was passed from sole to sole, along the lower limbs, across the trunk, for twenty minutes. The following rises of temperature were noted :—
>> Front of ankle 18·5° (from 94 to 104).
>> Popliteal space 10° (from 85 to 103·5).
>> Groin   1° (from 99 to 100).
>> Mouth   -   1° (from 98·2 to 99·2).
>> Wrist   -   No rise noted.

The subject felt the maximum heat in the ankles and the back of the knee. Other parts of the body experienced a sensation of increased warmth, but less so than when the current was directed along the upper limbs. As in the first experiment, the current was adjusted so that the heat could be tolerated in the narrowest parts without discomfort.

The difference in the temperature of the back and front of the knee was very evident, even to the touch. As in the case of the upper limbs, the difference is more evident when the knee is flexed than when it is extended. This is shown by the following experiments:—

> EXPERIMENT 8.—Knee *flexed* to right angle. Current directed from calf to calf. The following rises of temperature were noted :—
>> Front of knee   -   2° after 5 minutes, 3° after 10 minutes.
>>   (91 to 93).   (91 to 94).
>> Back of knee   9° after 5 minutes, 11° after 10 minutes.
>>   (94 to 103).   (94 to 105).

> EXPERIMENT 9.—Knee *extended*. The following rises were noted :—
>> Front of knee   -   6° after 5 minutes, 10° after 10 minutes.
>>   (91 to 97).   (91 to 101).
>> Back of knee   -   7° after 5 minutes, 14° after 10 minutes.
>>   (93 to 100).   (93 to 107).

When the soles rest on the electrodes and the current is passed along the lower limbs, the toes and front portion of the feet do not feel any warmth, even though the ankles become very hot. The difference is very apparent to the touch. If the current is passed from sole to sole of a subject whose feet are cyanosed a good ocular demonstration is obtained of the distribution of the heat. The toes and anterior portions of the feet retain their livid appearance, while the ankles and the parts of the feet immediately below gradually acquire a red hue.

When the diathermy current is directed across the trunk the subject feels heat in the skin where covered by the electrodes. The general sensation of warmth, which was felt to pervade gradually the whole body when the current was directed along the limbs, is not perceived unless the current flows for much longer than twenty minutes.

> EXPERIMENT 10.—Circular metal plated electrodes, 3in. in diameter, were placed on the trunk, one on the abdominal wall below the umbilicus, the other on the lower lumbar region. A current of 0·8 amp. was passed for twenty minutes. The following rises of temperature were noted :—
>
> | | | |
> |---|---|---|
> | Skin under abdominal electrode | - | 4° (from 95 to 99). |
> | Skin under lumbar electrode | - | 9° (from 92 to 101). |
> | Mouth - - - | - | 0·4° (from 99·6 to 100). |
> | Axilla - | - | 0·6° (from 99·2 to 99·8). |
> | Popliteal space - - | - | No rise. |

It is seen, in this experiment, that the temperature of distant parts, and the internal temperature (as registered in the mouth) showed a very small rise, considerably less than that noted after the current had passed for the same period of time along the limbs. As mentioned before, the rise of temperature of distant parts is due to the circulation of heated blood. The blood is heated most when the diathermy current is passed along the limbs, because it flows along the same general direction as the current, and is exposed to the heating action of the current for a relatively long time. When the current passes through the abdomen the conditions are different. There is no direct flow of blood across the trunk between electrodes placed back and front of the abdomen. It flows in all directions, its general course being longitudinal rather than transverse. The general direction of the diathermy current in Experiment 10 was transverse. Assuming that it travels direct from electrode to electrode, the blood would pass into and out of the path of the current before it was heated. If, however, the current takes a more circuitous path, its density would therefore be greatly lessened and its heating power diminished. In either case the current cannot heat the blood more than a trifling amount.

When the current is passed through the abdomen or chest, demonstration of the rise of temperature (if any) in the contained organs is, in the case of the normal subject, impossible. The organs are very vascular, and the proportion of circulating fluid to fixed tissue is, in them, larger than in the case of the tissues composing a limb. Therefore, heat generated in the abdominal or thoracic organs can be more quickly conducted away by the blood. If electrodes of large surface are used, of a size sufficient to cover the front and back of the abdomen completely, the density of the current will be greatly diminished, and, with the machines at present available, no rise of temperature will be noted, even in the skin.* If smaller electrodes are used a rise of the skin temperature can be brought about. If, however, the lines of flow of the current diverge on their passage into the trunk, the density of the current will fall and its power to generate heat in the abdomen will be greatly lessened. It is therefore unlikely that the temperature in the interior of the abdomen or chest will be raised directly, at any rate, raised sufficiently to affect an ordinary thermometer. Long continued passage of the current will, however, raise the temperature of the blood so that the abdominal organs will be heated, together with other parts of the body.

The following observations were made in order to ascertain whether (in the cases tried) any rise of temperature could be detected in the abdomen after passage of the diathermy current:—

> EXPERIMENT 11.—A patient, the subject of a former operation for pyo-nephrosis, had a sinus leading to the region of the kidney. One electrode was placed on the abdomen, the other on the back, so as to cover the surface marking of the kidney, A clinical thermometer was placed in the sinus. A current of 1·2 amp. was passed for twenty minutes. At the end of this time the thermometer indicated no rise of temperature, although the skin was made as hot as the patient could bear without discomfort.

> EXPERIMENT 12.—A thermometer was placed with its bulb in the posterior fornix vaginæ of a patient, and electrodes were placed on the pubes and lower hypogastric and gluteal regions. After thirty minutes the following rises of temperature were noted:—
>
> Posterior fornix 0·4° (99·2 to 99·6).
> Mouth   -   0·4° (98·4 to 98·8).

In Experiment 12 the temperature of the interior of the pelvis was raised, but not more than the internal temperature (as registered in the mouth); pelvic and oral temperatures rose *pari passu.* This may be explained in the following way: the current heated not only the fixed pelvic tissues but their contained blood and lymph. As a result of the heating of the circulating fluids the general temperature of the body rose gradually. The failure of the pelvic tissues to attain a higher temperature than that of the blood was due probably to the vascularity of the pelvic organs and the conduction of the heat from them by the blood.

The temperature of the pelvic organs can be raised (together with that of the rest of the interior of the body) by passing the current through other parts away from the pelvis. Thus, a current was passed from arm to arm, and the pelvic temperature rose 0·6° (from 99·4 to 100). The oral temperature rose a similar amount.

Path of the Diathermy Current in the Body.—The path which currents, oscillating with high-frequency, take in the body is not known with certainty. When they travel along metal conductors they are confined almost wholly to the surface. This restriction to the surface is spoken of as the "skin effect." The body, however, is a conductor of a different kind, viz., an electrolyte, and

---

* When the body is placed on a condenser couch, designed for use with the diathermy machine, larger electrodes can be used, and an appreciable amount of heat generated. This couch was described and illustrated in the present Journal, No. 169, August, 1914.

its power to conduct the high-frequency (and other) currents is due to the presence of the ions in the tissue fluids.

In their passage through saline solutions high-frequency currents do not show this preference for the surface layers. D'Arsonval passed a high-frequency current along a cylindrical conductor composed of 0·7 per cent. salt solution and found that the current, in the centre and at the periphery, did not differ sensibly in intensity.

The body, however, is a conductor of a most complicated kind. Not only is it composed of different tissues, each presenting a different resistance, but it is permeated with a network of vessels of different sizes, running in all directions and containing conducting fluids, viz., blood and lymph. There is, in addition, the skin, which, of all the tissues, presents the highest resistance.

When the current passes along a limb it does not confine itself to the skin. D'Arsonval showed that on passing a high-frequency current along the hind limbs of a rabbit, the deep tissues as well as the skin could be coagulated by the heat. An experiment by Maragliano showed that high-frequency currents penetrate the skin. A small electric lamp was placed in the thorax of a dog, with its poles connected to metal plates placed one in each pleural cavity. When electrodes were placed on the exterior of the chest and connected to a source of high-frequency current the lamp became incandescent.

We may conclude from this experience that the current passes through the skin under the electrodes. What its exact course is after passing through the skin cannot be said with certainty. It probably does not confine itself entirely to the less resistant superficial fasciæ after passing through the more resistant skin. If it did the skin should develop the same temperature on both sides of the limb. But it has been shown by the experiments that the temperature of the skin on the extensor region does not rise the same amount as the temperature of the skin on the flexor aspect.

In all probability, therefore, the current distributes itself throughout the tissues, less travelling by way of the more resistant tissues and *vice versa*. Further proof of the penetration of the current into the deep tissues can be demonstrated by the following experiment:—

EXPERIMENT 13.—The two palms, thoroughly moistened with saline, were pressed together, so that the themar and hypothemar eminences made good contact over as large an area as possible. Electrodes were placed on the back of each hand. A thermometer was inserted, so that its bulb lay in the shallow depression between the themar and hypothemar eminences. This depression was then obliterated by firm pressure together of the opposing palms. A current of 1·4 amp. was passed for six minutes. The thermometer showed a rise of 7° (95 to 102).

Further proof of the penetration of the current is afforded by the coagulation of tissue for some distance under the electrode when strong currents are used for surgical purposes. A large fungating mass of growth, arising from the neck of a patient, was traversed by the current. A circular electrode, ¾ in. in diameter, was placed on it, and a thermometer was thrust in the growth so that its bulb lay about 1 in. below the electrode. Another electrode, a large metal plate, was placed on the chest. On increasing the current the thermometer was seen to rise. A temperature of 130° F. was quickly reached, and could have been exceeded. (The object, in this case, was to raise the growth to the supposed minimum lethal temperature for new growths of malignant type.)

When the current is directed along a limb it is confined to a relatively narrow path. When, however, the electrodes are placed on the trunk, a number of paths are presented to the current. Whether its course is entirely confined to the region included between the electrodes, or whether it travels in addition along outlying regions, has not been settled, because of the difficulties that lie in the way of direct investigation. It may be said, however, that wide divergence of the lines of flow of the current would mean great lowering of density of the current, and little, if any, development of heat. In Experiment 10, it was found that a rise of 0·4° was obtained in the mouth and 0.6° in the axilla. It is not likely that this rise was due to the heating of the blood in the skin under the electrodes, where the current density was high, because the amount of blood passing through these small areas of skin was small, particularly as the electrodes were pressed against the body, and must have caused some compression of the vessels. It is more likely that the current took a more direct path in the trunk between the electrodes without much lowering of its density.

Practical Conclusions.—The above described experiments give some indication of the position in which to place the electrodes when it is wished to apply diathermy, for medical purposes, either to the whole body or to a region of it. If it is desired to raise the temperature of the whole body, the easiest way to do it is to pass the current along the upper limbs by way of electrodes grasped in the hand. If an internal temperature higher than 100° is desired, the wrists will become too hot if the electrodes are held in the hands. Plate electrodes should then be substituted and applied to the forearms.

When the current passes along the upper limbs, the latter are heated *directly* and attain the highest temperature. The trunk and lower limbs are heated *indirectly* by means of the circulating fluids. If the current is then passed along the lower limbs, the latter will be heated *directly* : the tissues which are less vascular and therefore less easily heated by the blood, are now traversed by the current and heated directly.

When it is wished to apply diathermy to a joint the electrodes should be placed on opposite aspects, one anterior and the other posterior, and afterwards one on each side when possible. If the current is passed longitudinally along a limb, the major portion will pass along the better conducting tissues outside the joint.

With regard to the feet and hands, one electrode should be placed on the sole or palm, the other on the dorsum of the foot or back of hand.

THE PLACE OF THE RADIOLOGIST AND HIS KINDRED IN THE WORLD OF MEDICINE.

By FRANCIS HERNAMAN-JOHNSON, M.D.

Radiologist to the French Hospital; Physician to the X-Ray Department, the Margaret Street Hospital for Consumption, etc.; late Consulting Radiologist, Aldershot Command.

IT is difficult to realise that less than a century ago the general physician held complete sway in the medical world. The ·local practitioner, when in doubt, called in a consultant who was but a glorified replica of himself : and before a surgeon of the period could obtain any cases, he had nearly always to secure the interest of some well known physician. Even then, he was generally confronted with a diagnosis already made, which he was not expected to question, and was more or less ordered to undertake such operative procedures as his colleague considered desirable.

The few surgical pioneers who, by force of character, were able from time to time to break through this constraint, did so almost at the risk of their lives ; for the early performers of abdominal operations had sometimes to be rescued from howling mobs, who pursued them with stones and cries of " belly ripper " !

The mortality rate from surgical operations was at that time so high that the popular opposition is to some extent understandable, especially when it is remembered that all operations were performed with the victim fully conscious ; and no increase of mechanical skill could have carried surgery to its present high place, apart from the discovery of anæsthesia and antiseptics.

At the present day the public divides " doctors " into two great groups —those who effect their cures mainly by the knife, and those who treat their cases by means of medicines taken by the mouth or injected under the skin. The order of precedence above given, and the exact phrases used, are employed deliberately, as intending to sum up the respective values which the man in the street attaches respectively to surgical and medical procedures.

The layman, of course, realises that there are " regional specialists," who concern themselves solely with the eye, or with the ear and throat, or it may be even with a single internal organ, such as the heart. But he looks upon such specialists as combined surgeons and physicians, so far as their own speciality is concerned.

The bacteriologist he hardly thinks of as a practising doctor at all, but rather as one who spends his time in a mysterious laboratory far removed from the personal contact of ordinary professional life.

That there has arisen, practically within the last twenty years, a great system of diagnosis and treatment worthy of being looked upon as an entity on a par with " medicine " or " surgery," is a fact recognised not at all by the public, only vaguely by the medical profession at large, and by no means fully appreciated even by its own votaries—the "radiologists" and "physio-therapists" of the present day.   Yet the methods which they specially employ have to do neither with the use of the knife nor the giving of medicines ; nor yet, as regards diagnosis, with the *tactus eruditus*, or with chemical or microscopical examinations.   On the other hand, the range of diseases which they can relieve or cure is quite as wide as that claimed by surgery or medicine.

The new department has suffered much from lack of a convenient nomenclature, both for itself and those who practise it.   "Radiology" appears to leave "Electrotherapeutics" in the cold ; and the latter term takes no cognisance of massage and remedial exercises.   Compound titles for the practitioners of these arts are ungainly mouthfuls ; for example, the term "Radio-physio-therapist," which recently appeared in an official document, is scarcely likely to come into general use.   And it will be noted that, despite its Teutonic profusion of hyphens, the title is misleading, as it suggests therapeutic activities only.

A name for the subject as a whole is difficult to find : the present writer does not pretend to know of any really satisfactory one.   Generally speaking, it may be said that anything ending in " 'ology " is not sufficiently wide.   We should rather seek an analogy in such terms as "Tropical Medicine," "Forensic Medicine," etc.   The term "Physical Medicine" has been pro-posed, and while it is open to obvious objections, it may perhaps serve.   This leaves us without any name, such as "physician" or "surgeon," to describe the practitioner of physical medicine ; but this is of less moment than might at first sight appear.   For in a sense every practitioner is a physician if he does not practise surgery ; and, secondly, the tendency of the day is for physicians and surgeons to attach some descriptive or limiting adjective or phrase to the ancient titles.   We have thus cardiologists and neurologists among the physicians ; and among the surgical experts, "abdominal" surgeons, "gynæcological" surgeons, proctologists, orthopædists, *et hoc genus omne*.

Among practitioners of physical medicine we find similar subdivisions—"Radiologists," "Electrotherapeutists," "Specialists in massage," etc.   And already there are even lesser divisions of subdivisions : experts in diagnosis as opposed to treatment ; experts in the treatment of certain diseases ; radium-therapists and even—one would suppose, from their writings—"ionists " or "galvanists."

Practitioners of physical medicine have possessed a "class consciousness" only for about a decade—certainly not for two ; the modern surgeon dates from the days of Lister, and may therefore be said to have half a century of tradition behind him. · We cannot therefore do better, in seeking an ideal for ourselves, than study the relationships which the best modern surgeons have established between themselves and the public on the one hand, and the rest of the medical profession on the other.

What do we expect from the most eminent surgeons? Certainly that they should be more than brilliant operators. We look for them to have a general knowledge of medicine in all its branches—not a technical knowledge, but a familiarity with principles. For instance, we should feel that a surgeon was ignorant who did not suggest vaccines in suitable cases, but we should not expect him to prepare them, or even to take sole responsibility for the size and frequency of the doses. Moreover, one does not require such a man to accept a diagnosis ready made, nor necessarily to perform the particular operation which he sets out to do. In fact, width of judgment is even more important than operative skill ; in the sense that a moderately good operator, of sound judgment and balanced mind, will do more good in a lifetime than the brilliant technician of narrow views. The first will lose a few cases that the second would have saved ; but his tale of useless operations, of shattered nerves and disappointed hopes will be, by comparison, small. The surgeon who knows the limitations as well as the possibilities of surgery, who knows when to call on the help of colleagues, both in diagnosis and treatment, yet is not led away by " stunts "—this is the man in whose hands we, who know medicine from the inside, would fain place ourselves in time of need.

We see then that the modern surgeon claims to exercise his unfettered judgment as to—

(1) Diagnosis.

(2) The nature of the operations he performs and the after treatment.

(3) The procedures which he recommends apart from operative interference.

A similar freedom should be claimed and exercised by the practitioner of physical medicine. For example, a case may be sent to him with a diagnosis of " frontal neuralgia," and a request for "ionization." Assuming that the condition is indeed neuralgic, it is his business to use whatever modalities his experience teaches him give the best results in such cases ; further than this, it is his duty to satisfy himself that the condition is really " neuralgic," and not the result, for instance, of sinus infection. A knowledge of X-ray diagnosis will often suggest procedures likely to throw light upon such cases ; and, when it is likely that X-ray investigation can help, the patient's doctor should be informed to that effect. How this is to be done tactfully it is not my purpose here to discuss, as that is a matter which concerns the relationship of consultants and practitioners in general.

Instances might be multiplied. A case which occurs to the writer was that of a middle-aged man who was developing a gradually increasing tendency to constipation, but otherwise seemed in perfect health. He was sent for " Bergonié stimulation to the abdomen " ; but an opaque enema revealed a mass in the sigmoid, which proved to be carcinomatous. Other examples are, " rheumatic shoulder," in reality a sarcoma ; " intercostal neuralgia," turning out to be of locomotor origin ; " sciatica," the result of pelvic tumour.

Now comes the important question as to how far the expert should concern himself with the general treatment of his patients. Certainly he should always know the exact nature of any other therapeutic measures which are being undertaken. If they are incompatible with his own treatment, he must see that they are discontinued. In the case of a rheumatic joint treated by the author, the patient's physician applied irritating liniments without consultation; result, a painful skin condition for which "the electricity" was blamed. A hæmorrhoid case, which failed to improve, was found to be taking an aloes pill daily. Such errors, as a rule, only need to be pointed out to be rectified. More difficult to deal with are cases where patients are receiving "routine treatment" for some correctly diagnosed disease. The chronic malarial patient, sent for help in the matter of headaches and for general "toning up," is found to be poisoned by quinine, which his doctor urges him to continue; the Graves' case, already pigmented by arsenic, and still taking it; the unhealed specific ulcer in a mercury intoxicated victim—what is one to do about these? If, as a physician (not as an —ologist) you believe these drugs are doing harm, get them stopped, or give up the case. One may sometimes be wrong, but there is no middle course.

Nor should one hesitate to recommend measures, apart from electrical treatments, which one knows to be of value. We all pick up individual "tips" in the course of our professional career, and they should be utilized, no matter to what special branch of medicine we ultimately devote ourselves. The use of large doses of salicylate of bismuth in the diarrhœa of exophthalmic goitre may perhaps be cited as an instance. The general practitioner is, as a rule, glad to try anything suggested; the consulting physician may require more careful handling! (I need hardly say that all the above measures, whether positive or negative, must be carried out with the co-operation of the practitioner in general charge of the case.)

Then there is the frequent necessity of calling in the help of other experts. There is no use in treating a dirty wound by light until it has been scraped clean by the surgeon; no sense in stimulating weakened muscles against a contracted tendon; no likelihood of complete success in cases partly hysterical unless the aid of the psycho-therapeutist is invoked. That this calling in is as yet too often not mutual must not cause us to neglect it.

Despite the necessity for the large measure of freedom above outlined, one limitation may be accepted, *i.e.*, a case may be seen with a view to diagnosis only. But, within this wide boundary, there must be no restriction, except, in private practice, what may be determined by the patient's circumstances. A commission to examine one kidney is quite inadmissible; and a request to investigate the whole urinary tract is by no means always sufficient. Every radiologist knows that the elucidation of the cause of some vague abdominal pain may call for all the resources of his art. An examination by the opaque meal and opaque enema, and separate examinations for gall stones, pancreatic calculus, renal calculus, and ureteral kink, may all be called for in a single case, and some of them may need to be repeated. It may be said that few private patients can afford to pay for such extensive investigations, which, if properly remunerated, would approximate to the cost of an operation. But they are either necessary or not. We must prove them necessary in hospital practice. In private those who can afford will pay, and for the others the Ministry of Health will no doubt make provision. The public must be educated to realize that a skilled diagnosis is every whit as important as the operation which is advised—or not advised—on the strength of it.

The custom of distributing X-ray prints broadcast, which was so prevalent some years ago, did much to make the public regard the radiologist as a sort of glorified tradesman who was paid for taking photographs. This view is still by no means obsolete, and occasionally one receives a peremptory demand to " send the photographs round to Mr. So-and-so "—about whose connection with the particular case one may never have heard. Now the chief *raison d'etre* of the modern radiologist is to see with his own eyes " living pathology " upon the screen ; to correlate clinical and radioscopic findings ; and to *interpret* the plates which he makes or has made for him. In every case, where distance is not a bar, such demands should be met by an offer to meet and consult with the doctor named. So far as my experience goes, such offers are rarely refused, and the result of their acceptance is a benefit to all concerned. When distance is a factor, prints may be sent, provided that their meaning is likely to be appreciated by the aid of an explanatory report. The finest detail cannot be reproduced in prints, and even as to the interpretation of a good negative there may be more than one opinion. In such cases, the patient and his doctor must accept the view offered as an *ipse dixit*, or call in another radiologist. It cannot be too strongly urged that the final reputation of an X-ray diagnostician is deter-mined neither by pretty pictures nor an engaging manner ; but by the general correctness or otherwise of the opinions which he gives. Wide clinical knowledge and skill in the interpretation of screen findings and plate appearances are essentials. The actual production of the plates may or may not be carried out by the radiologist ; if large numbers are concerned, it is certainly a gross waste of time.

Thus we come to grips with the problem of the lay operator. There are still some few radiologists who hold that even the switches on their apparatus are sacred, and that none save the initiate must touch them. Such men are often those whose real interests lie towards engineering or physical science. They were not happy in ordinary medical practice, and welcomed X-ray work, with its mechanics and physics, as a God-sent avenue of escape. They have done invaluable work in perfecting apparatus and technique ; but some of them make the mistake of wasting time in personally carrying out procedures long after they have become a routine, instead of leaving them to laymen, so that they themselves may devote their time to further progress.

The fact that intelligent laymen can produce plates as nearly perfect as present conditions permit cannot be gainsaid. To fight against their employ-ment at this late day is to emulate Mrs. Partington and her mop. What can be done and what should be done is to control the training, and, in so far as may be, the practice of such people—to secure, in a word, that they shall be competent, and that they shall not accept patients except in conjunction with a medical man.   Any attempt to carry restriction further than this is bound to result in failure.   For we cannot prevent any qualified medical man from dabbling in radiology any more than we can stop him from practising ophthalmology, or abdominal surgery, whether his knowledge of these subjects be great or little.   Whether this freedom is desirable or not on broad grounds it is difficult to say.   Restriction would undoubtedly reduce the harm done, but it would also prevent many cures, and sometimes rob the medical world of a genius.

It will be said, with truth, that in some cases the radiographer—the term is used as opposed to radiologist—will dominate the doctor who seeks his aid. At present we cannot help this ; but by educating both the medical and lay public we shall in time create an opinion which will no more allow a lay-operator to exceed his limitations that it would at the present time permit a chiropodist to amputate a leg, or a mid-wife to perform cæsarean section.

Physicians have their dispensers ; surgeons their dressers ; dentists their mechanics.   We hear of lay-inoculators, and even of lay-anæsthetists.   The whole trend of modern medicine is to delegate its more simple routine procedures to lay assistants.   So long as quackery is legally permitted, certain of these people will break away from their legitimate sphere and "set up" as independent practitioners.   The remedy is threefold :—

To organize and educate the various classes of lay helpers.

To see that their status, remuneration, and prospects are such as to make them contented.

To educate the public as to why such people are at one and the same time invaluable as helpers, and extraordinarily dangerous when they seek to practise independently.

The partial practice of radiology and electrotherapy by men with regional specialities is a subject which should be briefly referred to.   It is often the hard fate of the radiologist to work out some procedure which is first abused, then ignored, and finally adopted by men in other branches of the profession. The use of X rays in ovarian and uterine troubles is one instance ; the employment of electricity in weakened or paralysed muscles is another.   The gynæcologist has, to some extent, appropriated the one, the orthopædic surgeon the other.   To grumble is futile ; we should rather appreciate the compliment of imitation.   The general surgeon suffers from similar trials ; there is scarcely a case sent to him which might not equally well go to one of the professors of regional specialities.   Whether he operates upon the sinuses of the skull, or resects a joint, or removes the uterus and ovaries, someone will look upon him as guilty of trespass ; yet he continues to flourish.   The truth is that general surgery and special surgery appeal to different types of mind, both of which are necessary to progress.   So it is with the practice of physical medicine. No matter how many people utilize electricity, X rays, and radium, to a limited extent in their work, there will always be not only room, but urgent need, for the man who makes them his exclusive province.

In conclusion, I venture to sum up as follows the ideals for which, as a body, we should strive:—

(1) That we should seek a freedom of judgment and action equal to that of the best type of modern surgeons, and justify it, as they do, by a familiarity with all that pertains to the general progress of modern medicine.

(2) That we should gain a reputation for being as fully acquainted with our limitations as cognisant of our powers, and seek to impress upon the public mind our belief that in co-operation and combined treatment lies the key to progress.

(3) That we should welcome lay assistance, and seek to organize and guide it. It is too late in the day to make a mystery of taking plates, but the interpretation of them is ours for ever.

THREE CASES OF INJURY TO THE ASTRAGALUS.

By W. DALE, Captain R.A.M.C. (T.F), Radiographer to 14th General Hospital, B.E.F.

THE following cases were seen within two months of each other, and although the injuries were sustained on active service they were not gun shot

wounds. All were the result of severe injuries to the ankle joint and resulted in fracture of the astragalus, a sufficiently rare accident to render them worthy of record.

CASE 1.

No. 63268. Sergt. T———, R.E.

This man was blown out of a dug-out by the force of a shell explosion near it. He was unable to say how he fell or exactly how the injury to the ankle came about.

X-ray (Fig. 1) shows fracture of posterior inferior border of the tibia, comminuted fracture through centre of the astragulas, with dislocation backwards of the posterior fragment.

There has been rotation of this fragment on its transverse horizontal axis, the superior articular surface now looking directly backwards.

The space between the two main fragments is filled with many small comminuted pieces of bone.

There is slight displacement of the dislocated fragment inwards so that it now overlaps the inner border of the tibia.

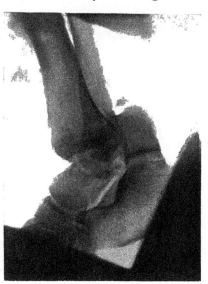

FIG. 1. CASE 1.

CASE 2.

No. 542694.   Pte. G————, Labour Company.

On June 6th, 1918, he was "blown up" by a shell exploding near him.   He landed on both feet at the bottom of a forty-foot well.   He unsuccessfully tried several times to climb up the well.

On admission he had very severe swelling and pain of left ankle and less pain and swelling of right ankle.

There was a fracture of internal malleolus of right ankle.

X-ray (Fig. 2) showed a comminuted fracture of lower 1 in. of anterior border of tibia and a comminuted fracture of the astragalus through the neck with complete dislocation backwards of posterior fragment.

This fragment has rotated on its antero-posterior axis so that the upper articular surface now looks directly inwards.

The interval between the two fragments of the astragalus is partially filled with much comminuted bone.

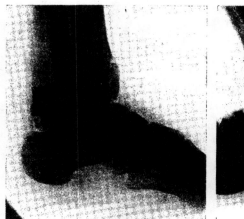 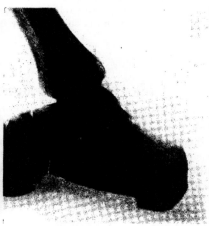

FIG. 2. CASE 2.   FIG. 3.—Normal ankle in full dorsi-flexion.

The points of especial interest are:—

(*a*) The different fractures of the tibia in these two cases.

(*b*) The rotation of the posterior fragment.

To explain (*a*) it is necessary to enquire into the probable mechanism of these fracture dislocations.

The fracture is caused, of course, by the approximation of the tibia to the os calcis.

To obtain fractures such as those described above the ankle must be in some degree of dorsi-flexion—the force being transmitted from the leg through the anterior inferior border of the tibia and neck of the astragalus to the remaining tarsal bones, but chiefly to the os calcis.

This tends to "squeeze" the posterior fragment backwards.   If the dorsi-flexion is sufficient there will be room enough for the passage backward of the posterior fragment without further damage.   This rarely happens.

What does happen is that the dislocated fragment on its journey backwards breaks off the posterior inferior border of the tibia, as in Case 1. Should, however, the original injury be severe enough to cause a fracture of the anterior inferior border of the tibia, then hyperdorsi flexion is permitted, and more room between the posterior border of the tibia and the os calcis is allowed. This enables the posterior fragment to travel backwards without causing further fractures. This is what has happened in Case 2. Fig. 3 is a normal ankle in a condition of full dorsi flexion.

(*b*) The question of rotation of the dislocated posterior fragment is very interesting. In referring to dislocations of the astragalus, Barwell[1] applies the term "tersion" and "version" to the rotation of the displaced bone. He distinguishes tersion rotation round a horizontal axis ; version rotation round a vertical axis.

Stimson,[2] in referring to fracture dislocations of the astragalus, says, "The fragment is also rotated so that its trochlear surface looks inwards and its fractures surface directed forwards and downwards."

In Morgan's[3] case the trochlear surface appears, from the skiagraph published, to look backwards and a little upwards. The mechanism of the rotation and its influence on reduction has not yet been worked out.

CASE 3.

For purposes of comparison with the foregoing cases, in which there was great displacement and comminution, the following case is of interest.

Here we have a simple transverse fracture through the neck of the astragalus and of the anterior lip of the articular surface of the lower end of the tibia, a very rare injury.

The history of the case is unfortunately unknown, as he was X-rayed and immediately evacuated during a "push."

The skiagraph shows an old fracture of the astragalus through the neck. Although many months old, in the stereoscopic plates taken there was seen to be non-union between the two fragments.

There has also been a fracture of the tibia, as described above. There are very considerable osteoarthritic changes around the ankle joint and there is distinct bony union of the anterior fragment of the astragalus to the os calcis.

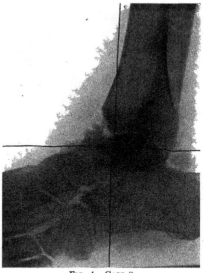

FIG. 4.   CASE 3.

My thanks are due to Capt. Geoffrey Jefferson, R.A.M.C., M.S., for his help and reference in this paper and on many other occasions.

REFERENCES

1. *Medico-Chirurgical Transactions*, 1883, Vol. LXVI, p. 35.
2. "Fractures and Dislocations," by Stimson.
3. *Archives of Radiography*, 1903-1904, VIII, p. 139.

A SATISFACTORY INJECTION MEDIUM FOR THE RADIOGRAPHY OF FISTULÆ.

By Neil Macleod, M.D. Edin., Shanghai.

THE purpose of these injections is twofold : 1st, to obtain a true estimate of their relations to bones and their extent, including those of branches and abscesses communicated with ; 2nd, to detect the presence and nature of foreign bodies if they are preventing closure.

Is a greasy medium like oil, paraffin oil, or vaselin, often recommended and used to hold the bismuth salt in suspension, a good one for the purpose ?

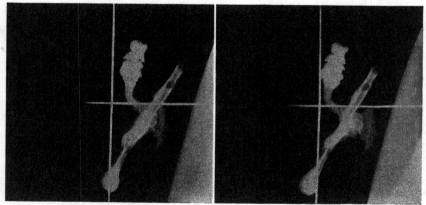

FIG. 1.

Fistulæ, with their branches often communicating with abscesses, all contain more or less pus which cannot be got rid of before injection. Can such greasy material be expected to mix with or become diffused through their purulent contents, or, will these latter be completely displaced by the former? Will greasy matter come into as close contact with the cavity boundaries to be outlined everywhere if there be pus present, as might be the case with an injection made with a non-greasy medium ?

These are not questions prompted by *a priori* considerations, but the result partly of experiments made to detect pus soaked cloth embedded in animal tissues, and partly from a careful consideration of how the unexpected result to be seen in Fig. 1 was obtained in the following case :—

In October, 1917, the writer was asked to radiograph a piece of reed, believed to have been in a man's leg for eighteen months, preventing the closure of a small wound on its outer side six inches above the heel. A radiograph was made, but, as expected, furnished no sign of reed or sinus.

Dr. Billinghurst, surgeon in charge of the case, then injected the fistula with a bismuth emulsion, the hospital pharmacienne being merely directed not to make it too thick to impede flow in the syringe, no special proportion of salt to medium or even the medium itself being indicated. Fig. 1 shows the result in a branching sinus containing what could be recognised as the reed. With the stereoscope the reed is seen to be foreshortened, making an angle with the plate of about 45 degrees. A bubble of air can be made out near its upper end, probably injected with the emulsion. The blunt-ended shadows at the bottom and top are *cul de sacs*, the fluffy shadow on the right of the reed leading to the opening in the skin plugged with cotton wool.

Five days later, before Dr. Billinghurst extracted the reed, it was again radiographed to determine whether any of the emulsion had soaked into the reed, possibly softened by so long immersion in pus, and whether such soakage could have accounted for the tube-like appearance it presented. No trace of tube or emulsion could be made out, from which it is probable that the appearance is due to mere displacement of the emulsion, as in the case of stomach hair balls.

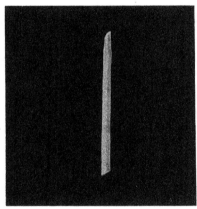

Fig. 2.

This appearance suggested the possibility of detecting similarly the presence of cloth in wounds, as was intimated by the writer in a note in the *British Medical Journal*, of 15th Dec., 1917, p. 791. Experiments were made with this object since that date, which, it is hoped, will be published later.

The emulsion used, in this case of the reed, consisted of oxychloride of bismuth, 1 part, and mucilage of acacia, 2 parts, both material and proportions chosen practically fortuitously, as previously stated. Whilst the earlier cloth experiments referred to were being carried out, an emulsion of 1 in 5 diluted with 5 parts of water was employed in two cases where the fistulæ themselves were only of importance, one of them as leading to a deep pelvic abscess of five months duration, into which a piece of drainage tube had slipped, the shadow of which it was desired should not be obliterated by that of the emulsion, and, the other of the two, an empyema discharging for nine months, the extent of which had to be estimated, and into which Beck's paste had been therapeutically injected. In both these cases the mucilage of acacia

injection apparently mixed with their purulent contents, furnishing a comparatively transparent shadow which disclosed the extent of the pelvic abscess and
the position of the drainage tube, both in relation to the pelvic bones and that
of the empyema cavity, with particles of Beck's paste scattered over the surfaces
of lung and chest wall—both seen in stereo projection. A radiograph of the
empyema case had been previously made after injection of as much of the
Beck's paste as could be introduced by the surgeon in charge of it, but only
disclosed large discrete masses of the paste, and failed to furnish an adequate
idea of the cavity extent.

These abscess cavity shadows, whilst dense enough to be distinguished in
the negatives, are not of sufficient density for satisfactory reproduction in
prints.

Fig. 2 is a photograph of the reed after extraction.

EXPERIMENTS ON THE DETECTION OF PUS SOAKED CLOTH IN ANIMAL TISSUES.

By Neil Macleod, M.D. Edin., Shanghai.

Prompted by the unexpected detection of a piece of reed in a man's leg,
recorded in the current issue of the Archives, the writer started experiments
with a view to similarly detecting cloth embedded in animal tissues. Whilst
these were successful in fresh masses of beef and liver, it became soon obvious
that bismuth injections of fresh human wounds would be too dangerous for
such a purpose, because of the injected material being easily driven beyond the
wound region into opened blood and lymphatic vessels and spaces between
tissue planes.

The enquiry, therefore, had to be confined to those cases where wounds are
walled in by inflammatory action, i.e., to fistulæ prevented from healing by the
presence of cloth. Instead of experimentally produced abscesses in the living
animal, after various methods of procedure were tried, the one to be described
was adopted, as, for radiographic purposes, it appeared to fit the case.

Fig. 1 is a radiograph of gauze and khaki cloth, each of which is structurally
recognisable. It was made in an air surrounding, the cloth being dipped in an
emulsion of bismuth oxychloride, 1 part to 5 of mucilage of acacia, diluted with
5 parts of water, a few drops of the emulsion being dropped on the gauze.
Radiographed through a leg just below the knee, the markings also could be
distinguished, whether the cloth or the limb was next the plate. This degree
of dilution failed to disclose the marking in pus soaked cloth embedded in beef.

To take the place of the inflammatory exudation limiting an abscess cavity, and to prevent injection into the neighbouring tissues, a membrane consisting of sausage skin was made into a sac, into the mouth of which was tied a short wooden tube representing a fistula. Filled with pus and containing a piece of pus soaked cloth, this artificial abscess was embedded in a mass of fresh beef. To prevent entrance of air into the sac interfering with the performance, the pus and cloth were introduced into the sac under water.

After experiments with various proportions of the bismuth salt in the emulsion made with mucilage of acacia, it was found that a proportion of 1 part of the former in from 3 to 6 parts of the latter succeeded, but that success was more dependent upon securing that not too thick a mass of the injected matter surrounded the cloth. At first sight this may appear difficult of control

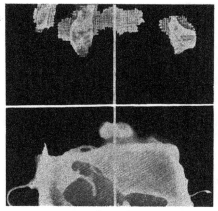

Fig. 1.

by the radiographer. Where the injection shadow proved too dense, obscuring the markings of the cloth, it was frequently found sufficient to allow the bulk of the injection to escape, when, even after gentle pressure with the hand increasing the escaped amount, the markings became obvious enough for recognition, as may be seen in Figs. 2 and 3, the former being radiographed before, the latter after escape of the injected material.

In certain cases where the serge-like pattern could not be made out, folds in the cloth betrayed its presence—these folds being verified on opening the sacs *in situ*.

In Fig. 2, as printed as well as in the negative, the dense shadow of the injection obscures completely the cloth signs in both sacs, the right one containing 1 to 6, the left 1 to 3 emulsion strength. By allowing the injection to escape aided by hand pressure, again radiographed, the result in Fig. 3 shows the cloth marks fairly well in the right sac of the print, whilst they were also visible more distinctly in the negative, and they could also there be made out faintly in the left sac.

Fig. 4 (stereo) shows the serge-like pattern in both the two lower sacs, the one with 1 to 3, the other with 1 to 6 emulsion strengths—better seen in stereo projection. Here, as in Figs. 2 and 3, it was not attempted to secure the same masses of injected matter in any two sacs. The masses are obviously unequal. After draining away the injection from both, and again radiographing, the result is seen in Fig. 5, cloth markings in the left sac (1 to 6), no markings in the right one (1 to 3) as printed, whilst in the negative they were to be made out in the right but not in the left sac.

The third (upper) sac in these two latter figures contained 1 to 6 emulsion *without* pus, cloth or tube (fistula). The lines in it are due to folds in the wall of the sac, not to be mistaken for cloth folds.

(Difficulties of war and after transport supply of plates from a source five to ten thousand miles distant, has unduly delayed completion of this paper and prevented the use of one plate in each experiment. The upper and lower halves of a plate, as seen in Figs. 2, 3, 4 and 5, where the transverse cross line is absent, had to be used for three experiments.)

Conclusions.

1st.—No attempt should be made to inject human *fresh wounds* with any bismuth or other injection for radiographic purposes.

2nd.—After injecting as much as can be introduced of an emulsion, strength 1 part of bismuth salt to 3, 4, 5 or 6 of mucilage of acacia, plug the opening and gently knead the area under suspicion, if that be possible, to facilitate mixture of emulsion and pus before radiographing.

3rd.—If cloth be suspected to be present, before radiographing remove the plug and drain away the injection by gentle hand pressure, at right angles to the plate, to secure possible flattening of the cloth and reduction of the emulsion mass.

4th.—The little extra effort thus involved in the radiographic examination of fistulæ containing pus soaked cloth will be amply rewarded if it result in its detection three times out of four, as was the case in the last dozen of these experiments.

5th.—Stereoscopic negatives should be invariably made if operating surgeons who have binocular vision are to have all the assistance the radiographer can give them in such cases.

(This 6th pronouncement is the result of the writer's experience between 1901 and 1907, before he had ceased to do surgical work. He has yet to make the acquaintance of a surgeon who prefers flat pictures to stereoscopic ones, even of fractures, after having had a few opportunities of comparing the two.)

Fig. 2.

Fig. 3

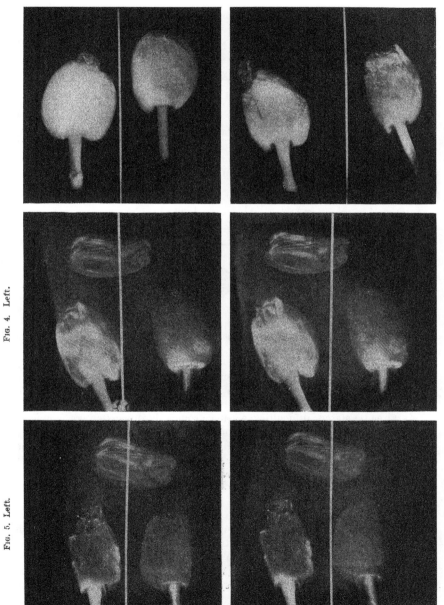

Fig. 4. Left.

Fig. 4. Right.

Fig. 5. Left.

Fig. 5. Right.

NOTE ON A METHOD OF RUNNING AN X-RAY TUBE ON THE "EARTHED" SYSTEM TO PREVENT LEAKAGE TO THE TUBE BOX OR HOLDER.

By Capt. J. A. Shorten, B.A., M.B., I.M.S., and Capt. T. W. Barnard, U.L.

In the Archives of Radiology and Electrotherapy, August, 1917, and August, 1919 (in conjunction with Captain Barnard), I discussed some of the problems in connection with running X-ray tubes on an "earthed" system. The experiments described in the two papers referred to were undertaken primarily to try to solve the difficulties experienced from leakage of high

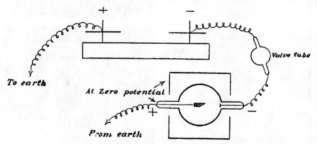

Fig. 1.—Diagram showing connections.

tension currents in damp surroundings. The possibility of earthing the negative pole of the coil and its many side issues having absorbed all our available leisure, it was only recently that we were able to proceed with the main investigation.

As already stated, difficulties arising from a high percentage humidity are often almost insurmountable, more especially when using tube boxes manufactured for dry climates, the main difficulty being leakage from the positive end of the tube to the tube box, so that with tubes of even moderate hardness it is difficult to get current through at all.

Apart from electrical connections there are two main ways of getting over this difficulty, viz.:—

1. By thoroughly heating the tube and box by means of carbon filament lamps hung inside the box. The lamps are attached to a special lid, which is replaced by the proper lid (with diaphragm) before giving the exposure. This was the plan adopted at Colaba War Hospital.

2. By keeping the whole tube box (with tube in position) in a drying box, removing it to give an exposure and replacing it in the drying box between exposures.

Both these methods, while fairly successful, are inconvenient and unsuitable to certain types of apparatus. We were, therefore, induced to try an electrical plan, viz., to earth the positive pole of the coil and allow the X-ray tube to pick up the current from the earth, thus running the coil on the negative side of the earth's potential. A reference to Fig. 1 will explain what happens.

From the above diagram it will be seen that the positive end of the tube and the tube box are at the same potential, therefore there can be no leakage to the tube box. Leakage might still take place over the surface of the tube, but once this becomes heated it will stop. This scheme makes possible the use of metal tube boxes, with absolute rigidity and the maximum of protection.

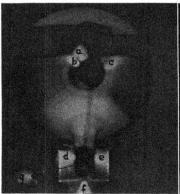 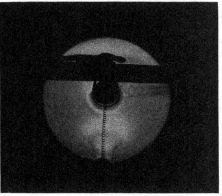

FIG. 2.—Photograph of an X-ray tube from the positive end while running with the negative pole of the coil earthed. Note the leakage at the points *a*, *b*, *c*, *d*, *e*, and *f*.

FIG. 3.—Photograph of an X-ray tube from the positive end while running with the positive pole of the coil earthed. Note complete absence of leakage.

Figs. 2 and 3 show the effect of the above system of connections on an X-ray tube at Colaba War Hospital, Bombay.

Tube: Mammoth (Siemen Bros.).
Alternative spark gap: 5½ inches.
Percentage humidity of atmosphere: 88.
Amperes in primary: 12.
Milliamperes: 4.

The photographs were produced by half-minute exposures, at a distance of four feet in the dark room, with the tube running under constant conditions as regards current in primary, etc.

From the above photographs it will be seen that there is no leakage to the tube box, either at the positive or negative ends, when the positive pole of the coil is earthed. The *positive pole* of the coil and tube can be freely handled as they are at zero potential. If the negative pole of the tube, or lead connecting the negative pole of the tube to the coil, be touched an "earth shock" is sustained, the current passing from the earth through the body to the part of the circuit touched. Similar precautions to those taken to prevent surface creeping at the positive end of the coil when the negative pole is earthed can be taken here to prevent damage to the negative end. From our short experience of the method we have noticed that there is not the same tendency to leakage in this case. As regards the behaviour of the tube, owing to the absence of the leakage at the positive end the fluorescence is much steadier, and the results in every way better. Theoretically, one would expect as much leakage at the negative pole as formerly occurred at the positive pole of the tube. But in practice there is little or none under exactly the same conditions. The reason for this apparent anomaly is that in the former case the leakage is of the point to plate variety, whereas in the latter case it is the opposite. We know that a current passes more readily from point to plate. This general principle may also explain the absence of surface creeping, etc., at the negative pole of the coil. It follows, from the above line of reasoning, that there will be less strain on the insulation of the coil than in the converse method.

It is also evident that the tube is now exposed to the full inverse potential of the coil. Some form of rectifying apparatus must therefore be used to protect the tube.

The method, of course, is unsuitable for use with the Coolidge tube, as it would intensify leakage from the battery circuit.

NEW TECHNIQUE.

RADIOGRAPHS DIRECT ON BROMIDE PAPER AND THEIR PLACE IN WAR ECONOMY.

By Captain Harold C. Gage, A.R.C., O.I.P.

Radiographer to the American Red Cross Hospital of Paris; Radiographer in Charge, Hôpital Militaire, No. 76 Ris Orangis (S. and O) and Supplementary Hospitals.

Limitations of Bromide Paper.—It should be understood from the beginning that the use of bromide paper to replace plates in radiography is limited. It is absolutely unsuited for fine detail and the diagnosis necessitating fine detail, such as injuries to joints, doubtful fractures, bone diseases, sequestra, etc. For it must be recognised beyond all doubt that a radiograph direct on bromide paper, or a print from a negative, viewed as it is by reflected light, can never show delicate gradations of tone and detail like a plate viewed by transmitted light. It is admitted, then, that plates (or films), are imperative for fine diagnostic work, but all war radiography is not of this kind. Civil practice is largely so, and, as a result, many radiographers are grossly prejudiced against bromide paper, and fail to see its use and advantages in certain branches of war radiography. Nevertheless, direct bromide radiographs have, beyond doubt, a field all their own from the point of view of efficiency and economy.

Indications for Use.—There are two large demands made on the radiographic service which bromide paper can admirably fill, namely, the demonstration of foreign bodies and of fractures.

At the advanced field hospitals many fluoroscopic observations are made for both these purposes—a search for foreign bodies, and an examination for the position and nature of fractures, and the alignment of fragments. A large percentage of such work is on the limbs, and the routine varies with different units   In many cases most of the fluoroscopic observations are followed by a plate, and a report made, upon which the subsequent operation and treatment are based. Evacuation of the patient follows, with a report (often

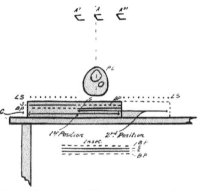

FIG. 1.—Stereo Radios Direct on Bromide Paper. Technique of Production. Single Copy.
A. Central position of tubes. A' A." Displacements right and left. PL. Patient's Limb. C. Stereoscopic Casette Carrier. LS. Lead Sheet. BP. Bromide Paper. S. Intensifying Screen. Inset. Position of screens and bromide paper for production of duplicates.

ambiguous and conveying little to the medical officer who receives the case), of the condition that led to the treatment or operation practised, such as resection, sequestrectomy, etc. What would the medical officer receiving a case not give to see the radiograph upon the evidence of which the treatment has been practised? What would not be gained in judgment, progress, and results, were the radiographic records complete in every case? Patients are perforce at times evacuated before their plates are dry; bromide radios can be blotted, and dry very quickly

I submit that here is the place for direct bromide radios. At the time of these first injuries in the shaft of the bones there are few fine details to diagnose; large sheets of bromide paper may be used, and this has the advantage of including the articulations at both ends, which will then disclose the nature and the degree of any displacement present. Antero-posterior and lateral views may be taken side by side on the same sheet. The development takes but a minute, and as the saving of time and labour at the front is

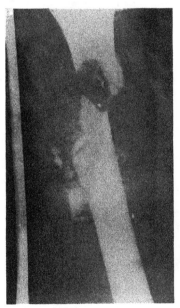

FIG. 2.—Radio for Position of Fragments. Femur. Bedside radiograph, taken with portable apparatus passing 2 ma. 42 mas. Penetration equivalent to 3½ in. spark-gap ; distance, 22 in.

important during a rush of work, this is a great gain ; moreover, if so desired, the time saved can be used to make prints from negatives, where plates have been necessary to decide as to the involvement of a joint. When so made these radios complete the records of the case by providing the earlier observations which are so frequently absent.

There are still many surgeons who prefer, in spite of the mathematical accuracy of improved localisation methods, to operate for the removal of foreign bodies by the information gained from antero-posterior and lateral plates; or it may be desirable, in conjunction with a localisation, to record the relationship of a foreign body to some bony landmark in a radiograph. For these purposes the use of plates is unwarranted extravagance, bromide paper giving in every respect the same information.

To follow our patient a stage further, the

lateral radiographs on the same sheet, as before mentioned, and in this way the results of treatment may be checked so as to give the best possible result in the alignment of the fracture.

When the time comes for final results, these can again be radiographed on bromide paper, so as to complete the papers of the case.

Where it is desired that one radiograph shall be retained and a second shall go with the patient's papers, two bromide radios can

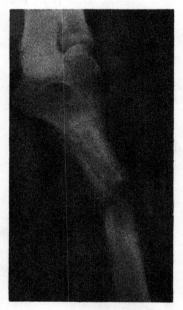 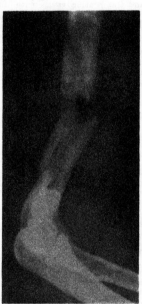

FIG. 3.—Radio of Humerus for Position of Fragments.　Antero-posterior and Lateral.
Taken in bed.　Portable apparatus passing 2 ma. 18 mas; equivalent spark-gap, 2½ in. ; distance, 17 in.

next demand on the department is to verify the position of the fracture on admission to a hospital; and should he be transferred to an apparatus for treatment by extension and suspension he will need to be radiographed in the apparatus as he lies in bed; it is well known that an extra kilo in extension pull, or a slight change of angle, may mean all the difference between a fair and an excellent result. For this work bromide paper is ideal; sheets may be used large enough to include the articulations, with antero-posterior and

be taken at the same time, as explained below under technique.

All these observations can be made, compiling valuable data and ensuring the best result obtainable, and at the same time the expenditure involved will be only a tithe of the cost of the plates that are saved.

From time to time radiographs will be needed to determine the presence of sequestra, osteomyelitis, etc.; for this work nothing short of the best plates and films will suffice.

Technique.—The bromide paper should be

the most rapid positive paper that can be obtained (of the carbon or contrast type), and a surface about the same as that of a plate is to be preferred to an enamel surface. The points requiring special attention are the following:—

Intensification Screen.—This should always be used, not only on account of the reduction of the exposure, but because the print is of a far better quality, being richer in detail and contrast.

Tube Penetration.—This should be about 15 to 20 per cent. less than the recognised penetration for plates. A tube too hard produces a flat and foggy print. Suitable penetration is an important factor.

Exposure.—This, of course, will vary with different papers; it should be approximately from $\frac{1}{4}$th to $\frac{1}{3}$rd of that required for a plate under the same conditions but without a screen. Over-exposure is to be avoided. The best exposure can be soon found with any special paper.

Development.—If metol hydroquinone developer is being used for plates, and it usually is so, it will answer perfectly for these prints; in this way no extra dishes or solutions are necessary. Some extra bromide is the only addition needed. Development is complete in from one to two minutes, and several prints can be developed at the same time, which should be appreciated when there is a rush of work.

Duplication.—If two copies are needed, two screens in the one casette at the same time will meet the case, and little difference can be observed in the resulting radiographs. It is not necessary to have special screens for the smaller sizes, as the bromide paper for radiographs of the long bones can be cut in halves lengthways and placed in the casette, without any risk of scratching the screen, as plates so used would do. If at a later date extra copies should be required, photographic copying on the same or a reduced scale may be resorted to. Intensification may be practised if a print needs strengthening. If so desired a print may be treated with wax and used to print from in the same manner as a glass negative. Such treatment is really superfluous, as excellent contact prints can be made without any preparation.

Stereoscopy.—Radiographs made with the usual technique of tube displacement can be viewed with a Pierre stereoscope, or if this useful little instrument is not on hand resort can be made to the mirror bisector principle. For the production of radiographs to be so viewed the rays pass, in the first exposure, through the bromide paper to the screen, and in the second through the screen to the bromide paper. For economy, in radiography of the long bones, half sheets may be used.

If duplicates are required, two screens and two sheets of bromide paper may be suitably arranged in the casette, so that the rays pass through one sheet of bromide paper to the first screen and through the second screen to the second sheet of bromide paper. The radiographs with a casette so arranged are taken

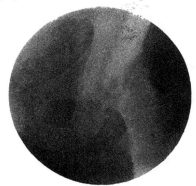

Fig. 4.—Direct Bromide Radiograph of Hip-joint. 65 mas; equivalent spark-gap, 4 in.; distance, 20 in.

according to the technique described elsewhere.*

The radiographs are afterwards cut, the left half of the first and the right half of the second form a stereoscopic pair, as do also the remaining two half sheets. If only one stereoscopic copy is needed a screen may be cut in halves and kept specially for the purpose; the half screens and the bromide half sheets are placed side by side in the casette, the paper lying on top of the screen on one side, and the screen on top of the paper on the other. The two halves are exposed in turns one half during each exposure being covered with lead, as explained more fully in the paper, referred to above (*). (See Fig. 1.)

* For further information as to Technique and Viewing, see Extract in *British Medical Journal*, No. 2961, Sept. 29th, 1917, or ARCHIVES OF RADIOLOGY AND ELECTROTHERAPY, June, 1917.

The arguments in favour of the use of bromide paper may be briefly summed up as follows: Glass is getting increasingly scarce, and old negative glass used over again produces an unsatisfactory plate. The breakage occupy less space and weigh less than six plates, a great economy of money, time, and material is effected, and the radiographs can accompany the patient and make his history complete. Large radiographs can be taken more fre-

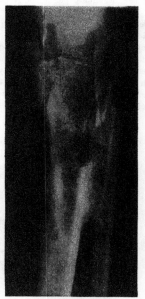 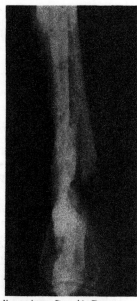

FIG. 5.—Antero-posterior and Lateral Direct Radiographs on Bromide Paper.
These pictures give an idea of the amount of detail that can be obtained. Sequestra, osteomyelitis, and rarefying osteitis are well shown.

of plates in transport and in the department is considerable: weight, packing, space, and labour of transport are serious questions, cost being last, but not least.

In contrast, 100 sheets of bromide paper quently to determine the position of a fracture, thus greatly increasing the efficiency of treatment and improving the results, since the cost at present renders the free use of plates for this purpose impossible.

REPORT OF SOCIETY.

ROYAL SOCIETY OF MEDICINE.

ELECTROTHERAPEUTIC SECTION.

(Summer Meeting at Oxford, June 28th, 1919.)

IN the unavoidable absence of the President of the Section (Mr. C. R. LYSTER), the chair was taken by Dr. A. E. BARCLAY, the President Elect.

The Rev. C. B. CRONSHAV, M.A., Treasurer of the Hospital, welcomed the members on behalf of the Management of the Radcliffe Infirmary.

Dr. TURRELL then gave an address in which he welcomed the members on behalf of the Electro-therapeutic Department of the hospital. Referring to their former visit in June, 1914, eight months after the installation of the department, he com-mented on the stimulus it had imparted to their work, and the useful effect it had in preparing the department to cope with the increased demand for electrotherapy at the Oxford hospitals which followed on the outbreak of war two months later.

Their department was the first, or at any rate one of the first, to be fully organised for the electrical treatment of the wounded soldier, and during the war more than 50,000 electrical treatments had been given, and more than 1,500 wounded soldiers treated free of expense to the Government.

Before dealing with the work of the department he proposed to refer briefly to the influence of war work on the development of electrotherapy. In his opinion its effect had been, with the exception of muscle and nerve work, to impede its development in general medicine and surgery. But the great benefits which electrical treatment had conferred on the wounded had drawn the attention both of the public and the medical profession to its great value and greater possibilities in the future. In former times their speciality had met with much opposition, the most formidable of which was the ridicule which some facetious persons endeavoured to cast upon it; for, as the celebrated Professor Challenger remarked, "The flippancy of the half educated was more obstructive to science than the obtuseness of the ignorant." A charge which was still brought against them was that they were continually on the change from one form of treatment to another; at one time it was ionic medication, at another diathermy, or static, or faradism, etc., which was the cure-all to be practised. In reply to this criticism he would point out that such a change of opinion was incidental to the development of any new science, and he would remind these critics of the dictum of the great Faraday, "In knowledge that man alone is to be contemned or despised who is not in a state of transition." As the result of its trial in the war electrotherapy could certainly claim to have made good, and such remarks as those alluded to were now very rarely heard.

The action of electricity in medicine might be viewed from two points: its direct, and its indirect action.

It might be contended that, as all vital processes were fundamentally electrical, by the suitable appli-cation of electricity it might be possible to regulate and control these processes. Such claims, however, must be based on that "specious image of the truth" hypothesis, and would belong to a philosophical rather than a practical discussion. He preferred to base claims for the benefits to be derived from electrotherapy on the far surer ground of its in-direct action. It might still be true that "Medicina est ars conjecturalis," but the action of electrical treatment, viewed from this standpoint, was clear, definite, and readily capable of demonstration. The indirect effects of electricity were due to the chemical changes, the heat, the muscular contractions, and the increased blood supply which resulted in the body from the application of the different forms of electrical treatment.

It would indeed be an extraordinary thing if the most powerful and most readily controlled and regulated agent in nature were incapable of being used with advantage in the treatment of disease. Each of the four forms into which electricity had been classified, by Sir Oliver Lodge, could be utilised in medicine. (1) The application of the current from the static machine was an example of the utilisation of electricity at rest; (2) galvanism illustrated electricity in locomotion; (3) faradism was obtained from electricity in rotation, or magnetism; and (4), from electricity in radiation or vibration, ultra-violet light radiation and radium- and radio-therapy were obtained.

The modern powerful static machine provided the means of exciting such vigorous muscular contrac-tions, that by its use muscular fibres could be so powerfully excited as to tear themselves away from adhesions caused by injury or disease, and by what he might term "auto-muscular massage," excited in this way, it was possible in only twenty minutes treatment to remove the fluid from a recent syno-vitis of the knee joint, or drain and diminish an enlarged prostate gland.

The time at his disposal obviously prevented him from dealing at any length with all the various electrical methods for the treatment of disease ; he would like, however, so far as time permitted, to pay special attention to two of these, ionic medi-cation and diathermy.

First of all, even at the risk of shocking some of them, he would like to attempt an exposure of what he termed the Phantasy of Ionic Medication. In his department it was held that this method of treat-ment, about which so much had been written and even more said, did not in reality exist. For two or three years they had entirely abandoned treatment on this principle. He wished to make it quite clear what he meant by ionic medication; he would define it as the attempt to obtain the specific action of certain drugs introduced into the deeper tissues by means of the electrical current.

It was commonly held that it was possible, by means of the electrical current, to introduce a drug such as salicylic acid into the interior of the body and there obtain the specific therapeutical action of that drug. That was the proposition that he wished emphatically to deny, and the contention that such a result could be obtained was so opposed to the fundamental principles of electro-chemistry that it was difficult to understand how such a theory could be so universally entertained.

First of all, this idea of ionic medication was entirely opposed to the teaching of Faraday, for he was led to formulate his theory of ions to explain the fact that the products of electrolysis appeared only at the electrodes and not in the interior of the electrolyte. For instance, if one took a glass jar, divided it into three compartments by two porous plates, and having filled each compartment with a solution of copper sulphate, placed a copper positive pole in one end compartment, and a copper negative pole in the other end compartment, after the passage of a galvanic current for some minutes, it would be found that the solution in the compartment with the positive pole was more concentrated, the solution in the negative compartment weaker, and that no change had taken place in the concentration of the solution in the middle compartment. It was clear that, when a drug was in an ionic state, it possessed entirely different properties to those it possessed before its dissociation into this form, whether it was an ion of hydrogen or of salicylic acid.

The experiments of the French and other observers had failed to detect the presence of salicylic acid, after ionic medication, deeper than the superficial layers of the skin. The ions present in the solution with which the pads were soaked served to carry the current through the epidermis, which in its dry state was very deficient in ions, the current was then carried by the faster and consequently more efficient hydrogen and hydroxyl ions, which existed in large numbers in the human tissues and rendered them so perfect an electrolyte. The experiments, such as the poisoning of rabbits, and the presence of iodine in the urine, after ionisation with these drugs, did not prove the deep penetration of their ions, but merely showed that they had been carried through the superficial layers of the skin; and then, having lost their electrical charge, had passed into the capillary circulation, and thence to the spinal centres in the one case, and the kidneys and the bladder in the other.

Chatsky's experiments with a potato were very instructive and were so simple that they could be readily demonstrated in the department. If a weak current be passed through a potato, a few drops of 2 per cent. potassium iodide having been placed in a small hole, scooped in the potato, in the interpolar path, after the passage of the current for a few minutes, the blue colouration characteristic of the action of free iodine on the starch of the potato would appear in immediate contact, and there only, with the positive pole. If, by the use of a cross shaped glass tube, a transverse current of sodium chloride solution were maintained during the experiment, no colouration would be found to occur at the positive pole, but a faint trace of iodine could be detected in the solution that had flowed transversely to the current.

Many other proofs might be quoted to show that drugs could not be conveyed to the deeper structures of the body by the electrical current and exercise their specific therapeutical action throughout their path. It was perhaps well that this was the case, for few supporters of the ionic medication theory took the trouble to sterilise their pads and solutions, or even to employ distilled water.

It had been the experience of the department that, provided a sufficient intensity of current was employed, and for a sufficient length of time, the result was the same whether the expensive solutions, such as potassium iodide and salicylate of soda, or the inexpensive solution of sodium chloride were used.

There were some electrotherapists who contended that, preceding ionic medication, a large dose of the drug which they wished to introduce should be administered by the mouth, with the idea that the current would then convey it into the tissues it was desired to treat. Let them consider for one moment what a very small proportion even 20 or 30 grain doses of sodium salicylate or potassium iodide bore to the body weight, and what an extremely minute amount of these drugs in the ionic state would be in the interpolar path at a given time compared with the large numbers of the more efficient hydrogen and hydroxyl ions, and then they would realise the improbability of any benefit resulting from such a procedure.

There was one more theory in regard to the action of the galvanic current which he would like to touch upon.

In 1907, Bouchet (*Journ. des Practiciens*, Feb. 9th, 1907) described a method for the treatment of gonorrhœa by introducing into the urethra a soft rubber catheter with many eyelets in it, through which the urethra could be irrigated with a 2 to 10 per cent solution of zinc sulphate or other drug, whilst a current was passed by an active platinum wire electrode in the lumen of the catheter and an indifferent electrode placed at a convenient place on the body. A theory had been recently propounded in respect to the action of this treatment which seemed to him to be rather far fetched. It was asserted that, because bacteria in a culture had been found to possess a definite electrical charge, and were attracted on the application of an electrical charge through the culture to the pole of opposite charge, therefore the gonococci, hidden away in the crypts and follicles of the urethra and prostate, were drawn from these recesses by the application of this treatment and grouped themselves round the active electrode. This theory reminded one of the charming of the rats by the Pied Piper of Hamelin:—

"And I chiefly use my charm
On creatures that do people harm,
The gonococcus, and newt, and viper;
And people call me the Pied Piper."

The beneficial effects resulting from this treatment were readily explained by the destructive action of the zinc, copper, or other oxychlorides, according to the solution used, on the germs and the diseased tissues in the immediate neighbourhood of the active electrode. The action of this treatment was in every way comparable with that of copper or zinc ionisation of endometritis, the excellent results of which were familiar to most electrotherapists.

It must not be concluded that they questioned the excellent results to be obtained from intensive and prolonged galvanism; so far from such being the case they regarded it as one of the most valuable of all electrical treatments, but with the above quoted explanations of its action they entirely disagreed. It was most important, if their treatments were to be rational and not merely empirical, that they should visualise as correctly as possible their mode of action. The ionic medication theory, apart from its being opposed to the laws of electrochemistry, was especially pernicious in leading to the extensive waste of such valuable and expensive drugs as potassium iodide, sodium salicylate, etc.

They believed the therapeutic effects of prolonged galvanism to be due to the direct and indirect results of the changes induced in the tissues by the prolonged passage of the current. The ionic interchange, taking place in the tissues whilst an electric charge was conveyed through them, must modify them and tend to increase metabolism throughout the whole interpolar path. Their daily experience showed them that the circulation of a limb was accelerated and its temperature considerably raised during and after the passage of an electrical current.

These changes doubtless were of a highly complex character, but they undoubtedly increased the nutrition and the resisting power of a limb, and it was due to such effects that the benefits of prolonged galvanism in such diseases as chronic rheumatism, neuritis, etc., were due. From such a view it followed that the galvanic current should be applied for as long a period as is convenient or practicable, and that the strength of the current should correspond with the toleration of the patient. In order to ensure the maximum toleration of current it was necessary that it should be administered by the least painful form of apparatus, and, bearing this in mind, he would like very strongly to recommend to them the water resistance introduced to this country by Dr. Ettie Sayer, from the clinic of Professor Leduc of Nantes. In favour of this apparatus they had in their department discarded all pantostats and wire wound resistances. Partly on account of the simplicity, safety, and cheapness of the instrument, but chiefly because their experience showed them

that patients tolerated about 25 per cent. more current than when the older forms of apparatus were used. The simple home made forms of this apparatus, costing only a few shillings, were far preferable to the costly and elaborate apparatus made on this principle by the instrument makers.

Diathermy was one of the most valuable methods used in their department. He had hoped to show them a new form of apparatus for this treatment, but owing to certain difficulties they had at present been unable to get it completed. Its principle was based on the valve tubes which had played so important a part in the development of wireless telegraphy during the war. By the use of these thermo-ionic valves continuous oscillations were obtained, and hence a higher degree of efficiency was yielded than by the widely spaced series of oscillations of the usual diathermy apparatus. The instrument would require two 400 watt valve tubes in parallel, costing about £14 each, and either an alternating supply with a step up transformer and two rectifying valves, or a 2,000 volt D.C. generator.

It was hoped by means of the higher efficiency of these valves to obtain a portable instrument, and so render possible the treatment by diathermy of pneumonia, in which its application was specially indicated, and other diseases which they were unable to treat at present owing to the difficulty of getting them to the department.

It was clear that the therapeutical effects of diathermy were directly due to the heat generated in the tissues by the oscillations of the high-frequency current. But they were apt to overlook the very important indirect effects of this heat on the organism. The experiments of Furstenburg and Schemel, of the Breyer Institute, showed that, when a small current of 300 ma. was passed through the abdomen, the temperature of the abdomen was raised half a degree above normal; but when the diathermy current was increased to 2 amperes, the temperature of the stomach fell to about ·3 of a degree above normal. Dr. Cumberbatch mentioned, at their meeting with the Electrical Engineers, that he found no rise of temperature recorded by a thermometer placed in a deep sinus during the passage of a strong diathermy current through the limb. These phenomena could only be explained by the heat regulating centres being brought into play, as the result of the heat generated in the deeper tissues by the passage of the diathermy current. By the operation of these centres the large abdominal and other vessels become relaxed and dilated, and in this way the effect of diathermy in its relief of spasm and pain can be explained. He, personally, had seen cases of spasm of the ureter, and the spasmodic pain of the menstrual period markedly relieved. In fact, he believed the relief of menstrual pain by diathermy to be one of its most valuable uses.

The method of indirect diathermy fulguration, which he described at a meeting of the Section in 1918, was very largely used in the department for the treatment of warts, epulis, nævi, rodent ulcer, etc. He would show them a case of very extensive hairy mole of the face which was in the course of cure by this method.

This case figured as a child in a well known book on skin diseases, but, with the exception of CO_2 snow, which failed to improve matters, no curative treatment had been adopted until the advent of this treatment.

He had to thank Captain Howard Humphris for a valuable practical suggestion in regard to the treatment of corns in this way; formerly, owing to the dryness of the skin in many corns, this method had not acted well in several cases. On Captain Humphris' suggestion, he thoroughly moistened the corns before treatment, and then found the method a satisfactory one in these cases.

He now proposed to show them, with the assistance of Captain Cooper, of Netley, Captain Iles, of Taunton, and Captain Morrell, of the Cowley Special Surgical Centre, six new forms of apparatus

(1) A very simple and inexpensive apparatus for rhythmically surging the static current.

(2) The apparatus with a practical demonstration of the method of Indirect Diathermy Fulguration.

(3) A new apparatus for surging the faradic current through a water resistance.

(4) The Ultra-violet Radiation from the Tungsten Arc, which they claimed to be by far the most effective form of giving this valuable treatment, would be shown by Captain Iles.

(5) Captain Morrell would exhibit the apparatus and would demonstrate the method in action of the Selective Galvanism of Lapicque. They attached great importance to the use of this apparatus, especially to its re-educative influence in recovering cases of nerve lesion.

(6) A Frimandeau Coil. This apparatus ingeniously utilises the magnetism of a faradic coil to interrupt the galvanic current. By its means an interruption of the galvanic current is obtained synchronous with the vibrations of the hammer of the coil. Thus, an interruption of the galvanic current of sufficient frequency and of adequate duration to excite a tetanic contraction in paralysed muscles can be obtained. Captain Cooper, who has paid special attention to this instrument, will exhibit it in action. He will also show you a new coil of his own design, based on the principle of Frimandeau, which he has very kindly brought with him from Netley. This coil gives an exceedingly high rate of interruption of the galvanic current.

Dr. Turrell, during the course of his remarks, strongly emphasised the importance of a closer relationship between the physicists and the electrotherapists. They often felt in their department the lack of assistance from the physicists, and in those hospitals where the co-operation of these experts had been secured great advantages had followed.

In their Section they all felt a deep sense of appreciation of the valuable assistance Dr. Russ had rendered them on the physical side of their work both at their Council and their Ordinary Meetings.

NOTES AND ABSTRACTS

Discussion on Dilatation of the Œsophagus without Anatomical Stenosis.—W. HILL (*Proc. Roy. Soc. of Med. Sect. of Laryngology*, March, 1919).—In well-marked cases of œsophagectasia the X-ray appearance is constant, the opaque meal being arrested at the phrenic level and not passing immediately into the stomach. The same appearance is, however, seen in fibrous stricture and other forms of true anatomic stenosis of the phrenocardiac gullet and the differential diagnosis can only be certainly made in all cases by endo-œsophageal inspection of the phreno-cardiac region by means of large-sized endoscopic tubes. When a soft rubber bougie of large calibre filled with mercury is seen under the fluorescent screen to pass without hindrance into the stomach, this test can be relied on as pointing to the absence of an organic stricture; but if the gullet presents a truncated and lobulated dilatation at the phrenic level, the nose of the bougie may fail to hit off the entrance to the phreno-cardiac gullet; the test then fails to differentiate between a functional and an organic stricture in this region, so that the superiority of the œsophagoscopic method as a certain means of diagnosis and applicable to all cases is evident.

Most physicians, surgeons and radiologists, it is stated, speak of the site of the stenosis being at the cardia; Hill believes from the X-ray findings that the arrest is at the level of the diaphragm, where the gullet is embraced by the crura, which constitute a potential extra-œsophageal sphincter. For this and other reasons, this observer has discarded the term "cardiospasm."

The various hypotheses of the cause of this condition are discussed, and it is stated that it is uncertain whether it is a primary or a secondary condition, and that none of the hypotheses is altogether satisfactory.

As functional stenosis has been been held to be due to paresis, it might be expected that the therapeutic application of electricity would supply some information. The faradic current, however, only acts on striped muscle which does not extend much beyond the upper third of the gullet, and the use of the galvanic current is contra-indicated in a moist tube like the gullet on account of the danger of electrolytic action. The sinusoidal current is safe, but in the only case tried it failed.

R. W. A. S.

Legg's Disease.—L. W. ELY (*Annals of Surgery*, Jan. 1919, pp. 47-51, with 16 radiograms.)—This disease, also called Perthes's disease, was, according to the author, described by Legg three years before Perthes, and thus it should rather be associated with the name of Legg.

The typical radiographic appearance consists in:—

(1) A flattening, broadening, and sometimes an apparent displacement of the epiphysis laterally, with one or more divisions of it and irregularity of ossification.

(2) An irregularity or even segmentation of the cartilage between it and the neck.

(3) Loss of bony structure in the neck, especially of its proximal and lateral part.

(4) Irregularity in contour of the upper part of the femur neck.

(5) Distortion of the head.

(6) Enlargement of the trochanter (occasionally).

(7) Irregularity of the acetabulum—not characteristic.

The marked difference between the radiographic changes and the comparative insignificance of the symptoms and physical signs is characteristic.

In the past it has often been mistaken for tuberculosis. The latter shows radiographically more involvement on the shaft side of the epiphysial line and less in the head of the bone and has not the same disproportion between the radiogram and the symptoms and physical signs. R. W. A. S.

Streptococcus Empyema.—W. H. STEWART (*Amer. Jour. of Roent.*, Feb., 1919, pp. 57-65, with 18 skiagrams).—In this infection, the pleural thickening and formation of adhesions are much more extensive than in cases due to other infections. In a certain number of cases, after empyema has been evacuated and the cavity become sterile, the lung fails to expand completely on account of pleural thickening and adhesions, leaving a cavity of varying size. Stereoscopic radiograms after the injection of some opaque substance has been found to be of value in certain cases with large cavities complicated by auxiliary sacculations.

In the differential diagnosis between pleural effusions and thickened pleura, the author says that the former, no matter how small, seldom remain stationary; even in old cases they usually slowly increase. On the other hand, pleuritic thickenings alone have a tendency toward slow but progressive diminution. In general also, the shadow of pleural thickening alone is rather more clear cut in detail than when fluid is present, as the latter produces a certain amount of haziness. All draining cases, unless contra-indicated, should be examined from time to time radiologically. If the information obtained is not complete, the cavity should be injected with an opaque solution or paste. For this, the author advises the following paste:—

Bismuth subnit.	... 25 per cent.	
Vaseline ...	... 73 ,, ,,	
Wax	... 2 ,, ,,	

Bismuth paste may be objectionable in large cavities, and for these a 15 per cent. neutral solution of thorium nitrate or a 20 per cent. solution of subcarbonate of bismuth in sweet oil, or liquid albolene, is recommended.

The article is illustrated by several radiograms showing the detail that can be got with these injections. R. W. A. S.

RÖNTGEN-SOCIETY.—MEMBERS OF COUNCIL; 1919-1920.

President: SIDNEY RUSS, D.Sc. (1919).

Past Presidents for last three years:

MAJOR C. THURSTAN HOLLAND (1916-17). MAJOR G. W. C. KAYE, M.A., D.Sc. (1917-18).
G. B. BATTEN, M.D., C.M. (1918-19).

Vice-Presidents:

J. HALL EDWARDS, M.R.C.S. (1914). PROF. A. W. PORTER, D.Sc., F.R.S. (1914)
PROF. J. W. NICHOLSON, M.A., D.Sc., F.R.S. (1919).

Hon. Secretaries: ROBERT KNOX, M.D. (1911), and R. W. A. SALMOND, M.D. (1919).

Hon. Treasurer: GEOFFREY PEARCE (1915).

Hon. Editor: MAJOR G. W. C. KAYE, M.A., D.Sc. (1919).

Council:

W. E. SCHALL, B.Sc. (1914).   A. E. BARCLAY, M.A., M.D. (1919).
G. H. RODMAN, M.D. (1915).   F. J. HARLOW, B.Sc. (1919).
C. HOWARD HEAD, ESQ. (1916).   W. MAKOWER, M.A., D.Sc. (1919).
C, R. C. LYSTER, M.R.C.S. (1916).   E. A. OWEN, D.Sc., B.A. (1919).
J. METCALFE, M.D. (1917).   J. RUSSELL REYNOLDS, M.B., B.Sc. (1919).
E. P. CUMBERBATCH, M.A., M.B. (1918). R. S. WRIGHT, M.I.E.E. (1919).

PUBLICATIONS RECEIVED.

Book.

Roentgen Interpretations. By HOLMES and RUGGLES. London: Hy. Kimpton.

Journals.

American Journal of Electrotherapeutics and Radiology, April, May, July, and August, 1919.

Archives d'Electricite Médicale et de Physio-therapie, Sept., 1919.

British Journal of Surgery, Oct., 1919.

Bulletin of the Johns Hopkins Hospital, Sept., 1919.

Bulletins et Mémoirs de la Société de Radio-logie Médicale de France, July, 1919.

Gaceta Médica Catalana, Sept. 30th, Oct. 15th, 1919.

Good Health, Oct., 1919.

Journals—continued.

Il Policlinico, July 15th, Aug. 1st, 1919.

International Journal of Orthodontia and Oral Surgery, Sept., 1919.

Journal of Cutaneous Diseases, Aug.-Sept., 1919.

Journal de Radiologie et d'Electrologie, Oct., 1919.

La Radiologia Medica, Sept.-Oct., 1919.

Medical Journal of Australia, Aug. 2nd, 1919.

Modern Medicine, Sept., 1919.

New York Medical Journal, Sept., 1919.

Norsk Mag. for Lægevidenskaben, Oct., 1919.

Rivista Italiana di Neuropatologia, Psichi-atria ed Elettroterapia, July, 1919.

Surgery, Gynæcology, and Obstetrics, Oct., 1919.

Ugeskrift for Læger, Oct. 9th, 16th, 1919.

NOTICES.

ARCHIVES OF RADIOLOGY AND ELECTROTHERAPY is published monthly.

The index for each volume, which ends with the May number, is supplied with the June number of each year.

Communications to the Editors should be addressed to " ROBERT KNOX, M.D., 38, Harley Street, W. 1."

Communications and illustrations from American contributors may be sent to Messrs. REBMAN COMPANY, 141-145, West Thirty-sixth Street, New York City.

All radiographs and photographs must be originals, and must not have been previously published. Drawings should be supplied on separate paper.

Owing to the scarcity of paper the Publishers are reluctantly compelled—as a temporary war measure—to reduce the number of free reprints of Papers to twenty-five.

Annual Subscriptions, payable in advance, 30/- including postage. Single copies, 3/- (postage 2d.) Single numbers and back numbers can be supplied on application.

Vol. XXIV—No. 7·   DECEMBER, 1919   No. 233

ARCHIVES OF RADIOLOGY AND ELECTROTHERAPY

THE OFFICIAL ORGAN OF THE

BRITISH ASSOCIATION OF RADIOLOGY AND PHYSIOTHERAPY

Editors.

ROBERT KNOX, M.D., Hon. Radiologist, King's College Hospital.

E. P. CUMBERBATCH, B.M., M.R.C.P., Medical Officer in Charge, Electrical Department, St. Bartholomew's Hospital.

SIDNEY RUSS, D.Sc., Physicist to the Middlesex Hospital.

IN COLLABORATION WITH

A. E. BARCLAY *(Manchester)*; BELOT *(Paris)*; H. MARTIN BERRY *(London)*; W. H. BRAGG *(London)*, N. BURKE *(Woodhall Spa)*; J. BURNET *(Edinburgh)*; W. J. S. BYTHELL *(Manchester)*; J. T. CASE *(Battle Creek, U.S.A.)*; A. ST. GEORGE CAULFEILD *(London)*; H. A. COLWELL *(London)*; FOVEAU DE COURMELLES *(Paris)*; GUNZBURG *(Antwerp)*; HALL-EDWARDS *(Birmingham)*; HARET *(Paris)*; HAUCHAMPS *(Brussels)*; F. HERNAMAN-JOHNSON *(London)*; W. F. HIGGINS *(Teddington)*; THURSTAN HOLLAND *(Liverpool)*; HURST *(London)*; KLYNENS *(Antwerp)*; LAQUERRIERE *(Paris)*; LAZARUS-BARLOW *(London)*; LEDUC *(Nantes)*; ALEXANDER MACKAY *(Edinburgh)*; REGINALD MORTON *(London)*; HARRISON ORTON *(London)*; W. OVEREND *(St. Leonards-on-Sea)*; PFAHLER *(Philadelphia)*; C. E. S. PHILLIPS *(London)*; GEORGE PIRIE *(Dundee)*; HOWARD PIRIE *(Montreal)*; A. W. PORTER *(London)*; R. W. A. SALMOND *(London)*; WERTHEIM SALOMONSON *(Amsterdam)*; S. SLOAN *(Glasgow)*; SOMERVILLE *(Glasgow)*; W. C. STEVENSON *(Dublin)*; W. J. TURRELL *(Oxford)*; HUGH WALSHAM *(London)*; ROBT. WILSON *(Montreal)*.

THE WORK OF THE BRITISH ASSOCIATION OF RADIOLOGY AND PHYSIOTHERAPY.

WE have great pleasure in submitting the first fruits of the above Association to the consideration of our readers. At the instigation of the B.A.R.P. the University of Cambridge has instituted a Diploma in Medical Radiology and Electrology. We feel that the main idea of the Diploma needs no further introduction, for from time to time statements have been made in our columns as to the desirability of some such happening, and the probability of its maturing; now we have simply to record that by a Grace of the University on 17th June, 1919, the Diploma initiation is complete.

What this is going to mean for the dual subjects of radiology and electrology in medicine time alone can show; but unless the outlook of those who have had the privilege of steering this little barque to port is entirely false, it will mean that the subject of Physical Medicine will take rank fitting to its importance in the domain of medicine and appropriate to the researches which have been made on the effect of radiation and of electric currents upon living things.

A knowledge of the facts is not likely to blind us all to the necessity for further investigation in these subjects. The Diploma will help towards this end ; it will, moreover, lead to a higher standard in the knowledge of these subjects on the part of medical men who specialise in them: Such a raising of the standard can but react in the most healthy way in the development of subjects which to many seem but in their infancy.

In conclusion, we would remind intending entrants for the Diploma that applications should be sent in as soon as possible to Dr. Shillington Scales for particulars of courses at Cambridge and to Dr. Robert Knox for those to be held in London.

UNIVERSITY OF CAMBRIDGE.

Regulations for the Diploma in Medical Radiology and Electrology (Grace 11 of 17 June, 1919).

1.   That a Diploma in Medical Radiology and Electrology be established.

2.   That a Committee on Medical Radiology and Electrology, hereinafter called the Committee, be appointed by the State Medicine Syndicate; the Committee to consist of the Regius Professor of Physic, the Cavendish Professor of Experimental Physics, and nine other members, of whom not less than six shall be members of the Syndicate; and that of the nine members three retire in rotation on the thirty-first day of December in every year, their places being supplied by three members appointed by the Syndicate before the end of full term in the preceding Michaelmas Term and that four members form a quorum.

3.   That it be the duty of the Committee to fix the number of Examiners in each year ; to nominate them for election by the Senate; to fix and announce to the Senate in the Easter Term of each year the time for the Examination or Examinations in the ensuing academical year ; to determine, subject to the approval of the State Medicine Syndicate, the payment to the Examiners ; to draw up and publish from time to time schedules defining the range and details of the subjects of the Examination; to recognise courses of study and places for clinical instruction, and to perform such other duties as may be assigned to them by the Senate.

4.   That the Committee be required to make an annual Report to the State Medicine Syndicate for communication to the Senate.

5.   That a candidate for the diploma shall either (*a*) present himself for examination or (*b*) submit for the approval of the Special Board for Medicine a dissertation. The dissertation may include or consist of any work already published by the candidate.

6.   That an Examination for the Diploma in Medical Radiology and Electrology be held once or, if the State Medicine Syndicate think fit, twice in the year.

7.   That the Examination be in two Parts : that the subjects in Part I be (*a*) Physics and (*b*) Electrotechnics ; in Part II, (*a*) Radiology (including Radiography and Radiotherapy), and (*b*) Electrology (including Electrodiagnosis and Electrotherapy) ; and that in each subject there be at least one paper and a practical or a clinical examination.

8.   That Part I be open to candidates who hold a recognised medical qualification and who produce evidence that after qualification they have for three months at least attended a course of lectures and of practical instruction recognised by the Committee both in Physics and in Electrotechnics : that Part II be open to candidates who are at the time of entering for the Examination duly qualified medical practitioners of not less than one year's standing, have attended a course of lectures on Radiology and Electrology for at least three months and have had at least six months' clinical experience and instruction in the electrical department of a Hospital recognised by the Committee. The course of lectures may be attended during the period of clinical instruction in the electrical department of a "recognised Hospital."

9.   That a candidate who has passed both Parts of the Examination to the satisfaction of the Examiners be entitled to a Diploma testifying to his knowledge of Radiology and Electrology in the following form :—

𝕶𝖓𝖔𝖜 𝖆𝖑𝖑 𝖒𝖊𝖓 by these presents that   hath been duly examined by   the Examiners on that behalf appointed by the Chancellor Masters and Scholars of the 𝖀𝖓𝖎𝖛𝖊𝖗𝖘𝖎𝖙𝖞 𝖔𝖋 𝖈𝖆𝖒𝖇𝖗𝖎𝖉𝖌𝖊 and hath approved himself to the Examiners by his KNOWLEDGE AND SKILL IN MEDICAL RADIOLOGY AND ELEC-TROLOGY to wit the diagnosis and treatment of disease by methods founded on clinical observations combined with radiological and electrological research In Testimony whereof the Vice-Chancellor of the said University by the authority of the said Chancellor Masters and Scholars hath hereto set his hand and seal the .   day of   one thousand nine hundred and   .
L S   *A.B.* Vice-Chancellor.

10.   That candidates who present themselves for examination be required to pay fees, to be fixed at the discretion of the Committee, subject to the approval of the State Medical Syndicate.

11.   That Candidates for either part of the Examination be required to send in their names to the Registrary, together with the requisite certificates, not less than three weeks before the day fixed for the beginning of the Examination, and that the fee be paid at the same time.

12.   That it shall be the duty of the Registrary to examine the certificates and to ascertain that no one is improperly admitted to the Examination.

13.   That a candidate who wishes to proceed to the Diploma under Regulation 5 (*b*) shall be required to send to the Registrary with his dissertation certificates (*a*) that he has been qualified for not less than ten years as a medical practitioner and (*b*) has been engaged for not less than five years in the practice of medical radiology and electrology in the Electrical Department of a public Hospital, the nature of such practice to be approved in each case by the Committee.

14.   That the certificates together with the dissertation submitted by the Candidate shall be sent by the Registrary, in the first instance, to the Special Board for Medicine who shall transmit it to the Committee, who if they approve the nature of the clinical practice required under Regulation 13 (*b*) shall appoint two or more Referees to examine the work submitted by the Candidate, to examine the Candidate, if it be thought necessary, on the subject of his work either orally or otherwise, and to report thereon to the Committee.

15.   That every candidate on sending in his dissertation shall pay to the Registrary a fee of ten guineas which shall be returned to him if the certificates of clinical practice required under Regulation 13 (*b*) be not approved by the Committee.

16.   That, if the Committee after considering the reports of the Referees approve the disser-tation submitted by the Candidate, they shall recommend to the Special Board for Medicine that the Diploma be granted to him, and shall send with their recommendation the reports of the Referees upon which their recommendation is based.

17.   That a candidate whose work is approved by the Special Board for Medicine on the recommendation of the Committee shall be entitled to receive a Diploma in the following terms :—

𝕶𝖓𝖔𝖜 𝖆𝖑𝖑 𝖒𝖊𝖓 by these presents that   whose dissertation has been duly examined by the Referees in that behalf appointed by the Committee on Radiology and Electrology of the 𝖀𝖓𝖎𝖛𝖊𝖗𝖘𝖎𝖙𝖞 𝖔𝖋 𝖈𝖆𝖒𝖇𝖗𝖎𝖉𝖌𝖊 has approved himself to that Committee and to the Special Board for Medicine of the said University by his KNOWLEDGE OF RADIOLOGY AND ELECTROLOGY and especially in the following branches thereof to wit   In Testimony whereof the Vice-Chancellor of the said University by the authority of the Chancellor Masters and Scholars hath hereto set his hand and seal the   .   day of one thousand nine hundred and
L S   *A.B.* Vice-Chancellor.

18.   That every candidate before receiving a Diploma under Regulation 5 (*b*) shall deposit in the Library of the Medical School a copy of his dissertation.

19.   That in the first instance the scheme for the Diploma be established for five years only.

COURSE OF STUDY FOR THE DIPLOMA.

The Course of Study for the Diploma extends over a period of not less than six months.

The Course of Study embraces (1) a Lecture Course with practical work ; (2) Clinical Instruction (*see* 8).

The Lecture Course :—
    Part I. (a) Physics; (b) Electro-technics (and Photography).
    Part II. (a) Radiology (Radio-diagnosis, Radio-therapy); (b) Electrology (Electro-
        diagnosis, Electro-therapy).

SYLLABUS OF SUBJECTS.

PART I.

(a) PHYSICS.

Electrostatics. Fundamental ideas of Charge—Laws of Attraction and Repulsion—Potential and
    Capacity—Frictional Electricity—Electrostatic Induction—Influence Machines.
Electric Currents. Distribution in Circuits—Magnetic Effects—Measurement and Detection of
    Electric Currents—Galvanometers—Ammeters—Ohm's Law—Generation of Heat by Elec-
    tricity—Electrolysis—Primary and Secondary Batteries—The transmission of Electricity
    through Solids, Liquids, Gases and Animal Tissues.
Electromagnetic Induction. Production of Induced Currents — Relations existing between
    Primary and Secondary Circuits—Induction Coils and Transformers.
Radiation. Heat—Visible Rays—Ultra-violet Rays—Sources and Methods of Production.
X rays Their Production—Their place in the Spectrum—Relation between Wave-length and
    Penetrating Power—Laws relating to the Absorption of X rays by various substances,
    metal, bone, tissues, fluids, etc.—Characteristic X rays—Scattering of X rays—Types of
    X-ray Tubes and Valves—Principles of X-ray Localisation and Stereoscopy—Protection
    against X rays.
Radio-activity. Properties of the different rays emitted by Radium and other radio-active
    bodies—The Laws according to which such rays are absorbed by different substances—
    Secondary rays excited by alpha, beta and gamma rays—Transformation of Radio-active
    substances.

(b) ELECTRO-TECHNICS.

Production of currents, direct and alternating—Sources of supply.
Construction and action of motors and dynamos—Action and construction of induction coils and
    high-tension transformers—Interrupters—Production of galvanic, faradic and diathermic
    currents—Theory of electric condensers—Nature of condenser discharges—Production of
    high frequency currents—Large Power Static Machines.
Photography. Arrangement of Photographic Departments—Theory of Photographic action and
    Image formation—Conditions for Development—Action of Intensifiers and Restrainers—
    Modes of printing—Enlargement.

PRACTICAL COURSE.

Simple Experiments in Electrostatics. Measurement of Current—Voltage—Resistance and
    Heating Effects—Experiments illustrating laws of induced currents—Use of Electroscopes
    and Electrometers for measuring Ionisation Currents due to X rays, Radium and Ultra-
    violet Rays—Induction Coils and Transformers—Methods of production of high vacua—
    Generation of Cathode and X rays—Measurement and Absorption of X rays and the Rays
    from radio-active substances—Preparation of Radium Emanation Applicators—Precautions
    in use of Radium and X rays.

PART II.

(a) RADIOLOGY.

General Anatomy and Histology with special reference to Radiology. Bones and Joints—
    —Epiphyses and Development of bones—The normal chest in Childhood and Adult
    Life—Abdominal Organs—Urinary Tract—Special Regions—Skull—Spinal Column—
    Pelvis—Teeth.
Morbid Anatomy with special reference to Radiology. Inflammation and repair, with special
    reference to bones and viscera—Atrophy and Hypertrophy—Special Infective Diseases, *e.g.*,
    tuberculosis, syphilis, actinomycosis—Developmental anomalies—Tumours, their classification
    and character — Diseases of special organs and tissues to include: classification and

differential diagnosis of diseases of bones and joints, fractures and dislocations, diseases of lungs and pleura, heart and circulatory system, gall bladder, liver, œsophagus, stomach and duodenum, small intestine, appendix, colon, rectum, kidney, ureter and bladder, skin.

Radio-diagnosis. Fractures of bones and dislocations of joints, diseases of bones and joints with differential diagnosis — Examination of lungs and pleura, heart and aorta, the alimentary system, the urinary system, skull and accessory sinuses—New Growths—Teeth— Radiographic technique—Localisation of foreign bodies.

Apparatus used in Radiography and Radio-therapy. Arrangement and Organisation of an X-ray department.

RADIO-THERAPY.

X-ray Therapy. Special considerations of apparatus—Measurement of Dosage — Methods of Filtration.

The action of X rays on normal tissues, pathological tissues, ferments, micro-organisms.

Treatment of diseases of the skin, tuberculosis, new growths, gynæcological conditions, diseases of the ductless glands, anæmias, leucocythemia, etc.

Histological changes in normal and pathological tissues produced by X rays.

Radium Therapy. Methods of application of radium and radium emanation and other radio-active substances. The principles of dosage, factors affecting the results of treatment.

The action of radium upon normal tissues, pathological tissues, ferments, micro-organisms.

The therapeutic value of radium emanation water and solutions of radium salts.

Histological changes produced in normal and pathological tissues by radium. Treatment of diseases of the skin, new growths, gynæcological conditions, diseases of the ductless glands, anæmias, leucocythemias, etc.

FORMS OF LIGHT AND HEAT TREATMENT.

(*b*) ELECTROLOGY.

Electro-therapy—History—The mode of action of Electricity on the body—Treatment of Disease —The different forms of Electric Current used in Medicine—Sources of Supply—The Body as a conductor of Electricity—The action of the direct current on the body—Ionisation, medical and surgical—The action of interrupted and other modified currents on the body—Use of these currents for purposes of stimulation of tissues—High frequency currents, their production, action and uses—Diathermy—Static Electricity, production, action and uses— Morbid conditions for which Electricity has therapeutic action.

Electro-diagnosis—Elementary Physiology of muscle and nerve—The use of Electrical currents for Diagnosis.

	£	s.	d.
Fee for Part I with practical work	10	10	0
Fee for Part II.	15	15	0

Note :—These fees do not include the six months clinical instruction in a hospital recognised by the University.

The courses in Cambridge are open to non-members of the University, subject to the condition that their names are enrolled for the purpose at the Registry of the University, and that they pay a fee of one-and-a half guineas in respect of each quarter during which or any portion of which their names are so enrolled (*Ordinances*, pp. 274-6).

	£	s.	d.
Fee for Part I of the Examination	6	6	0
Fee for Part II of the Examination	6	6	0
Fee for Dissertation	10	10	0

All applications for information respecting the course and examinations should be addressed to F. SHILLINGTON SCALES, M.A., M.D., at the Medical Schools, Cambridge.

UNIVERSITY OF CAMBRIDGE.

DIPLOMA IN RADIOLOGY AND ELECTROLOGY.

Courses of Lectures and Practical Work in Part I (*a* and *b*) will be given at the Cavendish Laboratory, Cambridge, beginning January 20th, 1920. *Lecturer :* J. A. Crowther M.A., Sc.D. (Cantab).

·Courses of Lectures in Part II (a) will be given in the Medical Schools, Cambridge, beginning April 26th, 1920. *Lecturers :* A. E. Barclay. M.A., M.D. (Cantab.), Royal Infirmary, Manchester (*Alimentary System*) ; W. Ironside Bruce, M.D. (Aberdeen), Charing Cross Hospital (*Diseases of Joints*); N. S. Finzi, M.B. (Lond.), St. Bartholomew's Hospital (*Radiotherapy, Radium Therapy,* *Œsophagus*); C. Thurstan Holland, M.R.C.S., L.R.C.P., Royal Infirmary, Liverpool (*Urinary System, Production of Skiagrams*); C. E. Iredell, M.D. (Lond.), Guy's Hospital (*Radiotherapy, Radium Therapy*); R. Knox, M.D. (Edin.), King's College Hospital (*New Growths, Liver and Gall Bladder, Technical Apparatus, Radium Therapy*); W. S. Lazarus-Barlow, M.D. (Cantab), F.R.C.P., Middlesex Hospital (*Effects of Radiation on Tissues*); W. Lindsay Locke, M.B. (Edin.), Guy's Hospital (*Intestines and Appendix*); Stanley Melville, M.D. (Brux.), St. George's Hospital (*Thorax*); E. Reginald Morton, M.D. (Toronto), London Post-Graduate College (*The Heart and Aorta, Orthodiagraphy, Technical Apparatus*); G. Harrison Orton, M.A., M.D. (Cantab.), St. Mary's Hospital (*The Lungs, Tuberculosis, etc.*); Sir Archibald D. Reid, K.B.E., C.M.G., M.R.C.S., L.R.C.P., St. Thomas' Hospital (*Stereoscopy*); Sidney Russ, D.Sc. (Lond.) Middlesex Hospital (*Biological Effects of Radiation*); F. Shillington Scales, M.A., M.D. (Cantab), Addenbrooke's Hospital, Cambridge (*X-ray Anatomy and Pathology, Technical Apparatus*); S. G. Scott, M.R.C.S., L.R.C.P., London Hospital (*Bone Diseases, Craniology*); E. S. Worrall, M.R.C.S., L.R.C.P., Westminster Hospital (*Injuries of Bones and Joints*).

Courses of Lectures in Part II (b) will be given in the Medical Schools, Cambridge, beginning January 19th, 1920. *Lecturers :* E. P. Cumberbatch, M.A., M.B. (Oxon), M.R.C.P., St. Bartholomew's Hospital ; C. E. Iredell, M.D. (Lond.), M.R.C.P., Guy's Hospital ; F. Shillington Scales, M.A., M.D. (Cantab), Addenbrooke's Hospital, Cambridge; W. J. Turrell, M.A., M.D. (Oxon), Radcliffe Infirmary, Oxford ; R. S. Woods, M.D. (Lond.), M.R.C.P., London Hospital.

NOTE.—The above list of lecturers and subjects is provisional only.

Applications for attendance at the above courses in Cambridge should be made early to F. Shillington Scales, M.A., M.D., Medical Schools, Cambridge.

The following Hospitals are recognized by the University of Cambridge for clinical instruction in the Radiological and Electrical Department : Addenbrooke's, Cambridge ; Charing Cross ; Guy's ; King's College ; London ; Middlesex ; St. Bartholomew's ; St. George's ; St. Mary's ; St. Thomas' ; University College ; Westminster ; Royal Free ; Cancer Hospital (Brompton) ; Hospital for Consumption, etc. (Brompton). This list will be supplemented as occasion may require.

The next examination will be held at Cambridge in July, 1920 (provisional date only).

Similar courses in Parts I and II, recognised by the University, will be given in London. Arrangements are in progress with the Fellowship and Post Graduate Medical Association for an emergency course of lectures in Part II (A and B) to be given at the Royal Society of Medicine. (Details of these Lectures will be published in the January number of the ARCHIVES.)

Applications for information and attendance at the courses in London should be made to Robt. Knox, M.D., 38 Harley Street, London, W.

UNIVERSITY OF CAMBRIDGE

DIPLOMA IN MEDICAL RADIOLOGY AND ELECTROLOGY

I submit herewith a Dissertation for the Diploma in Radiology and Electrology, which I declare to be my own work, and I submit the following particulars of my qualifications   The fee of ten guineas is sent herewith to THE REGISTRARY OF THE UNIVERSITY.

Signed......................................(Full Postal address)..

Date of application..............................Name in full..

Registrable qualifications with the dates and places when they were respectively attained.   (Ten years qualification required)..

I hereby certify that has been engaged for not less than five years, namely from 19 to 19 in the practice of medical radiology and electrology in the Radiological and Electrical Department of · Hospital, in the capacity of (Signed) Date

Note.—This certificate must be signed by the Medical Officer in charge of the department, or by the Chairman of the Hospital.

The above form, duly filled up and signed, and the fee of ten guineas, must be sent to THE REGISTRARY OF THE UNIVERSITY, CAMBRIDGE.

UNIVERSITY OF CAMBRIDGE

APPLICATION FOR ADMISSION TO THE EXAMINATION FOR THE DIPLOMA IN MEDICAL RADIOLOGY AND ELECTROLOGY

Name of Candidate in full............................Full postal address..........................

Registrable qualifications with the dates and places when they were respectively obtained.........

....

PART I.

I certify that attended a course of LECTURES IN PHYSICS given by me at from 19 to 19 ; and that he worked in the Laboratory for not less than hours.

Signed of Date

I certify that attended a course of LECTURES IN ELECTROTECHNICS AND PHOTOGRAPHY given by me at from 19 to 19 ; and that he worked in the Laboratory for not less than hours.

Signed of Date

Having fulfilled the requirements of the University, and having paid the fee of six guineas to the Registrary, I desire to be admitted to Part I. of the Examination in Medical Radiology and Electrology to be held 19 .

(Signed) Date

PART II.

FIRST CERTIFICATE.

I certify that has attended a course of LECTURES IN RADIOLOGY (including Radiography and Radiotherapy) from 19 to 19 .

Date. (Signed)

SECOND CERTIFICATE.

I certify that has attended a course of LECTURES IN ELECTROLOGY (including Electrotherapy and Electrodiagnosis) from 19 to 19 .

Date (Signed)

THIRD CERTIFICATE.

I certify that   has had six months Clinical Experience and Instruction in the Radiological and Electrical Department of   Hospital (*at least four times weekly*), viz. from   19   to   19   .

    Date   (Signed)   (In charge of the Department.)

Having fulfilled the requirements of the University, and having paid the fee of six guineas to the Registrary, I desire to be admitted to Part II. of the Examination in Medical Radiology and Electrology to be held   19   .

    (Signed)   Date

Certificates must be sent in to the Registrary, University of Cambridge, and the fee paid, not less than three weeks before the date fixed for the Examination. Notice of the time and place of the Examination will be sent to the Candidate in due course.

THE NEW DISCOVERY IN ASTRO-PHYSICS.

ONE of the results of the British expeditions, in May last, to observe the total solar eclipse is a great discovery. It is that the light from a star is deflected from its path by the gravitational force of the sun ; this is an entirely new experimental fact, for it has hitherto been accepted that light in free space is propagated in a rectilinear manner, and that a deviation or deflection of a ray of light only occurred as the light passed from one medium to another ; in other words, by the action of material substances. Professor Eddington and Dr. Crommelin, who were in charge of the expeditions at Principe Island and at Sobral in North Brazil, brought the evidence of the new discovery before the scientific world at a joint meeting of the Royal Society and the Royal Astronomical Society on November 6th.

It is only at times of a total solar eclipse that stellar light passing near the sun can be observed on the earth. Under ordinary conditions, stellar photographs allow accurate measurements to be made of the distances separating the images obtained on the photographic plates. If under the special conditions possible in an eclipse the light from some members of a group of stars is deviated from its ordinary course a photograph will reveal a shift in the position of the stars. The shift which the observers had to anticipate was an extremely small one, in no case greater than 2″, which is the angle subtended by a sixpence at a distance of about a mile, but accurate micrometer measurements have shown that an undoubted shift does occur in the position of those stars, the light from which comes sufficiently near to the edge of the sun.

Professor Einstein predicted that a ray of light should be deviated by gravitational force, and calculations made by him showed that the shift would be about 1·75″. The average value of the shift which has been observed is about 1·56″; it may, therefore, be stated that Einstein's prediction of the effect of gravitational force upon a ray of light has been fulfilled. This fact is a very significant one, both from the experimental and the theoretical view points. As Professor Eddington has remarked, it is almost the first new thing which has been discovered about the gravitational force for the last 200 years. In fact, since the genius of Newton bade the world look upon the gravitational force as one pervading the universe and holding material bodies in their positions, few fundamental things have been added which can be said to have raised the curtain upon the mystery of the nature of this force. Now it appears that the force of gravity acts not only upon material bodies but upon ether vibrations; not (as yet proved) upon ether at rest, but upon ether disturbances, such as rays of light, and presumably also radiation, such as X rays; but this is conjecture. So much then for the newly acquired experimental fact, over which there is little difference of opinion; a ray of light is bent by the sun's gravitational force.

When we allow ourselves to linger for a moment on the speculations to which this fact has given rise, we are on much less substantial ground. Professor Einstein predicted this extraordinary fact; his theory of relativity, of the true inwardness of which the writer is in outer darkness, has, however, predicted that the spectral lines of stellar light should, under the influence of the sun's gravitational pull, be shifted towards the red end of the spectrum. This prediction is not confirmed by the observers. In Professor Einstein's opinion his theory is true only if all his predictions are fulfilled; therefore it has to be concluded that the whole truth is not to be found in his theory. This may not be so comfortless a situation to those who have stood outside the threshold of relativity appreciation, as it must be to Professor Einstein himself.

Newton would surely not have been surprised if it had been shown in his day that the gravitational force could deviate a ray of light, for in his famous emission theory, light was supposed to consist of minute corpuscles emitted by the luminous body. Newton's theory of the nature of light was eventually superseded by the undulatory theory which supposed that light consisted of something resembling undulations or waves in the ether.

Clerk Maxwell predicted that light exerts a pressure upon surfaces when incident upon them. This prediction was amply fulfilled by experiment; a beam of light therefore has momentum, it certainly has velocity, therefore it also has something corresponding to mass; if it has mass then it should be influenced by the gravitational force. Clerk Maxwell therefore, we may reasonably suppose would not have been a stranger to the idea that a ray of light should be influenced by gravitational force. A surprise, therefore, to few theorists, and yet a very fine experimental fact, and one which reflects the greatest skill on the part of the observers. To try to know what the discovery means to the person who predicted it is perhaps to seek too much.

S. R.

NOTES ON A SPECIAL TUBE STAND FOR RAPID X-RAY STEREO-SCOPIC WORK.   CONSTRUCTED FOR THE CANCER HOSPITAL.

By C. E. HOLLAND.

THIS stand has been designed with the view of giving the radiologist a substantial and not too costly piece of apparatus which will meet his requirements, be simple to operate, and not be liable to be constantly getting out of order.

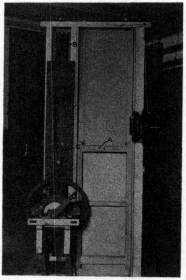

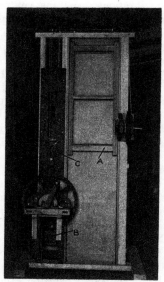

Front view of apparatus, showing the bar B in its top position, and the frame A in its lowest position, ready for working.

Front view of apparatus, showing the bar B in its lowest position, and the frame A in its top position; the second plate being in its correct place for exposure.

By one simple operation the two plates are successively brought into the proper position, the tube shifted the desired amount, and the two exposures made at the correct times. The operator simply turns a handle, and when working steadily at a suitable speed throws the moving parts into gear and the plates are exposed as follows :—

(i) The first plate is brought into position and an auxiliary switch in the primary circuit is closed.

(ii) The main switch in the primary circuit is closed for the desired time and the first plate exposed.

(iii) The first plate is moved away, the second plate brought into position, and the X-ray tube shifted the desired amount.

(iv) The main switch in the primary circuit is again closed for the desired time and the second plate exposed.

(v) A second auxiliary switch in the primary circuit is opened so that no further current can pass.

The present stand is constructed for use with the patient in a standing position, but the gear can be readily adapted for use with a couch or table if required.

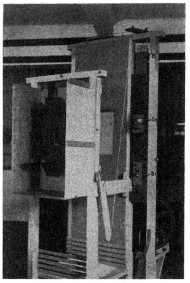

Back view of apparatus, showing the sliding frame for the tube; with its lead-lined case, and lever and cords for shifting the tube; the lever here has not been fitted with its stop, but is hanging free. This view also shows the two automatic switches S_1 and S_2.

The essential parts of the apparatus are as follows (see photos and reference letters):—

    (a) A sliding frame (A) to carry two casettes enclosing the plates and intensifying screens.

    (b) A sliding bar (B) connected either rigidly or by cords with the frame (A).

    (c) A spindle fitted with handle, circular switch for making the exposures, fly wheel, and connecting rod, operating :—

    (d) A sliding block (c) which gears in with the bar (B) by means of a pawl.

(*e*) A double sliding frame to carry the X-ray tube, arranged so that the tube shift can be made either vertically or horizontally as required, with a lever and cords or other suitable device to reduce the length of travel of the bar (B) to the required shift of the tube.

(*f*) Two auxiliary switches in the primary circuit, the first of which (s₁) is closed by the bar (B) as soon as it starts to move down from its initial position, and remains closed till the bar is returned to this position, when it automatically opens, and the second of which (s₂) is closed by hand before working the apparatus and is opened by the block (c) after the second plate has been exposed.

In the present case, in order to keep down to a minimum the floor space required, the frame (A) has been arranged to slide vertically, being connected to the sliding bar by means of flexible cords passing over pulleys on the top of the main frame of the stand.

The frame (A) and the bar (B) are partly balanced, the frame with the loaded casettes being kept slightly heavier than the bar, and a spring catch is fixed in the main frame so as to hold the bar accurately in its three positions and prevent its running backwards.

In the initial position the bar (B) is further held in its place by a wooden stop, which prevents the pawl in the sliding block from gearing in with the bar ; and as the fly wheel is rotated the block simply slides freely up and down in its guides.

When everything is ready and the operator is turning the handle steadily at the required speed, this stop is sharply withdrawn, preferably when the block is at the bottom of its travel. At the top of the next stroke the pawl falls into place in the bar and then draws it down for the full travel of the block, closing the auxiliary switch (s₁) and raising the frame (A), so that the first plate is in position for exposure.

The circular switch is then in the position i, shown in diagram I, and shortly after, in position ii, it closes the primary circuit, and keeps it closed till it reaches position iii, whilst the block (c) is still travelling up. The block then again gears in with the bar (B) and draws up the frame (A), so that the second plate is brought into position. At the same time a cord attached to the bar pulls over the lever that controls the shift of the tube. The second exposure is then made just as the first.

The bar (B) is now in its lowest position, and has allowed a small arm on the auxiliary switch (s₂) to fall forward, so that when the block (c) starts its next downward travel the pawl strikes this arm and opens the switch.

The block (c) then moves freely up and down in its guides till the operator has brought the handle to rest.

All the moving parts are started slowly from rest, taken up to their maximum speed, and gradually brought to rest again, so that there are no shocks at starting or stopping, and vibration can be reduced to a minimum.

Also, to assist in obtaining fairly steady speed of turning, a fly wheel of quite appreciable weight has been included.

It has been found that with the present apparatus the time covering the two exposures can be reduced to about a second without vibration, and with a stiffer framework and lighter moving parts this time can be considerably reduced if necessary, provided, of course, that the X-ray installation is of sufficient power to give the required rapid exposures.

The stand is fitted with an adjustable platform, which must be raised or lowered to get the patient into the exact position required. If desired, a fluorescent screen can be used whilst this is being done, after the plates in their casettes have been placed in their sliding frame, as the first plate is only brought into position just before it is exposed, and till then is protected by a thick lead screen.

Circular Switch.—The circular switch consists of two brushes bearing on

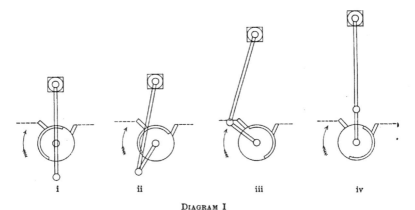

i   ii   iii   iv

DIAGRAM I

the periphery of an insulating cylinder, into which is let a metal sector, which electrically connects the two brushes for a part of each revolution.

The cylinder is mounted on the same spindle as the fly wheel, and is set so that the metal sector runs under the leading brush and closes the primary circuit shortly after the block (c) has reached its lowest position, and passes from under the backward brush and breaks the circuit before the block reaches its top position, as shown in positions i, ii, iii, and iv of diagram I.

The brushes are mounted on an insulating block, the leading one being fixed and the backward one adjustable, so that it may be set at varying distances from the fixed one, so as to regulate the length of the exposure, which will be greater when the brushes are close together, and less when they are far apart, as shown in diagram II, positions i and ii.

If θ be the angle in degrees subtended by that part of the metal sector from its back end up to the backward brush at the moment when its front end has just reached the leading brush, the time of exposure will be equal to the time of one revolution $\times \dfrac{\theta}{360}$.

If, for example, it is required to expose each plate for one-tenth of a second

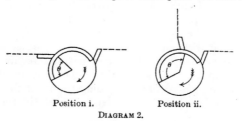

Position i.   Position ii.

DIAGRAM 2.

and to complete the two exposures within a second, the handle should be turned at $66\frac{2}{3}$ revolutions per minute, and the backward brush should be set so that the angle θ is $40°$, assuming perfectly steady speed of revolution. Of course, such accuracy will neither be required nor obtained in use.

[With heavy primary currents a good deal of sparking may occur at breaking, and a small carbon brush has been added to the main backward brush so as to take the spark. The brass brushes are only intended to be temporary, and more substantial ones will be put on later.]

Auxiliary Switches.—The auxiliary switches are never closed or opened

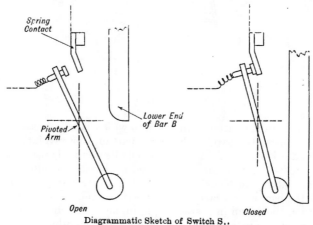

Diagrammatic Sketch of Switch S₁.

when current is on, and current is only on for a very short time, so that they can be of quite light and simple construction with only short break.

The switch (s₁) consists of a pivoted arm, which is pressed backwards by the bar (B) just after it starts to move down from its initial position, closing the switch and holding it closed until the bar is brought back to this original position, when it falls open by gravity.

The switch (s₂) is an ordinary hand switch with a projecting arm and pivoted end piece, arranged so that when the bar (ʙ is in its lowest position) this pivoted piece falls forward, and is then struck by the pawl of the block (ᴄ) on its next downward stroke and the switch is opened.

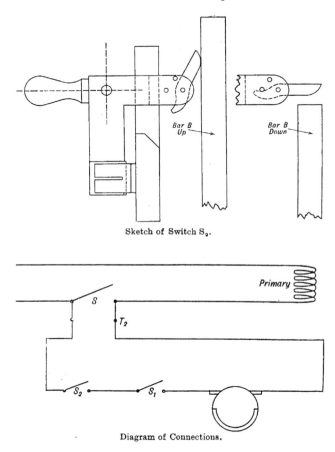

Sketch of Switch S₂.

Diagram of Connections.

A convenient method of connecting up is shown in the above diagram ; in which (s) is the usual single pole switch in the primary circuit used for making the exposures.

To its terminals two others (ᴛ₁ and ᴛ₂) are connected, and into these are run the leads going to the apparatus.

The switch (s) can then be used for screening and left open before exposing the plates. The auxiliary switches (s₁ and s₂) and the circular switch are joined in series, and, as the handle is turned, no current can pass in the primary circuit, except when all three switches are closed, as previously described.

Spring Catch.—The construction of the spring catch, with its holding off hook, is shown in the sketch below.

The only point to notice about this is that it is awkward to take to pieces and put in again ; the spindle (K) must be threaded backwards into place through the slides—there is just room to do this. It is unlikely that it will be necessary to take this out and in after it has once been correctly adjusted.

The hook is arranged to hold off the catch : simply pull back the milled head and let the hook fall into place.

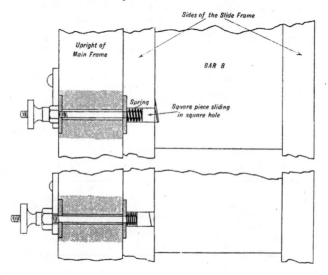

Tube Shift.—The shift of the tube is made by means of a lever, the shorter arm of which carries a plate with a row of holes near its upper edge, and the cord which draws over the tube is fitted with a small shackle, which is fixed in the hole that gives the desired shift. One cord is used for a horizontal tube shift and another for a vertical one. The shift can be varied over a range of about 4 to 10 centimetres. The longer arm of the lever ends in an eye, through which runs a cord, one end of which is fixed to the top of the sliding bar (B), and the other carries a weight just sufficiently heavy to keep the string taut, and too large to pass through the eye ; the cord passes over two small pulleys on the top of the main frame. During the first movement of the sliding bar, during which the first plate is brought into position, the lever remains in position against its fixed stop, the cord runs freely through the eye and draws up the weight so as just not to touch the eye. During the second movement of the bar, which brings the second plate into position, the eye at the end of the lever is drawn up through a vertical distance equal to the travel of the bar, and the tube is shifted.

The tube is mounted on a wooden board which slides vertically in guides fixed on a second board, which itself slides horizontally in guides fixed on the main frame of the apparatus.

When using a horizontal shift the vertical slide should first be firmly clamped in its central position on the horizontal slide, and when using a vertical shift the horizontal slide should be firmly clamped in its central position on the main frame.

When adjusting the cords for the tube shift, the tube should be accurately

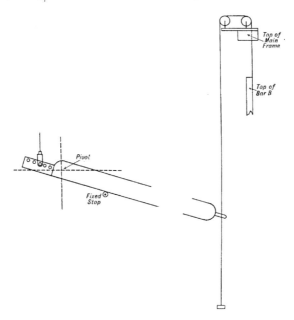

centred, both horizontally and vertically, the lever should be held horizontally, the shackle set in a hole about half way along the plate and the cord just drawn taut and fixed. This adjustment is made once for all for each cord, and need only be repeated in case the cord has stretched considerably or a new cord is required.

Method of Operation.—When working the apparatus proceed as follows :— See that the required tube slide is free and the other clamped, and fix the shackle of the correct cord in the plate in the hole which will give the required shift. Then move the slide over till the cord is taut and the lever drawn firmly against its stop, when the tube will be in the correct position for the exposure of the first plate.

Load the two casettes and place them in position in the sliding frame. Close the auxiliary switch (S_2) by hand. Turn the button on the block (c) so as to hold back the pawl, and draw back the spring catch that holds the bar (B) from sliding up; let the bar slide back till it is in its top position and then release the catch so as to hold it in this position. The frame carrying the plates will then be in its lowest position. Slip the long wooden stop into place. See that the auxiliary switch (s_1) has opened.

Adjust the patient in position, and screen if required, being careful to replace the tube in the position described above if it is centred for screening. Release the button on the block (c) so as to free the pawl.

Turn handle steadily until working at the required speed.

[The operator will, of course, not be able to maintain a perfectly uniform speed throughout the series of operations, but by turning firmly and as steadily as possible, a quite satisfactory result can be obtained, and the two exposures can be made very nearly equal to one another.]

Pull out the wooden stop sharply at a moment when the block (c) is in its lowest position—when the exposures will be made as previously described. Take out the casettes and remove the plates, when the apparatus will be ready for the next series of operations.

Use of Stand for a Slowly Moving Plate.—The sliding frame has also been adapted for use with a slowly moving plate, being slowly drawn upwards by a cord wound on to a pulley, which is turned steadily at a slow speed by means of a worm and wheel. This is simply worked by hand, but if it is found that the movement is not uniform enough, a small motor drive can easily be added later ; and if useful results are obtained other obvious improvements can be made.

To use the apparatus in this way, put the loaded casettes in the frame just as before, drop the frame to its lowest position, slip the loop of the winding cord over the hook provided for the purpose in the top of the frame and slowly wind it up. The bar (B) slides down with its own weight. The main operating handle must be left in such a position that the brushes of the circular switch are not connected together, and the hand switch (s) must be used for making the exposure.

The pulley on which the cord is wound is grooved in three steps of different diameters, so as to obtain a long range of plate speeds, while still turning the handle fairly fast so as to get a fairly uniform movement, or if a motor drive is added.

AN INHERITED ABNORMALITY.

By C. F. ODDIE, Radiographer to the North Stafford Infirmary.

THE patient was attending the massage department for flat feet, and one of the masseuses drew my attention to his hands, with the little stumpy one-jointed fingers.

I radiographed him from curiosity. He is a bright little boy of fourteen

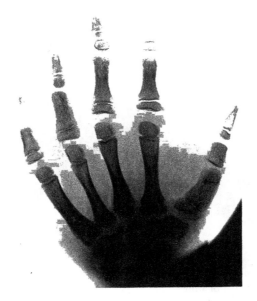

years old, and both his hands are like this. His mother—now dead—had similar hands, and four out of her nine children are similarly affected, the other five being normal.

CASE OF UNUSUAL FRACTURE OF THE OS CALCIS.

By C. J. GLASSON, M.D., M.R.C.S. Eng., L.R.C.P. Lond., Capt. R.A.M.C.,
o/c X-ray Dept., Netley, Hants.

PATIENT fell from ladder a distance of 14ft. and landed upon the point of right heel. There is a fracture of the upper and posterior surface of the os calcis with displacement of the fragment, the forward end to the inner side.

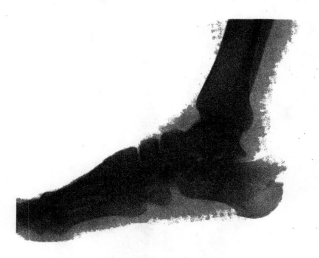

There is a transverse oblique fracture from the anterior portion to just in front of posterior third of upper surface, with dislocation forwards of the lower segment.

The tendo Achilles was not broken through, though some strands attached to upper and posterior point of os calcis were broken lifting the fractured piece upwards.

The upper piece was manipulated back into position. Patient did very well.

DETECTION OF A DIFFICULT FOREIGN BODY.

By ALFRED MARSH, Lt., R.A.M.C.

THE radiological examination of a man sent to me with a wound near the elbow which would not heal revealed nothing to account for it. I then tried a method I saw somewhere as useful in the differential diagnosis of T.B. of bone and thought it might also show up any non-metallic foreign body.

The illustration shows a foreign body very clearly. I said that it was wood and

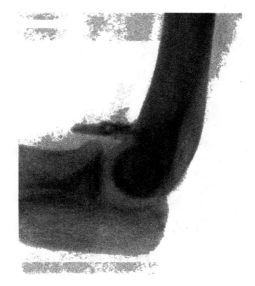

I could see the end of the splinter turned up where it had struck the bone, also a small knot in the bone. The surgeon was sceptical as to the "knot," but he cut down and removed a piece of wood exactly as described. The method will demonstrate cloth, etc., just as well. I simply inserted a small stick of No. 3 into the sinus, protecting the skin with cotton wool, removed the silver nitrate in one minute and took the radiogram.

NEW INVENTIONS.

SIMULTANEOUS FLUOROSCOPY IN TWO PLANES.

By H. C. GAGE, O.I.P.

Consulting Radiographer, American Red Cross Hospital, No. 2, Paris; Radiographer in Charge, Hôpital Militaire, V.R 76, Ris-Orangis, S.-et-O.

IT has been recognised for a long time that the reduction of fractures—especially simple may be left uncertain as to the accuracy of the alignment in one plane or the other. These difficulties are only avoided if it is possible to see both planes simultaneously, without any turning of the patient, and this can be done, without any very complicated apparatus, by means of the arrangement shown in the accompanying plates. These are from

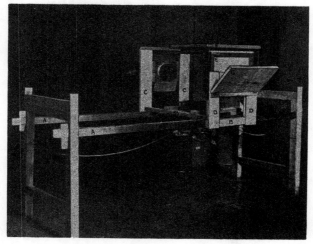

FIG. 1.

fractures which can be reduced by direct manipulation, and put up at once in plaster—is effected most satisfactorily under fluoroscopic control. The lateral view, however, particularly in the case of the lower limb, introduces a difficulty. With the ordinary under-table tube such a view can only be obtained by turning the patient over on to his side, and it is extremely difficult in such turning to avoid displacing the fragments. Moreover, if further manipulation is found to be necessary, the adjustment of the fragments in the lateral plane may throw them out in the antero-posterior plane, and the process will have to be repeated; and even then we

photographs of a rough home-made model, which will perhaps be more useful than drawings of a more elaborate design. The details could, of course, be improved upon, but under present conditions most radiographers probably find themselves under the same difficulty as the author in getting even the simplest piece of apparatus made, and that shown serves its purpose quite well.

The table illustrated is a simple wooden one, with a movable top of thin three-ply wood. On the horizontal bars, *A A* (Figs. 1 and 2), slides a rigid wooden framework, *B*, which carries, in addition to the under-table tube, uprights *C D*, just free of the table top on each side. Of these, *C* carries a second tube-holder, moving up and down in vertical grooves, while *D* carries two fluorescent screens, *E F*, and a hinged mirror, *G*. *E* drops into vertical slots, in which it can be fixed at the same horizontal level as the second tube; its fluorescent surface is outwards, and, with the mirror fixed at about 45 degrees, an observer looking downward sees the reflection of *E* side by side with the direct view of *F*. This arrangement enables the tubes and screens to be used at any distance along the table, and keeps them automatically in alignment. *F* is supported

ensure that no rays fall beyond the lead glass and protective framework of the screens.

In use the two X-ray tubes are connected in parallel to the high-tension circuit, so that both are in action simultaneously. The adjustments are, of course, very much simplified if two similar Coolidge tubes are used, as it then becomes a very easy matter to bring them to the same hardness and get the current equally divided between them. The small self-rectifying tubes are the most suitable. With gas tubes the necessary adjustment is

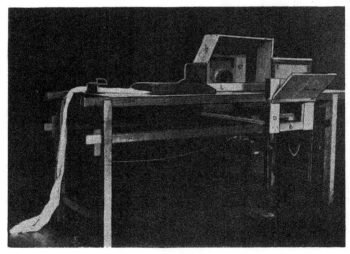

Fig. 2.

on two iron bars, hinged at *H* and *K*, so that they can be turned down out of the way when the screen is not actually in use (Figs. 2 and 3). The supports shown were designed for a pair of large screens, which were already in use in the department, but these are really unnecessarily large and clumsy; small screens of about 8 by 6 inches, on proportionately slighter supports, are all that is needed for examining the position of a fracture. For the protection of the observer, the mirror *G* and the frames *C* and *D* are covered by sheet lead, not shown in the illustrations. The diaphragms should be thoroughly opaque, and small enough to

rather more tiresome. It is best done by softening both tubes to a point a little below that which is required for use, and leaving the regenerating wires fixed at equal distances from the cathodes, such that neither can harden up much more than the other. If it is found practically impossible to get two tubes to keep equally hard, so as to give approximately equal illumination on the two screens, a high-tension switch can be inserted, and the tubes operated alternately. This is, of course, a little less convenient, but retains the main advantages of the arrangement.

The patient is placed on the table, as shown in Figs. 3 and 4, with the fractured limb on the same side of the table as *D* and *E*, and the and 4. To provide the counter-extension required in reducing an overlapping fracture, a small padded perineal support is used (*M*,

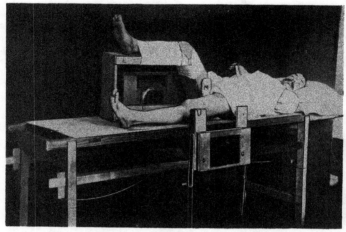

Fig. 3.

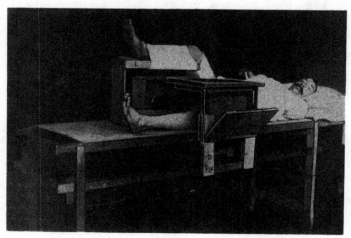

Fig. 4.

carrier *B* is adjusted so that the normal rays go through the fracture. In the case of the thigh or leg it is necessary to keep the sound limb off the table, and this is arranged for by the light wooden frame *L*, shown in Figs. 2, 3, Figs. 2 and 3), fastened to an iron clamp at the head of the table by webbing bands, which can be adjusted to any desired length. By mounting the support on a padded board (as shown in Fig. 2), on which the patient lies, we have the additional advantage of lifting the injured limb a little off the table, thus leaving room for manipulation, passing of plaster bandages under the limb, etc.

The fracture is first manipulated (if necessary) under as weak a light as can conveniently be used; the room is then completely darkened, and the two tubes activated, thus showing side by side the lateral and antero-posterior views of the fracture. Any required adjustment of the position can be effected without turning the limb, and the whole process is under direct fluoroscopic control. In the case of a toothed fracture, where the shape of the fragments

often makes it very difficult to bring them into alignment, the position of the teeth and the manipulation necessary to avoid them are readily appreciated. Either plaster or splints can be applied while the patient lies on the table, and if splints of wood or aluminium are used the final result can be again checked before the patient leaves the radioscopic room.

In this way the surgeon is able to get the best possible result, and is under no uncertainty as to the position ultimately obtained.

I should like to express my thanks to my assistant, Miss Slater, for drawing up this account for me at a very busy time.

REPORTS OF SOCIETIES.

RONTGEN SOCIETY.

An exhibition of prints illustrative of the employment of the X-ray is being organised by the Rontgen Society, who have accepted an invitation of the Royal Photographic Society to provide a collection of such prints, to form an exhibition at the Royal Photographic Society's House, 35, Russell Square, W.C., from January 6th to February 7th, 1920.

The Exhibition will be open daily (Admission Free) from 11 a.m. to 5 p.m., and on the evenings of January 6th and January 13th till 9 p.m. On the former date an elementary lecture, on "The X rays Approached from the Popular Standpoint," will be given by Dr. George H. Rodman, F.R.P.S., and on January 13th, a discussion will be opened by Major G. W. C. Kaye, O.B.E., M.D., D.Sc., on "Some Aspects of Radiology."

Both lectures will commence at 7 p.m.

AMERICAN ASSOCIATION OF ELECTROTHERAPEUTICS & RADIOLOGY.

The members elected for the year 1919-1920 are as follows:—

President: William Martin, M.D., Atlantic City, N.J.

Vice-Presidents: Virgil C. Kinney, M.D., Wellsville, N.Y.; William T. Johnson, M.D., Philadelphia, Penn.; S. St. John Wright, M.D., Akron, Ohio.; Mary Arnold Snow,

M.D., New York, N.Y.; John H. Burch, M.D., Syracuse, N.Y.

Treasurer: Emil Heuel, M.D., New York, N.Y.

Secretary and Registrar: Byron Sprague Price, M.D., 17 East 38th Street, New York, N.Y.

Board of Trustees: One year—J. Willard Travell, M.D,, New York, N.Y., and Frederick DeKraft, M.D., New York, N.Y. Two years —Frank B.Granger, M.D., Washington, D.C., and Frederick H. Morse, M.D., Boston, Mass. Three years—William L. Clark, M.D., Philadelphia, Penn, and Edward C. Titus, M.D., New York, N.Y.

Abstract of Papers from American Association of Electrotherapeutics and Radiology.

ACTION OF ELECTRICAL CURRENTS ON DUCTLESS GLANDS AND OTHER TISSUES.

By FREDERICK DE KRAFT, M.D., New York City.

THE author enumerates, as benefits derived from the application of the high-frequency currents, the checking of toxins, the promotion of metabolism and the improvement of the nutrition of the body as a whole, and cites cases in his own practice and reported by other physicians in which the exhibition of thermal penetration resulted in restoration of normal function in endocrine structures showing faulty metabolism.

Dr. De Kraft recommends the use of the resonator effluve from a large static machine in selected cases, using the bipolar method, first placing a metal plate attached to the tesla over the abdomen, and applying the effluve from the oudin gradually over every part of the back, then placing the plate on the back, and applying the effluve on the front of the body, thus producing rhythmic contraction of large muscle masses, and bringing about the resultant increase in tissue change, and improvement in muscular tone.

In cases of obesity accompanied by impaired circulation, feeble heart action and intestinal flatus, Dr. De Kraft finds that the static wave current to the abdomen corrects these conditions, reduces the weight, and tends to restore correct metabolism.

REPORT OF THE COMMITTEE ON HIGH-FRE-
QUENCY AND INDUCED CURRENTS.

Dr. FREDERICK DE KRAFT, Chairman.

The contention of H. C. Stevens that muscle wasting after paralysis is really due to fatigue from the incessant fibrillary action of the muscle is mentioned, and the benefit to be derived in these cases from the action of diathermy, with its quieting effect on fibrillary contractions, is pointed out. Debédat's report on the muscular development of rabbits under exercise by means of the rhythmic faradic current is cited, as is also Bier's report of the regeneration of muscle tissue in two cases, in one of which the regeneration was apparently of true functioning muscle (in the vastus externus of a child). This regeneration was attributed to an unusually abundant supply of lymphatic exudate, and it therefore suggests the use of diathermy with its ability to control the local lymph supply as a potential aid in future cases.

Leiner's investigations showing a large preponderance of smaller dextral diameters of the stylo-mastoid foramen, and the probable explanatory relation of that fact to the prevalence of dextral Bell's palsy is reviewed, and the observation made that the use of diathermy in the early stages would tend to remove the superficial vaso-constriction and the deep-seated venous engorgement, and prevent atrophy of the muscular fibre by quieting fibrillary contraction. The static wave current, by promoting vascular drainage would materially aid in preventing the swelling of the nerve trunk within the foramen, and that the galvano-sinusoidal or galvano-faradic-sinusoidal current would aid in the restoration of function after the subsidence of the acute inflammatory process.

SOCIÉTÉ DE RADIOLOGIE MÉDI-CALE DE FRANCE.
Séance, du 14 Octobre, 1919.

Un cas de corps étranger des voies respiratoires. — Le Dr. Ledoux-Lebard rapporte l'histoire d'un malade qui ayant avalé une pièce dentaire, munie de deux dents au cours d'une quinte de coqueluche, mais n'éprouvant aucun symptôme, fut considéré comme l'ayant expulsée par les voies naturelles sa coqueluche ayant guéri, il est repris quatre mois plus tard, de toux non coqueluchoïde avec expectoration sans bacilles. Un premier examen radiologique fut négatif. L'A. ayant en l'occasion de voir à son tour ce malade, mit en évidence sur un cliché oblique la pièce dentaire, etc. la localisa au niveau de la bifurcation de la trachée, accrochée à l'éperon trachéal et plongeant dans l'origine de la bronche gauche. Une bronchoscopie pratiquée par le Dr. Dufourmentel vérifie ces conclusions et permet de ramener la pièce par trachéotomie.

Diagnostic radiologique d'un calcul du péritoine confirmé par l'opérat. — Le Dr. Lejeuner présente ce cas concernant une malade prise brusquement d'accidents péritonéaux, avec syncopes. Le point douloureux siègeun peu à gauche de la ligne médiane et para-ombilicale. Sur la demande du Chirurgien on fait un examen. radiologique de la région urétérale gauche et l'òn constate qu'il existe centre la colonne lombaire et l'os iliaque gauche une opacité qui d'après l'avis de l'A. est non seulement calculeuse, mais autorise par son aspect particulier le diagnostic de concrétion du péritoine. Plusieurs clichés permirent de constater la mobilité de l'opacité ce qui confirmait le diagnostic posé et l'intervention chirurgicale permit de constater la véracité du diagnostic.

Biloculation d'estomac d'origine extrinsèque. — Les Drs. Aubourg et Ehren preiss rapportent l'obs. d'une malade qui présentait une biloculation et une déformation du bis-fond de l'estomac. L'intervention a montré qu'il s'agissait d'un lipome diffus de l'épiploon qui fut réséqué. Après l'opération l'aspect de l'estomac était redevenu normal.

Montage des soupapes sur bobine alimentant des Coolidges Standart.—Le Dr. Maingot présente un mode de montage de soupapes à gaz raréfié groupées en deux séries de deux. Les soupapes constituent un groupé de deux séries comprenant chacune deux éléments. Les deux séries sont en parellèle. Un fil connecte le milieu de chacune des deux séries. La rigidité électrostatique est la même qu' avec deux soupapes en série, le réglage est plus facile car les soupapes se supplé ent entre elles.

Dilatation congénitale de l'œsophage.—Le Dr. Aubourg présente les clichés du thorax d'un malade du service du Dr. Bezançon. L'examen radiologique donnait la figure d'une pleurésie médiastine. L'autopsie faite par le Prof. Letulle a montré qu'il s'agissait d'une énorme dilatation de l'œsophage. Les détails clini-ques et anatomo-pathologiqnes de cette obser-vation ont publiés été à la Société anatomique (Juillet, 1919).

Le Secrétaire Général : Dr. HARET.

REVIEW.

Radio-Diagnosis of Pleuro-Pulmonary Affections. By Dr. F. BARJON (Lyons), translated by Dr. J. A. HONEIJ (Yale). Published by the Yale University Press, New Haven, U.S.A.; Humphrey Milford, Oxford University Press, London, 1918. (French Edition, 1916.) 183 pages, 79 illustrations. Price 10s. 6d.

The monograph on diseases of the pleura and lungs, which has been written by Dr F. Barjon (Lyons) and translated by Dr. Honeij (Yale Medical School), is one which should appeal very strongly to three classes of readers. The general practitioner, who will find in it useful information which will help him to appreciate the value of radiographic examinations in these chest conditions, and which will help him to decide in which case he should recommend such an examination. The specialist in chest diseases, who has not especially studied the question of radiological examinations, and who is apt to think that the older methods of examination are such that radiography is rather a luxury than a necessity. The X-ray expert, who is too often under the impression that an X-ray examina-tion is the first and last word in diagnosis, and that physicians with their methods of auscul-tation and percussion, their history of the case, and possibly the examination of the sputum in addition, are simply mere camou-flage.

The author is an eminent physician; it is apparent, from a mere superficial look through his book, that he is equally an eminent radiologist, at any rate as far as the thorax is concerned. The expert radiologist, who is not at the same time a physician, would not venture to give the importance to certain X-ray appearances which the author insists are of the greatest importance; and such X-ray findings and the deductions to be drawn from them can only be made by either a man who is both an expert physician and radiologist, or by two men working in intimate conjunction, the one a physician and the other a radiologist.

We would more especially draw the attention of our readers to the diagnosis of pleurisy of the hilus, and the remarks of the author as to the X-ray signs in such a condition; and to the value laid upon the X-ray indications in cases of phthisis in which it is proposed to create an artificial pneumothorax. In its main construction, after an introduction and a chapter on the methods of examination, the book is divided into four parts, of which one deals with the pleura, one with the bronchi, one with the lungs, and one with the projectiles of war and their effects. The illustrations are typical and well chosen; the diagrams are excellent. The translation from the original French is obviously done very well; the substance is easily read and easily under-stood. All radiologists who have to make chest examinations should most certainly make themselves acquainted with the substance of this book. C. T. H.

NOTES AND ABSTRACTS

The Discovery and Extraction of Projectiles from the Lung by the Method of the Electro-Vibreur.—R. GREGOIRE and J. BERGONIÉ, (*Arch. d'Élect. Méd.*, December, 1918).—It is often advisable to remove these foreign bodies from the lung, but whereas the original estimation of their position can and must be done by means of X rays, the actual finding of the missile at operation is not so simple.

The two ordinary methods available are operation under the X-ray screen, which has obvious objections, and with the use of compass instruments which are most unsatisfactory in practice. The authors give details of cases illustrating the several kinds of operative conditions that have to be dealt with, and showing how the work is hastened and simplified by the use of the electro-vibreur. The chief use of this instrument is, of course, that it gives the actual position of the bullet or fragment of shell at the moment of operation, no matter how it may have moved since the X-ray localisation was performed. Further, it is used in a fully-lit operating theatre, and can be guided by the surgeon himself, is simple to work, and requires no geometrical or arithmetical calculation.

The optimum conditions for success are described as follows:—

A piece of shell or a ferro-nickel cased bullet (shrapnel ball cannot be detected) weighing five or more grammes, lying not too deeply below the surface, a powerful and skilfully used vibreur, a fairly thin subject, a sensitive palpating hand.

When the subject is fat or the foreign body lies very deep, the same effect results, that is, its distance from the vibreur is too great for vibrations to be produced. In the case of the deep-seated bullet, if the lung is free from adherence it can be palpated when the surgical pneumothorax is established, and the bullet easily felt; but when the lung is adherent palpation becomes impossible. It is now possible in these cases in effect to prolong the vibreur into the wound and so bring the bullet within range, and produce palpable vibrations.

This is done by an addition to Bergonie's original vibreur apparatus of a magnetic extension which is described as a sealed tube of glass, thoroughly sterilisable, and packed with a soft iron core.

In cases where the wound is too deep, or the body wall too thick, to allow of success with the ordinary vibreur, the surgeon can prolong the vibreur into the wound by means of this magnetic extension, and so obtain the desired result.   N. B.

The Continuous Current in the Treatment of War Wounds.—R. CASMAN (*Archives d'Élect. Méd.*, Nov., 1918).—The preliminary cleaning up and the final suturing of a wound are purely surgical, and matters of precision; the intervening stage of disinfection of the wound is a problem for all, and is no simple matter, as infection is a thing of caprice, and its treatment does not in practice lead so simply to success as do the experiments "in vitro."

The difficulty lies in the irregularity of the surface of the wound, with its minute pockets and crannies, and in the coagulating effect of most antiseptics.

In 1917 the author began to treat furuncles, after removal of the core of pus and debris, by ionisation, using metallic mercury as the ionising substance. The result was successful in that one treatment led to thorough cleansing and sterilisation of the cavity, which was then sutured on removal of the black scab resulting from the treatment.

He next began to treat ordinary war wounds with the continuous current, using sulphate of zinc as a soluble salt wherewith to apply zinc ions to the depths of the tissues forming the walls of the wounds. By careful packing of the wound with layer after layer of gauze impregnated with the 1 in 1,000 solution, and using moderate pressure, perfect contact can be obtained with all parts of the wound, so that no unsterilised portions are left. The result of this treatment has been that wounds have been rendered sterile in one sitting, and three days later the scab resulting from the zinc treatment has been removed and the wound sutured. N. B.

A Rare Case of Intrapulmonary Projectile.—
E. Salsac (*Arch. d'Él., Méd.*, Nov., 1918).—
The author shows a plate of, and describes the case of a man who was bombarded by fragments of wood and metal from a case of grenades which exploded close to him. A long carpenter's nail was seen lying in the lung, close to the hilum, and 60 millimetres from the anterior chest wall.

It had been there six months and was causing no symptoms or trouble of any kind, nor was there any sign of reaction on the part of the lung or pleura. It was successfully extracted by operation. N. B.

A Stretcher Carrier for Radiological Examination.—P. de Ferry and Jaubert de Beaujeu (*Arch. d'Élect. Méd.*, Nov., 1918).—
In an advanced medical formation it is necessary to avoid all loss of time, to reduce the sufferings and fatigue of patients to a minimum, and to manage with a restricted personnel. The authors describe their use of two upright supports on which the stretcher is placed direct for examination of the patient, without any difficulty of moving him from stretcher to table and back. By this means a patient can be brought into the operating theatre after all preparation and after X-ray examination without ever being moved from the stretcher on which he is carried into hospital. N. B.

Intermittent Currents of Low Tension in the Treatment and Electro-diagnosis of Nerve Degeneration.—F. Morin (*Arch. d'Electricité Méd.*, Nov., 1918).—The author in this, his final and posthumous publication, completes the observations made by him in an article in the same Journal in Dec., 1914.

His method of measurement is, first of all, to find the milliamperage of current necessary to provoke a little more than a minimum contraction when using a metronome interrupter, then with the same intensity of current to find what duration of stimulus is needed, with the Leduc interrupter, to obtain approximately the same contraction.

The result of treatment in the cases quoted, nerve lesions due to gun shot wounds, and one case of Landry's paralysis, show in the main

that with serious nerve injury and R.D. a prolonged stimulus is needed—of the order of ·08 sec.—equivalent to the chronaxie of the muscle of the snail. All the cases improved, and the duration time was reduced towards ·001 sec. in each instance.

Two other points were noted incidentally ; the effect of cold, and of fatigue as a result of treatment, in prolonging the necesssary duration time.

In all cases Na Cl and the — ve electrode was applied to the wound scar, and the author remarks that it is almost banal to mention the rapid resolution of scar tissue that was observed. He considers that the Leduc current is generally superior to rhythmic galvanism in treatment of these conditions, both by result of treatment and by the fact that it provides a measure of the condition at all stages, but that it has the drawback occasionally of rapidly producing fatigue effects. N. B.

Surgery, Gynecology and Obstetrics (October, 1919, p. 325).—Emil Beck and G. W. Warner publish an article entitled " The Intentional Removal of Skin and other Tissues overlying Deep-seated Inoperable Cancer, a Necessity for Effective Treatment with X-ray or Radium." The importance of this paper, a preliminary contribution, is that the authors have endeavoured to make an advance in the treatment of what has hitherto been looked upon as quite hopeless conditions. Essentially recognising the fact that superficial malignant growths respond well to radiotherapy, and recognising also that after an operation, if the wound is closed, the skin, the fat, and the subcutaneous tissues offer a very effectual filter to radiation, Beck recommends, in these hopeless cases of malignant disease, secondary or otherwise, after removing as much as is possible, not to close the wound but to leave it entirely open, and to apply to the whole area either X rays or radium, and to allow the wound to heal under this treatment. His argument being that he thus converts a deep seated growth into a superficial one.

The physical properties of radiations are discussed, and the comparative density of different thicknesses of aluminium are compared with that of skin, fat, and muscle.

The report of a few cases thus treated, with the photographic illustrations, is such as to give rise to thought. All the cases quoted are such as would be looked upon as past the aid of any method of treatment, such as had nothing except misery and death to look forward to. The method of treatment indicated is one which may have great possibilities.

C. T. H.

Roentgenological Diagnosis of Cholecystitis and Adhesions.—LEWIS J. FRIEDMAN, M.D. (*New York Medical Journal*, Feb. 8th, 1919).

—Acute cholecystitis is seldom met with in private X-ray practice. The chronic type is the one most commonly referred for diagnosis, because of its resemblance to lesions of the gastric, pyloric, and duodenal regions.

It is clinically impossible to state definitely whether there are stones in the gall bladder or not. With modern perfected technic, gall stones can be shown in about 85 per cent. of cases. It is only when the gall bladder is diseased that an increase of density of this organ can be brought out. If several plates be super-imposed, and held before a strong diffused light, the bladder outline may be traced. Anatomically, the gall bladder lies in very close relationship to the first part of the duodenum. From an analysis of two illustrative cases given, as well as from similar ones coming under his observation, the author concludes that definite evidence of chronic cholecystitis can be inferred from the presence of the following landmarks: Defect in the prepyloric region due to spasm, distortion or defect in the first and second portion of the duodenum (eliminating organic lesion), and increase in the density of the gall bladder area. The presence of choleliths can be assumed in practically every case of chronic cholecystitis. J. McK.

On a Case in which a Machine-gun Bullet was Embedded in the Wall of the Heart, With observations on the cardiac movements of the bullet during systole and diastole, and the translation movements during respiration and changes in bodily position.—C. J. BOND, E. V. PHILLIPS, and W. JEVONS (*Jour. of the R.A.M.C.*, Sept., 1918, pp. 229-235, with 7 diagrams).—Taking advantage of a case

with a bullet embedded in the heart wall, these observers have recorded :—

1. The effect of alterations in bodily position on the position of the heart.

2. The effect of respiratory movements on the bullet shadow.

3. The intrinsic movement of the bullet during cardiac systole and diastole.

R. W. A. S.

A New System of Localisation and Extraction of Foreign Bodies in the Brain: A Preliminary Note.—J. N. FERGUSSON (*Brit. Jour. of Surg.*, Jan., 1919, pp. 409-417, with 6 Figs.).—For the description of this ingenious device a perusal of the original article is necessary. R. W. A. S.

Some Cases of Urinary Disease in Children.—R. THOMPSON (*Brit. Jour. of Children's Dis.*, Nos. 172-174, Vol. XV., pp. 81-91).—Discussing renal calculi, the author states that these may occur at an early age, and that for the ultimate cause of their formation we may have to go back to very early life. From a large number of autopsies at Guy's Hospital an interesting fact becomes apparent. In the pelvis and kidney substance, especially the former, uric acid, sand, concretions, or even very small calculi, may be found after death from marasmus, or an acute infectious disease, with which considerable wasting has been associated. The author believes it is not unreasonable to assume that these concretions may be the origin of larger stones and the formation of definite calculi.

It is pointed out that the epiphyses of the transverse processes of the lumbar vertebræ may not appear either at the same time or symmetrically, and if there be only one present, perhaps in the third or fourth lumbar vertebra, and there be symptoms of renal colic, a wrong diagnosis may be made unless an opaque catheter be passed. R. W. A. S.

Severe Radio-dermatitis after three Examinations.—CHAILLOUS and LAQUERRIÈRE (*Jour. de Radiol. et d'Elect.*, Dec., 1918, pp. 103-105).—This condition followed on three radiographic examinations, lasting in all nearly an hour, and persisted in spite of various treatments for nearly three years.

At the end of that time, intravenous injections of solutions of copper sulphate of the strength 1 in 200 and copper sulphate ointment were tried. In two and a half months the ulcerated area had healed, the abscesses no longer recurred, pain almost completely disappeared, and the pain on movement was relieved.

These observers think that the almost specific action of the copper sulphate in this case is worth recording. R. W. A. S.

CORRESPONDENCE.

To the Editors of ARCHIVES OF RADIOLOGY AND ELECTROTHERAPY.

SIRS,

It may interest Members of the B.A.R.P. to know that the effort we are making to place radiology and electrology on a proper footing in this country has its counterpart abroad. A recent number of *La Radiologia Medica* gives an account of the movement in Italy, of which the following is a precis :—

The Council of the Italian Society of Radiology, at its meeting at Genoa in May, discussed the necessity of a proper recognition of the position of radiology in any scheme of University reform. There is no field of medicine or surgery in which radiology does not provide valuable assistance in diagnosis or treatment. This had begun to be recognised in war; it is just as true in peace. The technique is complicated, the possibilities are complex and far-reaching, the dangers are also great. Proper teaching in the essentials of the science should therefore be given to all students of medicine, so that the average medical man can have an adequate understanding of the scope and utility of radiology, and so call it to his aid at the proper time for the benefit of his patients. But this teaching will not be provided by the scheme propounded by "Riforma Medica," which combines in a small group of subjects, subsidiary to the general studies, a number of branches of science which bear to each other little or no relation : serumtherapy, dietetics, meccanotherapy, electrotherapy, radiology, etc. Further, it is suggested that this impracticable conglomeration of subjects should be taken in the third year of studies, when the students have acquired not even the elements of diagnosis, and cannot possibly appreciate the diagnostic or clinical possibilities of the methods shown to them. Although it is already burdened with divers subjects, this Council considers that the last two years curriculum could yet be expanded to include a sufficient course of instruction in radiology, provided such course is eminently practical and wastes no time on useless theoretical lectures. In any case it is convinced that radiology must be taught efficiently and adequately by practical radiologists, and as a necessary and compulsory part of the medical curriculum, and has charged the holders of the existing Chairs of Radiology to press the matter on the attention of the Ministry of Public Instruction.

At the same time Professor Ghilarducci has presented a memorial to the Faculty of Medicine of Rome, showing with clear and strong statement of the arguments the necessity of an improved position for radiology and electrology in the University studies, and urging the Council of the Faculty to express an opinion in favour of the necessary reform.

Allusion is made to the strong movement already on foot in America and England with the movement gaining impetus and spreading to other countries, the time cannot be far distant when radiology and electrology shall come into their own.

Yours, etc.,

NOEL H. M. BURKE.

Woodhall Spa,

Oct. 7th, 1919.

"PROTECTIVE SANDWICH."

To the Editors of ARCHIVES OF RADIOLOGY
AND ELECTROTHERAPY.

SIRS,

For some considerable time I have been employing a very simple and most efficacious form of mask when treating certain skin areas with radium or X rays, and I can recommend it to others. It consists of three layers, viz., lead, cardboard, and Z.O. plaster, in this order. The lead is rolled to a thickness of about 1 mm.; the cardboard, about the same thickness, is glued on to this lead, and then on to the cardboard is glued the wrong side of the Z.O. plaster, so as to leave the adhesive side exposed. This proves a very neat "sandwich," and can be cut into any size, and can be moulded into any shape. All that is necessary is to gently heat the plaster and to apply it to the part. It adheres firmly, and does not move if properly adjusted. It has proved of especial use in treating rodent ulcers of the face.

Yours faithfully,

HERSCHEL HARRIS.

Sydney, N.S.W., Australia.

August 25th, 1919.

PUBLICATIONS RECEIVED.
Book.

Electrical Treatment. By WILFRED HARRIS. Third Edition, 1919. Cassell & Co., Ltd.

Journals.

American Journal of Electrotherapeutics and Radiology, Sept., 1919.

Archives d'Electricite Médicale et de Physiotherapie, Oct., 1919.

British Journal of Dermatology and Syphilis, July-Sept., 1919.

Bulletin of the Johns Hopkins Hospital, Oct., 1919.

Bulletins et Mémoirs de la Société de Radiologie Médicale de France, Oct., 1919.

Gaceta Médica Catalana, Oct. 31st, 1919.

Good Health, Nov., 1919.

Hospitalstidende, Oct. 15th, 22nd, 29th, 1919.

Il Policlinico, Aug. 15th ; Sept. 1st, 15th; Oct. 1st, 15th, 1919.

Journals—*continued.*

International Journal of Orthodontia and Oral Surgery, Oct., 1919.

Journal of Cutaneous Diseases, Oct., 1919.

Journal de Radiologie et d'Electrologie, Nov., 1919.

Le Radium, July-Aug., 1919.

Medical Journal of Australia, Aug. 23rd, 30th ; Sept. 6th, 13th, 27th ; Oct. 4th, 1919.

Medical Science, Nov., 1919.

Modern Medicine, Oct., 1919.

Norsk Mag. for Lægevidenskaben, Nov., 1919.

Proceedings of the Royal Society of Medicine, Aug., 1919.

Rivista Italiana di Neuropatologia, Psichiatria ed Elettroterapia, Aug., Sept., Oct., 1919.

Sunic Record, No. 9.

Surgery, Gynæcology, and Obstetrics, Nov., 1919.

Ugeskrift for Læger, Nov. 6th, 13th, 20th, 1919.

NOTICES.

ARCHIVES OF RADIOLOGY AND ELECTROTHERAPY is published monthly.

The index for each volume, which ends with the May number, is supplied with the June number of each year.

Communications to the Editors should be, addressed to " ROBERT KNOX, M.D., 38, Harley Street, W. 1."

Communications and illustrations from American contributors may be sent to Messrs. REBMAN COMPANY, 141-145, West Thirty-sixth Street, New York City.

All radiographs and photographs must be originals, and must not have been previously published. Drawings should be supplied on separate paper.

Owing to the scarcity of paper the Publishers are reluctantly compelled—as a temporary war measure—to reduce the number of free reprints of Papers to twenty-five.

Annual Subscriptions, payable in advance, 30/- including postage. Single copies, 3/- (postage 2d.) Single numbers and back numbers can be supplied on application.

Vol. XXIV—No. 8   JANUARY, 1920   No. 234

ARCHIVES OF RADIOLOGY AND ELECTROTHERAPY

THE OFFICIAL ORGAN OF THE

BRITISH ASSOCIATION OF RADIOLOGY AND PHYSIOTHERAPY

Editors.

ROBERT KNOX, M.D., Hon. Radiologist, King's College Hospital.

E. P. CUMBERBATCH, B.M., M.R.C.P., Medical Officer in Charge, Electrical Department, St. Bartholomew's Hospital.

SIDNEY RUSS, D.Sc., Physicist to the Middlesex Hospital.

IN COLLABORATION WITH

A. E. BARCLAY (Manchester); BELOT (Paris); H. MARTIN BERRY (London); W. H. BRAGG (London), N. BURKE (Woodhall Spa); J. BURNET (Edinburgh); W. J. S. BYTHELL (Manchester); J. T. CASE (Battle Creek, U.S.A.); A. ST. GEORGE CAULFEILD (London); H. A. COLWELL (London); FOVEAU DE COURMELLES (Paris); GUNZBURG (Antwerp); HALL-EDWARDS (Birmingham); HARET (Paris); HAUCHAMPS (Brussels); F. HERNAMAN-JOHNSON (London); W. F. HIGGINS (Teddington); THURSTAN HOLLAND (Liverpool); HURST (London); KLYNENS (Antwerp); LAQUERRIERE (Paris); LAZARUS-BARLOW (London); LEDUC (Nantes); ALEXANDER MACKAY (Edinburgh); REGINALD MORTON (London); HARRISON ORTON (London); W. OVEREND (St. Leonards-on-Sea); PFAHLER (Philadelphia); C. E. S. PHILLIPS (London); GEORGE PIRIE (Dundee); HOWARD PIRIE (Montreal); A. W. PORTER (London); R. W. A. SALMOND (London); WERTHEIM SALOMONSON (Amsterdam); S. SLOAN (Glasgow); SOMERVILLE (Glasgow); W. C. STEVENSON (Dublin); W. J. TURRELL (Oxford); HUGH WALSHAM (London); ROBT. WILSON (Montreal).

DIPLOMA NOTICE, vide p. 252.

PERIHILAR BRONCHOPNEUMONIC PSEUDOLOBAR PHTHISIS.

By WALKER OVEREND, M.A., M.D.

IN perihilar tubercle—sometimes incorrectly called hilus tuberculosis—the foci of disease may be (a) small in size, disseminated and *nodular* ; (b) they may be larger and *nodal*, producing a characteristic dappled appearance on the radiogram. In some instances the nodal shadows become aggregated and then combined by intervening less dense opacities, consisting of condensed tissue often containing dilated and thickened tubes ; (c) in others there are extensive tracts of *pseudolobar* homogeneous consolidations approaching in aspect those present in pneumonia and pneumonic phthisis. If the lesion is on the right side its evolution may be influenced by the position of the small upper fissure, and the type might well be termed interlobar pneumonic. The distinction is probably immaterial ; at least it may be justified at certain phases of the disease only.

Perihilar disease, whether uni- or bilateral, may be secondary to apical lesions of a *minor* or *latent* character which for some reason have been reactivated ; very often, however, both apices, so far as clinical and radiological examination can ascertain, are normal.   Occasionally there may be impaired breath sounds, granular or interrupted breathing at one apex with some diminution of one supraclavicular isthmus.   But these are, generally, merely the persistent signs of a *latent* or *arrested* tubercle, and are no criteria of activity whatever.   In the perihilar types, which show tracts of pseudolobar disease, symptoms such as cough, pyrexia, emaciation and anorexia may become conspicuous before the diagnostic signs appear, or such radiographic shadows may be associated with quiet phases of the disease when both clinical signs and symptoms become minimal.   Of the five examples described below, No. 5 might be classed as bronchopneumonic *nodal*, although in certain situations in the left lung the shadowing is now quite uniform.

1. Amelia R——, æt. 35.   *Clinical:* in the right upper lobe percussion note impaired, a few crepitations.   In the left upper lobe expansion diminished: there is tubular breathing above, becoming amphoric near the nipple : cardiac apex not found.   *Radiogram 1:* on the left side there are many rounded opacities (bronchopneumonic nodal), connected by less dense indurations : an irregular cavitation extends as far as the supraclavicular apex,   On the right side a narrow band of disconnected induration from the hilum running outwards towards the axilla, and containing small cavities and dilated tubes : the right phrenic leaflet is much higher than the left.   There are a few opacities in the right middle lobe.   The disease on the right is older and becoming arrested.   The right extreme apex is free.   This patient contracted influenza during the winter of 1918, with a fatal result.

2. Regina R——, æt 16.   *Clinical:* has suffered from cough for 18 months : expectoration + : tubercle bacilli + : right lung, percussion note impaired : crepitations right apex : harsh breath sounds behind with increased whisper : temperature, 96°–98°.   *Radiogram 2 :* a unilateral bronchopneumonic pseudolobar infiltration, spreading along the right interlobe with irregular excavation (arrows) above and below it, near the hilum.   The lesion extends along the bronchi to the supraclavicular apex, where excavation also has ensued.   The left lung is practically free.   The heart, aorta, and trachea deviated slightly towards the right.

3. James S——, æt. 26 : family history + : cough + : expectoration + : hæmoptysis small, on several occasions : night sweats — : 97·6°–99·6° : Tbc. after several examinations —.   *Physical signs:* indefinite : a few doubtful crepitations observed on two occasions between vertebral border of scapula above the spine and the vertebral column.   Classed B, June, 1917.   *Radiogram 3 :* shows several round bronchopneumonic foci, nodal, outside the right hilum in the interlobar region, with some surrounding induration and thickened tubes or congested vessels running fan-wise towards the axilla.   *Radiological diagnosis :* right interlobar phthisis.   Ten months subsequently re-examined.   *Clinical:* cough + : Tbc. now + : emaciation + : night sweats + : has had an *attack of pleurisy* on right side.   *Radiogram 4 :* there is now a single perihilar cavity (arrows) in the right interlobar region, which is "silent" to the stethoscope and communicates with several bronchi : dilated tubes in the middle lobe surrounded by bands of infiltration apparently becoming fibroid : diminished interspaces on the right, and enlargement of right paratracheal glands.   A thin infiltration towards the right base.

4. Robert C——, æt 40 (10.9.17).   *Clinical:* patient had an attack of rheumatoid arthritis four years ago : now complains of morning cough, with slight expectoration : a small hæmoptysis occurred for the first time four days ago : a few scattered catarrhal sounds in the right lung, but there are *no definite physical signs.*   *Radiogram 5 :* posterior, shows a band of infiltration containing small cavities in the right interlobar area : involvement of the middle lobe: *lateral scoliosis*, convex to the right.   *Diagnosis:* right interlobar phthisis.   *Second examination* (12.3.18).   *Clinical:* crepitations (?) both apices (crackles), distant tubular breathing over right middle lobe : weight slightly increasing.   *Radiogram 6.*   There has been a dissemination from

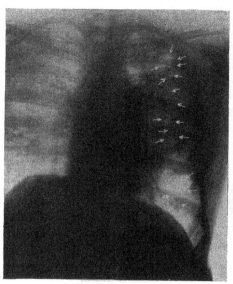

RADIOGRAM 1.

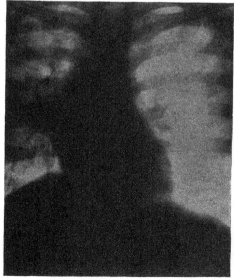

RADIOGRAM 2.

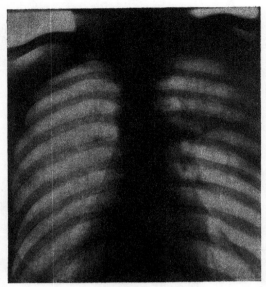

RADIOGRAM 3.

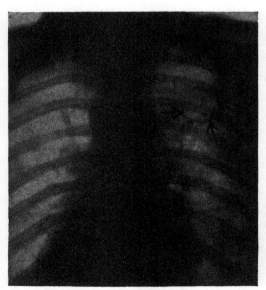

RADIOGRAM 4.

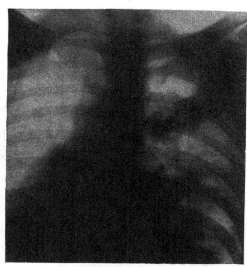

RADIOGRAM 5.

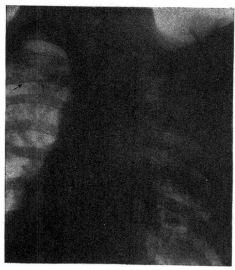

RADIOGRAM 6.

the interlobar cavities, which foci now appear to be undergoing fibroid metamorphosis. The disease has now become unilateral *disseminated fibroid*. The old excavation at left apex is visible. The patient is now following his employment. Scoliosis appears to be frequent in these unilateral forms.

5. Alice W——, æt 20.   *Clinical:* anæmic : cough for six weeks : expectoration scanty : hæmoptysis — : emaciation (?) : night sweats + : dyspnœa + .   The chest is long, emphysematous : crepitations (?) at apex : catarrhal sounds behind : supraclavicular isthmus on each side equal (4½) : Radiogram 7 shows a left perihilar tuberculosis extending to the summit of upper lobe : some left hilar and perihilar excavation : right basal tubercle : two large calcareous opacities (arrows) in right lung, and a small basal pneumothorax (arrows).   Partial pneumothorax as

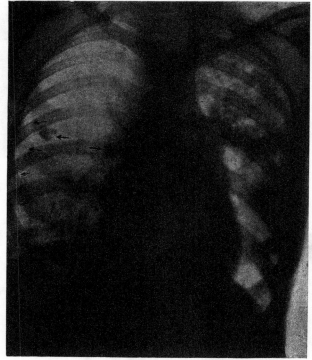

RADIOGRAM 7.

visualised by radiology in quiet tubercle often occurs *in connection with a subpleural calcareous focus,* and it is generally free from fluid.   The condition in the upper left reminds one of the Laennec's grey infiltration, which is due to a caseating lobular chronic bronchopneumonia.

General Remarks.

The above illustrations show that perihilar fibrocaseous tubercle may be almost exclusively unilateral.   If bilateral the pulmonary lesions are not, as a rule, contemporaneous ; one may be subacutely progressive, whilst the other is manifestly quiescent, even retrogressive.   They arise in connection with hilar or perihilar glands on the same side, and may produce either discrete disconnected nodes or broad homogeneous infiltrations. At times the disease may arise from apical lesions—presumably, from their radiological aspect, semi-quiescent — in the same or in the opposite lung, when bacilliferous material, issuing from a cavity, is scattered broadcast throughout the bronchi and fastens upon the perihilar area. During its subsequent evolution, cavities may form in the perihilum, and a second dispersal of aerial foci may proceed from them which may be partial—affecting the diseased side only— or it may be general. In Radiogram 3 the interlobar dissemination is discrete, and probably has spread by way of the lymphatic tracts. The evacuation of the deep perihilar cavity (Radiogram 4) is not yet complete ; but, in this case, there has been up to the present little deposition of foci in adjacent parts of the lung.

The disease advances in the upper lobe towards the axilla ; in the lower lobe towards the costophrenic sulcus, finally, in each case, producing a cuneate tract of infiltration with its apex situated at the hilum. In the left upper lobe, on account of the absence of the superior fissure, the opacity may be fan-shaped (Radiogram 1). As the lesion marches centrifugally it becomes more and more superficial, until in certain areas the characteristic tuberculous râle becomes audible to the stethoscope. In the earlier stages, when symptoms form the chief clinical feature, post-tussive inspiratory crepitations may be audible (a) *at the sides* of the chest, between the axillary lines above the level of the nipple; (b) *in front*, on the left side in particular, in the parasternal area within the second and third interspaces, and (c) *behind*, at the level of the hila or a little higher, between the vertebral border of the scapula and the spine, also (d) along the interlobe on the right, or (e) at the base of the lung. Mistakes may be made by the clinician, who thinks only of apical crepitations, and does not auscultate the fissures, the axilla, and the base. When the disease progresses towards the summit, crepitations (œdema ?) are occasionally conducted towards the apex, before any radiological evidence is forthcoming as to the existence of disease in that area. Pleuritic pains in the axillary regions, and right basal effusion, are not infrequent. The latter is more likely to occur when the middle and lower lobes are invaded. Basal effusions may be met with in middle age, which recur several times after tapping, and may conceal perihilar discrete foci in the middle and lower lobes. At this period of life they may be accompanied by serious cardiac embarrassment and alarming dyspnœa, which necessitate a partial evacuation of the fluid.

Perihilar bronchopneumonic infiltration, when bilateral, may therefore occupy the wings of the chest, or it may approach the apex in the one, and the base in the other lung ; there may be an obvious protrusion of the middle intermammary region of the chest, especially in women, and the more marked the deformity the more likely is the disease to be semiquiescent or arrested. Such disfigurement may be termed *annular emphysema*. There is a greater tendency in this type to fibrosis and chronicity than in the purely apical variety. The prognosis is more serious in the cavitary forms, and, *cæteris paribus*, the younger the age of the patient; when the foci are small and disconnected, the prospect is brighter than when continuous tracts of infiltration are visible on the radiogram. In the strictly unilateral forms the outlook is also more favourable. Finally, this essentially chronic type appears to be more closely connected with the flat chest (*thorax aplati*, or *paralyticus*), whether congenital or acquired, which, when it becomes emphysematous, still remains practically flat, merely bulging, if at all, in the lower middle and basal parts of the lung.

SPECIAL POINTS IN THE TECHNIQUE FOR THE RADIOGRAPHY OF THE CLAVICLE AND THE LATERAL ASPECT OF THE RIBS FOR THE DETECTION OF INJURIES.

THE radiography of special parts of the body frequently calls for the exercise of ingenuity on the part of the radiographer. When the screen method is used the details of the technique are simplified, for then it is possible to place the part under examination into the most favourable position for radiographing it. The plate is then placed in position, the screen replaced over the plate,

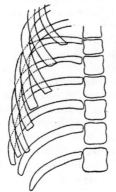
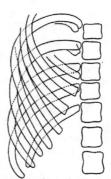

FIG. 1.—Usual A.P. position.　　　　FIG. 2.—Patient tilted as in Fig. 3.

and the exposure is made. It is possible to watch the part during the exposure and so ensure that the part required is X-rayed under the best possible conditions. In the majority of instances this will be found to be the most reliable method. There are, however, workers who prefer to do the radiography with the tube above the patient, or it may be that screening is not possible on account of the condition of the patient; then it may be necessary to work from above.   Screening in these cases may still be possible by means of a fluorescent screen placed under the top of the couch with the fluorescent side

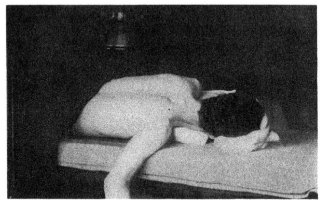

Fig. 3.—Patient tilted to obtain view of anterior portion of ribs as in diagram (Fig. 2).

facing directly downwards.   A mirror set at an angle of 40 degrees will enable the operator to ascertain if the plate is in the proper position.*   Another method which will always ensure the radiography of the correct position is to have a cassette constructed with a central director attached to it.†   The part required

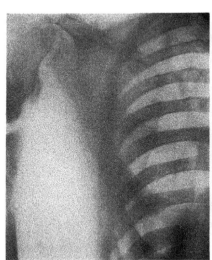

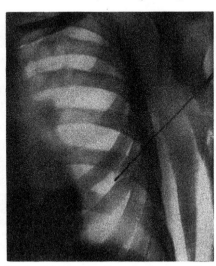

Fig. 4.—Print from radiograph taken with patient in usual A.P. position. Fracture of lateral aspect of the ribs not seen.

Fig. 5.—Print from radiograph of same patient lying on face and tilted as in Fig. 3. Fracture well seen.

* Described by Mr. Gage, ARCHIVES, June, 1917.

† Campion's method of utilizing the central radiation is also very useful, ARCHIVES, Sept., 1918.

is placed over the centre of the plate, the central ray is arranged by means of the director so that it will reach the centre of the plate. The full details of this cassette will be shown in a later communication.

I am indebted to Sister Edmunds, who was in charge of the X-ray depart-

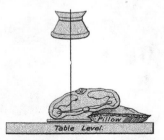

Fig. 6.—Diagram showing direction
of ray for obtaining improved view
of anterior portions of ribs.

ment of the Ruskin Park extension of the 4th London General Hospital, for the drawings and photographs which illustrate the special points in the technique described, and also for the radiograms which show the results obtained by using the technique as described.

The position described for obtaining a view of the lateral aspects of the ribs will be found to be particularly useful in a number of cases. These are

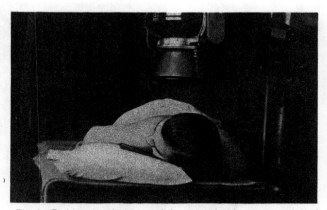

Fig. 7.—Position of patient for whole length of clavicle and sterno-clavicular
articulation.

always troublesome cases with which to deal, and frequently a fracture of the ribs may escape detection if the radiologist depends entirely upon the antero-posterior position alone. All cases of injury to ribs should be, when possible, carefully scrutinised by the screen method in several positions. The oblique position in front of the tube is very useful; the patient can readily be manipulated into the required position for radiographing the part.

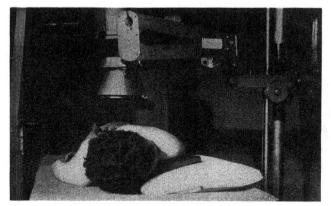

FIG. 7.—Position of patient for whole length of clavicle and sterno-clavicular articulation.

As is shown in the diagrams, it is possible to get the oblique position when using the tube above the patient.

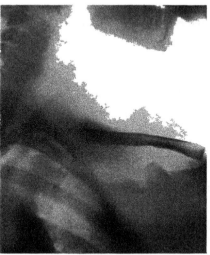

FIG. 8.—Radiograph showing whole length of clavicle, with sterno - clavicular articulation obtained from position (Fig. 7.)

Diagram (Fig. 1) illustrates view of ribs in usual antero-posterior position, patient lying face down and the tube above the table.

If the patient is tilted, as in the photograph (Fig. 3), the view of front ribs obtained is as in diagram (Fig. 2). The advantage of this is obvious, as a much greater length of each front rib is obtained, and a lateral fracture which might easily be missed in position (Fig. 1) would certainly be seen in the position described (Fig. 2).

Prints from radiographs (Figs. 4 and 5) prove this, though the tilt is more particularly useful where there is suspected injury to lower anterior portions of the ribs.

A patient was sent up with a sinus below the axilla. An antero-posterior radiograph was taken (see Fig. 4) with no injury detected. The examination

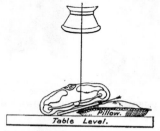

FIG. 9.—Diagram showing direction of ray for obtaining sterno-clavicular articulation.

was repeated with probe in sinus and patient lying on face, tilted as described above, with the satisfactory result shown in print (Fig. 5). Fig. 6 shows the position in cross section.

In radiographs for the whole length of the clavicle, showing sternal articulation, this position is useful, the patient's body being then tilted on the other side, as in photograph (Fig. 7). The radiograph obtained is seen in print (Fig. 8), and when taken stereoscopically this position gives a very good picture.

Diagram (Fig. 9) illustrates this position in cross section.   R. K.

DIPLOMA OF RADIOLOGY AND ELECTROLOGY.

PARTICULARS OF LECTURES TO BE HELD IN LONDON.

The Course of Lectures in Radiology and Electrology qualifying for the examination for the Diploma at Cambridge University will, by arrangement with the Fellowship of Medicine and Post-Graduate Medical Association, be delivered at the Rooms of the Royal Society of Medicine, 1, Wimpole Street, W. 1. The Lectures will be given on Mondays and Wednesdays at 5.30 p.m.

The first Lecture will be delivered by Dr. Turrell, of Oxford, on February 2nd. Subject: "The History of Electrotherapeutics." For those wishing to take the Diploma the fee for the course, Part II, is £15 15s., as already announced in the ARCHIVES, December, 1919, p. 213, with the additional enrolment fee of 10s. 6d. to the Fellowship of Medicine and Post-Graduate Medical Association, but members of the Fellowship Post-Graduate Course are invited to attend any of the lectures advertised. A detailed syllabus will be issued shortly, and all information can be obtained from Miss M. A. Willis, Secretary to the Fellowship of Medicine and Post-Graduate Association, 1, Wimpole Street, London, W. 1. The lectures and practical work in physics will be given at University College, Gower Street, W.C. 1, commencing on February 3rd, at 5.30 p.m.

TWO CASES OF CALCIFIED OVARIAN TUMOURS.

Radcliffe Infirmary and County Hospital, Oxford.

January 22, 1916. Gertrude H., unmarried, age 27. Under Dr. Mallan, and operated on by Mr. A. P. Dodds Parker. Cyst removed, weighing 1 lb. 12 ozs.

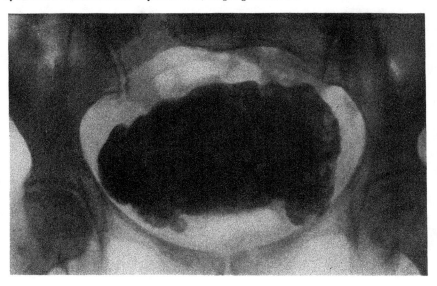

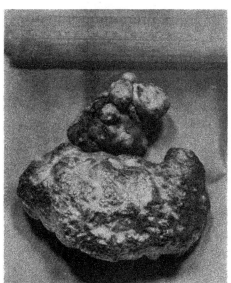

Photo of tumour after removal.

December 12, 1918. Emily H., age 56. Under Dr. Collier. Bladder and kidney were to be X-rayed for ? calculi. Operated on by Mr. Whitelocke, and a very dense calcified ovarian tumour removed. See photo.

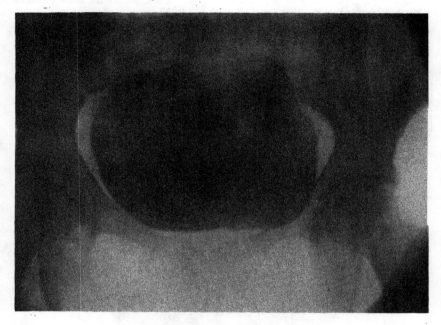

COMMUNICATION ON THE RADIOTHERAPY OF UTERINE FIBROIDS,

With the Results of 400 Cases, personally observed, the Mode of Action of the Treatment, and the Indications for its Adoption.

By Dr. Béclère, Physician to the Hospital of St. Antoine,
Member of the Academy of Medicine.

From *Journal de Radiologie et d'Electrologie*, Tome III, No. 10.

THE Congress of Gynæcology and Obstetrics was held at Brussels on September 27th, 1919. This communication is the sequel and the complement to that which I made in London in August, 1913, at the Twenty-seventh Congress of International Medicine, before the united Sections of Gynæcology and Radiology.

I now bring forward the statistics of sixty cases of uterine fibroids, which, since 1908, I have myself radiated in my private clinic, the progress of which I have been able to follow up more completely and for a longer time than is the case with hospital patients.

At the present time the total number of observations which I have made under these conditions has been raised to nearly 500, but the more recent of these have not undergone the test of time. The statistics, therefore, that I bring before you only refer to 400 cases of fibroid that I have treated, including those reported in London.

This communication comprises three parts: the facts observed, their bearing on the still disputed mode of action of Roentgen rays, the practical indications which result from these observations.

Conditions and Results of Treatment.—In view of the impossibility of reporting in detail on 400 observations, I pass briefly in review the age of the patients treated, the volume of the uterine tumours, the accompanying functional disturbances, the technique and the duration of the treatment, its dangers, its action on the metorrhagias and the dimensions of the fibroids.

Age of the Patients Treated.—From the point of view of age the 400 cases are tabulated as follows :—

Patients of 55 to 56 years	.	.	9	cases
,,	50 to 54 years, inclusive	.	89	,,
,,	45 to 49 ,,	,,	.	130	,,
,,	40 to 44 ,,	,,	.	126	,,
,,	35 to 39 ,,	,,	.	31	,,
,,	30 to 34 ,,	,,	.	15	,,

The percentage is as follows :—

Patients of 50 years and upwards	.	24·5 per cent.
,,	40 to 49 years	.	.	64 ,,
,,	30 to 39 years	.	.	11·5 ,,

Dimensions of the Uterine Fibroids.—In regard to their situation, their dimensions and volume, the 400 cases treated are divisible into two groups, according as they admit of abdominal palpation or not.

The first group, where vaginal examination reveals the uterus more or less enlarged, deformed, and nodulated, but where it does not rise above the symphysis pubis, comprises only 62 cases.

The second group, much more important both in number and interest, comprises the remaining 338 cases, characterised by the fact that the uterine tumour is accessible to abdominal palpation, either alone or combined with vaginal examination, and is raised more or less high above the symphysis pubis.

The following is the percentage of the two groups :—

Intrapelvic fibroids	.	.	.	.	15·5 per cent.
Fibroids admitting of abdominal palpation	84·5 ,,

For the estimation of the volume of the uterine tumour, precise measurements are to be preferred to the comparisons ordinarily used. When the tumour can be palpated it is easy to measure with sufficient accuracy, in centimetres, the distance of its upper extremity from the symphysis pubis ; one can also measure its transverse diameter, and even, in certain cases, the antero-posterior dimensions of the abnormally protruding abdomen. It is important in taking these measurements that the patient should be recumbent on her back, and perfectly flat. It is absolutely essential, moreover, that the bladder should be emptied immediately before the examination.

In the 338 cases in which the tumours were palpable the measurements were made under these conditions. Before the treatment the upper extremity of the uterine tumour was raised above the symphysis pubis:—

From 25 to 30 centimetres in   9 patients, that is, in 2·66 per cent. of the cases.
   ,, 20 to 24   ,,   25 ,,   ,,   7·39   ,,   ,,
   ,, 15 to 19   ,,   51 ,,   ,,   15·88   ,,   ,,
   ,, 10 to 14   ,,   111 ,,   ,,   32·84   ,,   ,,
   ,,   5 to 9   ,,   104 ,,   ,,   30·76   ,,   ,,
   ,,   1 to 4   ,,   38 ,,   ,,   11·29   ,,   ,,

Accompanying Functional Troubles.—In the majority of the patients in question the predominant symptom was more or less copious metorrhagia, more or less prolonged, more or less regular in its appearance. In many cases the loss of blood necessitated the repeated use of the tampon. Many were profoundly anæmic, and in some cases the estimation of hæmoglobin fell below 50 per cent.

On the other hand, in a considerable number of cases the periods maintained, or only slightly exceeded their usual loss. The noticeable size of the uterine tumour, its very apparent prominence, its rapid increase, the compression it exercised on the neighbouring organs, especially on the bladder, necessitating in some cases the frequent use of the catheter, such were the principal reasons which frequently induced the patients to come to me for treatment.

Technique and Duration of Treatment.—As regards technique, I continue to employ the method of weekly séances, and this necessitates the use of moderate doses. For many reasons I prefer this to the method of monthly and intensive radiation, which is preached in Germany, and recommended also in our country by a certain number of radiotherapeutic physicians.

Each weekly séance essentially consists of two successive radiations, the one to the right, the other to the left of the median line of the abdomen, immediately above the horizontal rami of the pubis. Occasionally, when the uterus is retroflected, when the fibroid occupies the cavity of the sacrum or the neck of the uterus, a third radiation is directed on the sacral region. Finally, if the dimensions of the tumour demand it, the surface of the abdomen is divided not only into two, but into three, four, and up to six circular areas which, turn by turn, serve for the port of entrance of the irradiations. Each irradiation is localised to a circular surface of 10 cm. in diameter, by the aid of a cylinder of lead glass opaque to X rays. A thin disc of wood is interposed between the localising cylinder and the abdominal wall ; this depresses, levels the surface, and distributes over a considerable area the weight of the cylinder, and serves, by a gentle compression, to reduce the distance between the ovaries and the skin. The focus of the emission of the rays is, according to the size of the tube in use, from 18 to 22 cm. above

the irradiated surface. The tube used in nearly all the cases was a Thur-
nessen, with a Villard osmo-regulator, furnished with a platinum or iridium
anticathode ; a current of 1 milliampere was used. It has now been replaced
by a Coolidge tube, which, working at the same voltage, allows of the same
dose being given in a third of the time. With this new tube each radiation
lasts a maximum of 5 minutes, instead of the 10 to 15 minutes treatment given
with the former tube. On two points only have I modified my original
technique. For a long time I employed a filter of 1 to 2, then of 2 to 3 mm. of
aluminium, now I employ a filter of 5 mm. of aluminium.

I have to a like extent increased the radiation itself, so as to give, as nearly
as possible, a penetration equivalent to that measured by a spintermeter of an
equivalent spark-gap gradually increased from 15 to 20 cm. As regards the
dose, measured by means of the Sabouraud-Noire reaction, after the rays have
passed through the filter, it usually has not exceeded, at each séance and for
each of the areas treated, 3 Holzknecht units, and at most has reached to
3½ units.

Under these conditions the treatment has demanded :—

4 to 11	séances with	38	patients.
12 to 14	,,	202	,,
15 to 20	,,	109	.,
21 to 30	,,	45	.,
31 to 50	.,	6	.,

Moreover, in 60 per cent. of the cases, the treatment has not required more
than 12 to 14 weekly séances, and has not lasted more than two and a half to
three months.

Dangers of Treatment.—The only real danger of radiotherapy is an excessive
dose provoking cutaneous reactions, either in the form of acute dermatitis or
slow trophic lesions. All the other mishaps of which it has been accused are
imaginary. The cutaneous lesions can be avoided by a good technique and
some experience.

Twice only, when I first started the radiotherapy of fibroids, and these
were the first and third cases I treated, at a time when I was not employing
filters of sufficient thickness, have I failed to prevent the onset of a slow
ulceration of the abdominal wall. One of these cases supervened four, and
the other seven years after the conclusion of the treatment. In the one case
the cure necessitated the excision of a small piece of the injured integument;
the other case was cured in three months by simple poultices. Since then
I have not observed any accidents.

Therapeutic Results.—The two principal results obtained have been the
suppression of the metorrhagia and the reduction in the volume of the tumours.
These results have been obtained without any suffering and without any
change in the patients' mode of life.

Action on the Menorrhagia.—Four times only, to my knowledge, has radiotherapy failed to avoid surgical interference, it was then called for on account

of the profuseness of the hæmorrhage. It seems to me that to-day, with the perfected technique at our disposal, radiotherapy should be capable of dealing with even such cases as these. In every other case the treatment has resulted in the disappearance of the metorrhagia and the suppression of the menstrual function ; and this suppression, when it has been accompanied by the appearance of what are popularly termed the "hot flushes" characteristic of the menopause, has been the signal for the suspension of the séances. In some cases, before their disappearance the metorrhagias have become more profuse. Putting on one side the patients in whom the flow of blood, either on account of its continuity or its irregularity, is indistinguishable from true menstrual hæmorrhage, this table states how many times the periods have appeared after the commencement of the treatment before they have been suppressed.

The menopause has supervened:—

Without fresh appearance of the periods in		3	patients.	
After 1 appearance of the periods in	.	61	,,	
After 2 appearances of the periods in	.	128	,,	
,, 3 ,, ,,	.	89	..	
,, 4 ,, ,,	.	29		
,, 5 ,, ,,	.	9		
,, 6 ,, ,,		8		
,, 7 ,, ,,		5		
,, 8 ,, ,,		4		
,, 10 ,, ,,		2		

Thus, in the majority of cases the periods were suppressed without having appeared more than two or three times after the start of the treatment.

This menopause, prematurely provoked, was usually definitely established. Nevertheless, in 48 patients, it may be in 12 per cent. of the cases treated, the suppression of the periods was only temporary, and they recommenced after a cessation of variable duration. Most often this reappearance took place after some months, in exceptional cases after a year or two years, or even in one case after three years and a half. The recommencement of the treatment resulted after a few séances in establishing a new menopause. In nine of these patients there was another relapse after some months interval, and even in three cases there was a third relapse. But finally, with repetition of the treatment, the menopause was always definitely established.

Action on the Uterine Tumours.—In every case treated not only was the growth of the tumour arrested but its size diminished. In the case of the intrapelvic tumours this decrease in size was often estimated by the tests applied as a third, a half, or two-thirds of the original dimensions; in some cases even the uterus was regarded as having returned to its normal size. The diminution, however, did not admit of measurement. On the other hand, I actually measured with suitable precautions, usually at a séance of instruction, the palpable tumours. In 278 cases, where the results were accurately noted, I found, at the end of the treatment, a lowering of the upper limit of the fibromatous uterus from the symphysis pubis, as indicated in the following table:—

From	1 to 2	centimetres in	12	patients.
,,	3 to 4	,	42	,,
,,	5 to 6	,	73	,,
,,	7 to 8	,,	82	,,
,,	9 to 10	,,	52	,,
,,	11 to 12	,,	26	,,
,,	13 to 14	,,	10	,,
,,	16	,	1	,,

The reduction of the transverse dimensions was not less than that of the vertical dimensions, and, in those cases where the abdomen was very prominent, I have noticed a very appreciable diminution of its antero-posterior diameter.

Attention ought certainly to be drawn to this remarkable decrease in the size of the tumour, it is so marked and so rapid ; it is an actual resolution of the tumour.

This reduction in the size of these uterine tumours commences with the first séances, it is appreciable usually at the third, perhaps even at the second séance. Week by week the upper limit progressively recedes to the symphysis pubis. In the more favourable cases it recedes about a centimetre a week.

The Mode of Action of the Treatment.—According to current opinion Roentgen rays, in the radiotherapy of uterine tumours, act exclusively on the ovaries ; they bring about a " dry castration " as the result of which the fibroids decrease in size, in the same way as they diminished after the surgical castration extolled by Hegar and Battey. This opinion prevails in Germany, and from thence is propagated abroad.

Nevertheless, in France, where the radiotherapy of uterine fibroids originated in 1904, Foveau de Courmelles, who was the first to publish a communication on this subject, together with a number of other medical radiotherapists, including Bordier, Laquerriere, Guilliminot, Jaugeas, Haret, Beaujard, Ledoux-Lebard, d'Hallum, and others whose names I have forgotten, rightly remarked that the reduction in size of fibroids treated by radiotherapy occurred earlier, and to a more marked degree, than the reduction which occurred as the result of the menopause. They also showed that this reduction took place before the periods were suppressed. Wetterer, of Mannheim, made similar observations. Moreover, all these authors are agreed that the Roentgen rays have a direct action on the fibroids apart from their action on the ovaries.

In regard to this my observations not only confirm theirs, but, unless I am mistaken, this method of weekly séances and the taking of measurements at each séance, affords such a mass of precise evidence as to admit of no doubt that in the first instance radiotherapy acts directly on the fibroids. To these incontestable proofs I would add one other, not less capable of demonstration. I have seen radiotherapy effect an important reduction in the size of the palpable fibroids of three patients, whose tumours continued to increase for some years after the cessation of their natural menopause.

To sum up, the radiotherapy of uterine fibroids is one of the most important of the uses of X rays in the treatment of neoplasms. Its principal *rôle* is to induce the destruction and disappearance of the neoplastic cellular elements of which the fibromata consist; this is the direct effect of this form of treatment and is the earliest manifestation of its action.

It is, however, nearly always necessary to continue the radiations up to the point of the destruction of the normal cellular elements of the primitive ovarian follicles. It is on this point that the menstruation affords valuable information.

When the treatment is suspended after the cessation of the periods and the appearance of the hot flushes which characterise the menopause, the uterine tumours usually continue to decrease, sometimes much more slowly than during the treatment.

But if, after a more or less long interval the periods reappear, this return is very frequently accompanied by a revival of the activity of the fibroid, and it again increases in size. This increase in size, according to many convincing observations, even precedes the return of the periods, but is itself preceded by the premature disappearance of the hot flushes. The ovary is a gland of internal secretion and a trophic centre of the whole genital apparatus ; it consequently exercises a very important stimulating action on the development of neoplasms of the uterine muscular substance. It is for this reason that I recommend that patients, especially those below the menopause age, should not wait until the periods return before they resume treatment, but that they should submit themselves for a fresh examination if the hot flushes prematurely cease. In a similar manner the discovery that the uterine tumour has increased in size is an indication for the immediate resumption of the treatment.

Indications for Treatment.—In the treatment of fibroids the field of action of radiotherapy depends on whether it is regarded as a means of sterilising the ovaries, or whether it is regarded as a means of destroying the neoplastic elements of the tumour.

In the eyes of those holding the first opinion radiotherapy is principally, and almost exclusively, called for in the treatment of the metorrhagia caused by small fibroids occurring in women over forty years of age.

In all the other cases they prefer extirpation, except when surgical interference is contraindicated for some such reason, as age, obesity, bad general state of health, extreme anæmia, affections of the heart, aorta, lungs, liver, or kidneys, old or recent phlebitis, etc. ; in such cases they allow that radiotherapy is a justifiable experiment and a last resort. As a matter of fact, in all such cases where surgical interference is for one or other of these reasons contraindicated radiotherapy brings about a cure.

The results obtained have greatly enlarged the list of indications for radiotherapy in the treatment of fibroids.

I hope that I have shown you that radiotherapy acts directly on the fibroids, arresting their development and leading to a reduction in their size, that it is as efficacious before as after forty years of age, that it is as efficacious on the large as on the small fibroids, that it is as efficacious when the courses are normal as when there is metorrhagia.

I ought to add that the details and technique of this method of treatment, still undergoing change and improvement, have long ago reached a high degree of perfection. I do not ignore that therapeutic successes, obtained more rapidly than those in these statistics, perhaps in an extraordinarily short time, have been obtained. May we not look forward to arriving at the time, in the near future, when every medical radiotherapist will be able to obtain similar results? Moreover, I believe that I am justified in this general conclusion:

Apart from certain conditions, which imperatively call for surgical interference, radiotherapy is applicable to all uterine fibroids.

ROENTGEN-RAY TREATMENT OF A CASE OF EARLY ACROMEGALY.

By J. H. Douglas Webster, M.D., M.R.C.P., Ed.

Hon. Radiographer, Manchester Ear Hospital; late Radiographer, No. 29 General Hospital, B.M.F. ; late Officer in charge, X-Ray Dept., Nell Lane Military Hospital, Manchester.

The Roentgen-ray treatment of exophthalmic goitre has advanced to an assured position in the last few years. By irradiation sclerotic changes can be produced in the thyroid, as subsequent operation in some cases has proved ; and the clinical results in the large majority of cases are so excellent that it has become superior to any alternative method of treatment in its " speed, safety and agreeableness."

In acromegaly, however, the Roentgen treatment at present rests almost entirely on a theoretical basis. But it should be eminently a disease suitable for Roentgentherapy, especially in its early stages, when the anterior lobe of the pituitary would show merely a simple chromophil hyperplasia, and before secondary tumour-like formation, local pressure damage, and much skeletal change have been produced.

I was encouraged to begin Roentgen treatment of the following case through some previous knowledge of acromegaly (its pathology I discussed briefly in my M.D. thesis (1907)) and through success in my first cases of the X-ray treatment of exophthalmic goitre in 1911-12.

The patient, N. H., aged 28, a barmaid, unmarried, first came under observation in February, 1913. She complained of severe headache, attacks of " queer feelings," pains in the hands, and amenorrhœa. The amenorrhœa and headache began about four years before : about three years before she had first begun to require larger sizes of boots and gloves. For the last two years not a day had been free from headache : for the four months before consulting me it had been continuous and she said, "almost maddening" in violence at times. She had consulted six or seven doctors in a Midland town, and taken a large variety of blood tonics and headache remedies without avail.

She had had no previous illnesses of importance.

Her mother was alive and well: father died early from heart disease. One sister died of phthisis, age 26. Two brothers alive and well.

PRESENT CONDITION (Feb. 16th, 1913).

The headache is chiefly in the right forehead and temple, also at the vertex, worse on lying down usually, sometimes appearing to waken from sleep. The right eye often pains if used for near work. Her temper has changed; she has become moody and irritable, with fits of depression. "Queer feelings" come over her, a general feeling of formication, then a "wave" passing up to the head and neck, which feel full almost to bursting, passing off with free perspiration, the whole lasting only a few minutes. (I have witnessed two such attacks. The pulse was not altered. During the attack she suffers from a paralysing sensation of dread. These are probably the "vaso-vagal" attacks described by Gowers. The possibility of "uncinate fits" was considered, but she had noticed no numbness of hands during an attack, nor any smell or taste aura.) She has had as many as five attacks of this kind daily; they began six months previously and averaged two or three a week. She has had occasional severe epistaxis, being wakened from sleep once by this.

Height, 5 ft. 5 in. Weight, 13 st. 5 lb. Weight used to be about 10 st.

She is a typical acromegalic in an early stage: the facial pallor, lower jaw, nostrils, eyelids, and hands are all characteristic. Hair is luxuriant, thicker than before. Skin moist: no dermatographia. Temperature, 97·4 F.

Head, 18 cm. long, 16 cm. broad, height from external meatus 21cm. Teeth oppose at the back, lower incisors project, and spacing present. Tongue large. No post-nasal protrusion. Hands, circumference at metacarpo-phalangeal joint 22·6 cm. right, 22·4 left; breadth 10. right, 9·8 left. Maximum circumference of mid-finger, right 8·0 cm., left 7·6 cm.

Blood pressure, systolic, 100-105 mm. Hg. Blood, 90 per cent. Hb. Eosinophiles 3 per cent. Pulse 75-85. No kyphosis, nor evident enlargement of heart, liver or spleen. Eyes, right eye exophthalmic, whole right forehead is protuberant. Distant and near sight satisfactory. Both optic discs show well marked papillitis. Fields of vision : right eye shows considerable temporal retraction for white, and great irregular contraction in colour fields. Left eye, some temporal colour contraction.

Reflexes : right knee jerk unduly brisk, left normal.

Glandular symptoms. Carbohydrate tolerance, no diabetes present, and 300 gm. sugar (over ½ lb) produced no glycosuria. Thyroid enlarged, particularly right lobe. Amenorrhœa for the last four years. No adrenal symptoms (pigmentation, etc). Thermic reaction to anterior lobe injection was not tested. Radiographs showed enlargement of the sella turcica to 2·2 cm. by 1·6 in depth. (Average 1·5 by 1 cm., Cushing, *loc. cit.*)

Radiographs of the hands show slight phalangeal tufting and exostosis: most of the enlargement being, as usual, in the soft tissues.

TREATMENT.

The patient was advised that her illness was a serious one, and appeared to be progressive, and that the best treatments were operative or X-ray applications. Absolutely refusing to consider operation, irradiations were commenced.

She had in all 16 treatments, with hard filtered rays from temporal and fronto-temporal areas, the first 11 at weekly intervals, then fortnightly, latterly at monthly or longer periods.

The effect was remarkable. The severe headache was rapidly relieved, and soon entirely disappeared. The "queer feelings" almost entirely left her: from two or three weekly they dropped to about one a month. The irritability and depression almost completely left her. She lost about half-a-stone in weight. The most striking changes were in the eyes, the optic discs returned practically to the normal, while the fields of vision (especially for red) greatly enlarged. The right eye still presented some irregular contraction, chiefly inferior temporal. Apart from one or two bromide powders there was no treatment beyond the irradiation.

LATER HISTORY.

The patient removed and was lost sight of, till she was heard of again, after nearly two years, from Liverpool; her condition, subjectively and objectively, had become aggravated again, and I had the opportunity of being present when Professor Thelwall Thomas operated on her on February 3rd, 1915, by the naso-sphenoidal route.

COMMENTS.

The case in 1913 was an early progressive one, but evidently not early enough for arrest to be attained with the one course of treatment, and there were already mixed signs—it was a dyspituitarism, for the predominant signs were those of hyperpituitarism, but some due to infundibular under-activity were present. For a succinct recent account of the various structure and functions of the pituitary and its pathology Schäfer's "Endocrine Organs," 1916, pp. 74-117, may be referred to. Harvey Cushing has given a detailed analysis (*loc. cit.*). The complicated possibilities of present or past increased or diminished activity of one or of both lobes, together with the presence or absence of local pressure phenomena, are very numerous and difficult to classify; and the complexity of the subject is increased when widespread glandular changes co-exist. What the *essential* factor in the production of a pituitary giant or an acromegalic is still eludes our analysis, but for polyglandular cases at least some general developmental, nervous or chemical cause or causes must be at work, perhaps similar in nature or mode of action to whatever binds the chromaffin system together in health.

In acromegaly, as in exophthalmic goitre, "formes frustres" are met with; similarly, in recently progressive cases under treatment, it will often be found a matter requiring careful consideration when to stop treatment—when a sufficiently approximate balance has been established between hyper- and hypo-activity of the gland. Specially uncertain must this be in the case of the complex hypophysis; and in its case the matter is also more complex in that the simple chromophil hyperplasia causing the skeletal overgrowth tends to a secondary chromophope angio-sarcomatous tumour formation, the local pressure symptoms of which might benefit by irradiation, even though there were no longer any hyperpituitarism present. Thus, in late cases of acromegaly, as in other pituitary tumours, irradiation may be of benefit; but it is in the very early progressive cases that the best results may be confidently expected.

I have only been able to find two references in the literature to cases similarly treated. (There are others in which pituitary tumours have been irradiated with benefit.)

Gramenga treated a case by X rays directed from the palate, for an hour twice a month. The case was a very advanced one, a woman aged 45: amenorrhœa had been present for 13 years. After eight treatments headache had disappeared, and the ophthalmoscopic signs had become almost normal. In some months the patient returned, and again a good result followed. Still later the patient returned, but in such a condition that further irradiation was impossible.

Béclère has reported briefly a case of a giantess, aged 16. Operation had been proposed to relieve her headache and severe visual troubles, but irradiation weekly for ten weeks from fronto-temporal areas gave her total relief from the headache, and tripled the field of vision of the right eye in two months.

Williams has reported a case of pituitary tumour treated beneficially by irradiation: a woman aged 37, with severe headaches, nausea, dizziness and vomiting, two months diplopia, and constant "awful feeling." There was "slight haziness of the optic papilla, the arteries of which were very small." The headaches disappeared and there was general improvement.

Terrien and Darier have articles on visual troubles of pituitary origin which I have not been able to verify.

At Professor Forssell's Roentgen clinic, at the Serafimer Hospital at Stockholm, a few cases of acromegaly have had irradiation with benefit, but no report has been made on them yet.

The subject obviously is one on which many further observations are required. In any case it is not to be expected that pituitary gigantism and acromegaly will yield so readily to irradiation as exophthalmic goitre ; but they should theoretically be the most likely pituitary conditions to do so ; and results such as the above suggest that in Roentgen irradiation there may yet be found a safe and permanent means of arrest of processes which unchecked can produce such profound and widespread destructive changes.

REFERENCES.

Béclère, A. "The Radio-therapeutic Treatment of Tumours of the Hypophysis, Gigantism and Acromegaly." *Arch. Roent. Ray*, 1909-10, XIV, 142.

Cushing, H. "The Pituitary Body and its Disorders." (Lippincott), 1912.

*Darier, A. "Optic Nerve Atrophy, Hypophysis and Roentgen Rays." *Amer. Jour. Ophth.*, St. Louis, 1916, XXXIII, 144-152.

Gramenga, A. "Un Cas d'Acromégalie traité par la radiotherapie." *Rev. Neurolog.*, 1909, XVII, 15.

Schäfer, E. A. (Sir). "The Endocrine Organs." (Longmans), 1916.

'Terrien, F. "Le traitement par les rayons X des troubles visuels d'origine hypophysaire." *Arch. d'Ophth.*, Paris, 1916, V, 257-85.

Webster, J. H. D. "A Case of Unilateral Cerebral Hyperplasia with Acromegaly . . . and . . . Unilateral Gigantism." *Jour. Path. and Bact.*, XII, 1908

Williams. T. A. "Case of Subsidence through Radiotherapy of a Neoplasm in the Region of the Hypophysis Cerebri." *N. Y. Jour. Nerv. and Ment. Dis.*, XLII, 159, 1915.

*Reference not personally confirmed.

THE FETISH OF THE CENTRAL RAY.

By MARTIN BERRY, M.D., Captain R.A.M.C.

Radiologist, Royal Herbert Military Hospital, Woolwich, etc.

SUFFICIENT has been written on the subject of localization during the past five years to fill many large books. It is not the intention of the present writer to add appreciably to the bulk of this material, but merely to indicate one point which appears to have been overlooked.

FIG. 1.

Localization of a foreign body resolves itself in essence into taking two views from different points and then discovering its position, either by mathematical calculation or by the use of accessory apparatus.

The usual instructions for localization commence by directing the operator to so place the tube that the central ray is vertical and at right angles to the plate, and passes through the foreign body to be localized.

The tube is now to be displaced through a measured distance, parallel with the plane of the plate, on each side of its central position, and an exposure made with the tube at each of these two points.

The familiar diagram, shown in Fig. 1, is now consulted and localization performed by its aid. Here A, B, are the two positions of the tube ; C, D, are the corresponding shadows of the point x, and Y z is a line perpendicular to the planes A B and C D passing through the point x. In this case Y z also represents the magical central ray.

An elementary knowledge of geometry now shows that the intersection of the two straight lines, A C and B D, between the parallels A B and C D gives us two similar triangles, A B X, C D X, and from this we obtain the equation:—

$$\frac{A B}{C D} = \frac{X Y}{X Z}(1)$$

Now, since we have measured A B and Y Z before making the exposures, and we measure C D after the plate is developed, we have all the factors requisite to obtain the measurement X Z, which is the distance of the foreign body from the plate.

The above procedure is familiar to anyone who has ever performed a localization, and is only introduced here as the basis for what follows.

It is sometimes difficult or impossible to ensure the passage of the central ray through the foreign body, *e.g.*, if two or more foreign bodies are present the central ray cannot pass through each unless a corresponding number of localizations are performed on separate plates. Also, it may be necessary to localize under circumstances precluding screen observation, which is essential to ensure coincidence of foreign body and central ray.

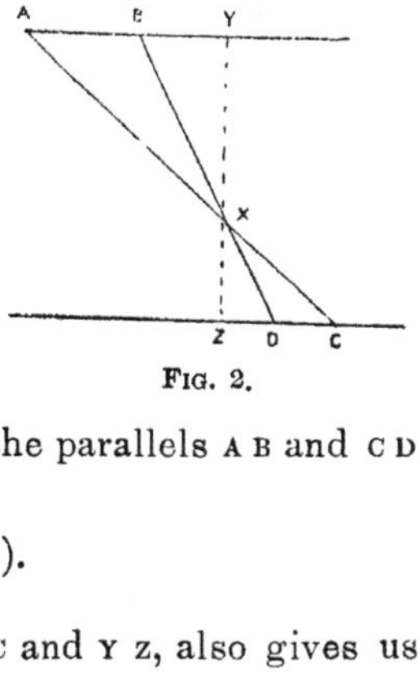

Now glance at Fig. 2, whose lettering corresponds to that of Fig. 1. Here it is obvious that the line Y Z, perpendicular to A B and C D, and passing through the point x, by no means represents the central ray.

Fig. 2.

Just as in the construction of Fig. 1, the intersection of the two straight lines A C and B D between the parallels A B and C D gives us similar triangles,

A B X, C D X, therefore $\frac{A B}{C D} = \frac{A X}{C X}(2)$.

But the intersection of the two straight lines, A C and Y Z, also gives us similar triangles, A Y X, C Z X, therefore, $\frac{A X}{C X} = \frac{X Y}{X Z}(3)$.

Combining (2) and (3) we get $\frac{A B}{C D} = \frac{X Y}{X Z}(4)$, which is precisely the same as equation (1), obtained when the central ray passed through the foreign body.

From this it is obvious that the accuracy of depth localization is not affected, whether the central ray passes through the foreign body or not ; in fact, it is quite immaterial where the tube is centred so long as the measurements A B, C D, Y Z can be obtained.

But there is one more point to be considered. In Fig. 1 it will be seen that the point x is projected on to the plate at z, in the same vertical line, and therefore, if a skin mark be made at the point over or under which the tube is centred, the foreign body will be found vertically under or over the mark. In Fig. 2 no such condition obtains, and we must consider how to give the surgeon such a surface mark for his guidance. The only requisite is to know where the tube is centred. For this purpose a small metallic marker is affixed to the skin surface over or under the spot selected for centring. A plumb line will show the coincidence of central ray and marker, without any necessity for screening, and the marker will leave its image on the plate and give us a point from which to take measurements.

In Fig. 3, T represents the central position of the tube, casting a shadow of the foreign body x on the plate at s, which is midway between the two shadows of x in the displaced positions of the tube. M is the spot over or under which the tube has been centred and the metallic marker placed. Y z is the perpendicular through the point x.

Now the construction of the figure gives us two similar triangles, T M s, x z s, therefore $\dfrac{T M}{M S} = \dfrac{X Z}{Z S}.$

But T M is the known distance from focus spot to plate, M s can be measured on the plate, and x z has already been obtained from equation (4), therefore we

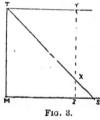

FIG. 3.

can easily calculate z s. By deducting z s from M s we get M z, which gives us the point z in relation to M. The point M, having been marked on the skin surface by the metallic marker, we can now make a more permanent mark at the point z, and inform the surgeon that the foreign body will be found under or over this point at the depth already ascertained ; localization is thus as precise as though the mystic central ray had passed accurately through the foreign body.

The foregoing method may seem to involve much calculation, but it is very simple, and the whole procedure, both for obtaining the depth of the foreign body and a skin mark for the point beneath which it lies, can be compressed into a single short table. This is proved by reference to Fig. 3.

From the similar triangles T Y X, s z x $\dfrac{T Y}{S Z} = \dfrac{X Y}{X Z}.$

By equation (4) $\dfrac{A B}{C D} = \dfrac{X Y}{X Z}$, therefore $\dfrac{A B}{C D} = \dfrac{T Y}{S Z}$.

But T Y = M z (opposite sides of a rectangle), therefore $\dfrac{A B}{C D} = \dfrac{M Z}{S Z}$ (5).

That is to say, the point z is obtained by dividing the line M s in the proportion of A B to C D. We have already seen in equation (4) that the point x is obtained by dividing the line Y z in the proportion of A B to C D ; therefore this proportion is the sole requisite for exact localization.

A B being the tube shift, which is measured before exposure, and C D the shadow shift, which is measured on the plate, we can now proceed to construct a table for proportionate division, as follows, assuming that the tube shift is 6 cm. (60 mm.).

Shadow Shift.	Fraction.	Shadow Shift.	Fraction.	Shadow Shift.	Fraction.
1 mm.	... $\frac{1}{61}$	11 mm.	... $\frac{11}{7}$	21 mm.	... $\frac{7}{7}$
2 ,,	. $\frac{1}{31}$	12 ,,	... $\frac{1}{5}$	22 ,,	... $\frac{11}{41}$
3 ,.	... $\frac{1}{21}$	13 ,,	... $\frac{14}{3}$	23 ,,	... $\frac{23}{83}$
4 ,,	... $\frac{1}{18}$	14 ,,	... $\frac{7}{37}$	24 ,,	... $\frac{2}{7}$
5 ,,	... $\frac{1}{13}$	15 ,,	... $\frac{1}{5}$	25 ,,	... $\frac{1}{17}$
6 ,,	... $\frac{1}{11}$	16 ,,	... $\frac{1}{16}$	26 ,,	... $\frac{13}{43}$
7 ,	... $\frac{7}{67}$	17 ,,	... $\frac{17}{7}$	27 ,,	... $\frac{9}{2\pi}$
8 ,,	... $\frac{1}{7}$	18 ,,	... $\frac{3}{16}$	28 ,,	... $\frac{7}{37}$
9 ,,	... $\frac{3}{23}$	19 ,,	... $\frac{19}{10}$	29 ,,	... $\frac{22}{83}$
10 ,,	... $\frac{1}{7}$	20 ,,	... $\frac{1}{4}$	30 ,,	... $\frac{1}{5}$

Provided that the tube shift of 6 cm. be adhered to, the table can now be used for any distance between focus spot and plate as follows :—

Measure the displacement of the shadows on the plate and look down the table until that figure is reached in the column marked "Shadow Shift." Opposite to this figure is a fraction, which represents the proportion of focus to plate distance indicating the distance of the foreign body from the plate. Now measure the line M s from the image of the marker to the point midway between the two shadows of the foreign body, and from this measurement subtract the same fractional part as was used to obtain the depth of the foreign body, and thus we arrive at the point under or over which the foreign body is situated.

This is no mere theoretical argument, but has stood the test of many actual localizations, and has been especially useful in cases where it was not advisable to remove the patient from his bed. It is offered in the hope that it may be of equal use to others in similar circumstances.

ERRATUM.

ARCHIVES, December, 1919, p. 217, line 21 from top, for " stellar" read " solar."

ELECTROCUTION OF A RADIOLOGIST.

EARLY in December the daily press announced that a well known French X-ray specialist, Dr. Auguste Jaugeas, had been electrocuted whilst carrying out an ordinary X-ray examination of a patient. Messrs. Watson & Sons, X-ray apparatus manufacturers, give the following account of how the accident occurred: "Dr. Jaugeas was making a screen examination at a hospital in Paris. The equipment consisted of a small high tension transformer, working from alternating current, without a rotating rectifier and with a radiator type of Coolidge tube. The X-ray room was very small, and the high tension wires from the transformer to the tube were hanging in the form of a loop. Dr. Jaugeas was making a fluoroscopic examination, and had his hand upon the wheel of the tube stand, which was of metal, for the purpose of adjusting the height of the tube. The tube stand was not 'earthed,' and the result of the movement of the tube was to bring one of the hanging wires in contact with the stand, causing a direct short-circuit from the main through the transformer to Dr. Jaugeas, who fell with his hand still grasping the tube holder, which he pulled down with him ; the floor was of concrete, which made matters worse." It should be understood that with the ordinary X-ray apparatus, which is in constant use in this country, there is no danger of an accident of this kind to either the patient or the operator. The small American type of transformer in use was one in which the secondary high tension wires are in direct connection with the primary current. With an apparatus of this kind it is imperative that examination couches, screening stands, and so on, should be earthed, and if this had been done the accident could not have happened. With this type of apparatus it is also essential that the wiring should be such that any short-circuiting is impossible. Unhappily, both these precautions had been omitted.

The risk of such an accident is very remote if precautions are observed. Messrs. Watson & Sons, with commendable promptitude, issued a leaflet, entitled "Dangers in the X-ray Room," which sets out clearly the precautions necessary to ensure the safety of operators.

This leaflet has been circulated to all radiologists and hospital departments, but in case it may not have reached all who are interested we take the liberty of giving it further publicity in the current number of the ARCHIVES :—

DANGERS IN THE X-RAY ROOM.

1. All metal parts of the Outfit, such as the Switch Table, Couch, Screening Stand, Tube Stand, and particularly the Tube Box and handles controlling the movements and diaphragm, should be efficiently earthed. For this purpose a flexible cable is preferable to a rigid wire, which may break or become disconnected. The earth wire should be connected to a water supply pipe, a drain pipe or an earthing plate. Wooden floors are safer than concrete for the operator. Concrete should be covered with some suitable material, such as wood or thick linoleum. Rubber-soled shoes may prevent a nasty accident.

2. When operating X-ray Tubes there should be no slack wires ; all connections should be taut and kept so by a spring.

3. Whenever possible use heavily insulated wires, but even these should always be treated with the same precaution as a bare wire, as the insulation deteriorates in the course of time.

4. All connecting wires and High Tension Apparatus must be out of easy reach or guarded so that assistants or patients cannot inadvertently touch them.

5. It is most important that overhead wires should be examined from time to time, and precaution should be taken so that a live wire cannot fall on the patient or operator. With this end in view, it is a good plan to place across the X-ray room several bare wires connected to earth and at right angles and below the High Tension overhead wires, so that should one of these break it is brought into contact with an earthed wire.

6. Periodically examine all wires leading from the High Tension Apparatus to the overhead High Tension Cables, and if necessary duplicate the method of fixing.

7. Great care should be taken that all fuses carry only the maximum current required by the apparatus, so that any overload or earth leakage will immediately blow the fuse.

8. When using the Coolidge Tube Installation, where the metal extremities of the tube may be close to the patient, it is desirable to provide a cover of metallic gauze, which is connected to earth, so that an involuntary movement may not cause the patient to receive a spark. All metal applicators should also be earthed. Sand-bags will be found useful for checking the involuntary movement of patients.

9. In those X-ray rooms which are without a water supply, a special earth plate should be fixed in the ground and an earth wire run round the room so that several earth connections can be easily made.

10. Avoid an arrangement which allows of two pieces of apparatus being simultaneously connected to one High Tension source.

11. Never touch the High Tension Trolley rods without first shutting off the current.

12. Do not instal the apparatus in a room so small that it becomes dangerous to move about.

13. Always have a colleague or assistant, if possible, who is familiar with the position of the main switch.

14. When examining and testing an installation do not be satisfied with merely shutting off the main switch on the apparatus but also switch off at the main supply.

Apart from the above suggestions great care must be exercised in working because it is impossible to foresee every contingency, and accidents may occur which are not provided for in the above notes.

Workers are reminded that the above precautions only refer to High Tension Currents, and that, in addition, there is constant danger from primary and secondary radiations unless there is adequate protection. The occupants of a room above or below the X-ray room may be unwittingly subjected to radiation unless proper steps are taken. The X-ray Tube should be completely surrounded by lead sheet, not less than 2 mm. thick (preferably more), leaving only the smallest necessary aperture for the beam of rays utilized to emerge.

The need for thorough protection from high and low tension currents is very great, and all who are responsible for the safety of workers in X-ray and electrical departments will feel with us that the time has come when thorough inspection by electrical experts is essential in all of those departments. The Board of Trade, or some other authority, should take the matter up and appoint an expert, who should visit all X-ray and electrical departments in hospitals and private institutions, with a view to ensuring that the work be carried out under conditions of absolute safety.

We deplore the loss of a distinguished radiologist, who had taken a leading place in the literature of the subject, and we offer our deepest sympathy to the relatives of Dr. Jaugeas in time of grief, rendered all the more terrible because of the tragic circumstances which led to his death.

We also sympathise with our colleagues in France and the French School of Radiology in having lost a most distinguished member, whose work, great as it has been, was only beginning, and from whom a great deal of still more valuable work was expected.

NOTES AND ABSTRACTS

The Value and Limitations of Radium in the Treatment of Cancer.—RUSSELL H. BOGGS, M.D., Roentgenologist, Allegheny General Hospital (*New York Medical Journal*, March 22nd, 1919).—The position of radium as a modern therapeutic agent in the treatment of malignancy is here outlined with clearness and moderation. Like all new remedies, radium has suffered from the extravagant claims put forward by the inexperienced, leading in many cases to disappointment and scepticism, but nowadays its value in the treatment of malignant growths has been definitely established, and while we must not lose sight of other methods, since the best results are often obtained by a judicious combination of the different therapeutic agencies, radium holds its own as a curative measure and as a palliative procedure.

The haphazard use of radium is to-day discouraged. The radiotherapeutist should possess a thorough knowledge of its physical properties and its physiological action, without which accurate dosage is impossible. His opinion as a skilled and experienced technician should be as much valued as that of the expert surgeon.

The radium treatment of epithelioma has been such that many conceive it to be the most efficient we possess. Four classes of epithelioma are considered : First, the lesion which can be cured by one application of radium with the proper dose; second, the lesion which is so situated that glandular involvement is likely to take place or has already occurred, and in which the roentgen rays should be employed as an adjunct to treat adjacent glands; third, those cases in which the local application of radium supplemented by X rays will act only as a palliative measure; and fourth, those cases in which excision is justified, to be followed by radiotherapy.

Epithelioma of the upper part of the face, not involving cartilage or bone, is more amenable to treatment than in any other location; in early cases one application will usually effect a cure. In epithelioma of the lower lip, results obtained by efficient treatment by radium, supplemented by X-rays to the adjacent glands, have proved equal or superior to those obtained by surgery. Over 90 per cent. of early superficial cases are cured without producing any deformity, and more advanced cases are cured, and hopeless cases receive retardation and palliation than by any other method.

Roentgenisation of the lymphatic glands should always supplement radiumtherapy. A cure is never obtained unless the disease in the lymphatics is completely eradicated. Cancer cells are from three to seven times less resistant than normal tissue, depending upon the type of lesion. The squamous type requires two to four times more radiation than the basilar form.

Carcinoma of the mouth and throat, when ulceration has invaded the muscle tissues, is very resistant to radium treatment, and large doses sufficient to produce a marked reaction require to be given. This can then be followed in a few weeks by electric coagulation to destroy the lesion.

In carcinoma of the uterus, radium is indicated as a palliative for inoperable and recurrent cancers; also for operable cases constitutionally contra-indicated, and for prophylaxis after surgical removal. Where recurrence takes place, as a rule the patient suffers little in comparison with those who had no radium treatment. In hopeless cases the cessation of discharge, so offensive in character, is a remarkable feature.

In carcinoma of the breast, there are only a comparatively few patients who receive benefit from operation, and these only the very early cases. Of the total number of cases, it may be stated positively that radium and X rays have done far more than surgery alone. If a more comprehensive study of the glandular involvement and the metastases should be made by both the surgeon and the radiotherapeutist, the surgeon would not operate in certain cases and the radio-therapeutist would give more efficient treatment.

It is greatly to be deplored that so many cases of inoperable carcinoma receive so little attention when their condition is pronounced hopeless. A great many would certainly receive considerable palliation and prolongation of life from radium. As the writer puts it, treatment of hopeless carcinoma in the past has been with morphine; to-day it should be radiotherapy.   J. McK.

The Pathology of Œsophagectasia (Dilatation of the Œsophagus without Anatomic Stenosis at the Cardiac Orifice).—I. Moore (*Proc. Roy. Soc. of Med., Sect. of Laryngology*, March, 1919).—Moore has compiled notes and references relating to a unique series of specimens collected from various hospitals. Very careful drawings of these have been made and their reproduction forms an important part of this contribution.   R. W. A. S.

Internal Hernia.—M. R. J. Hayes (*Med. Press*, April 9th, 1919, pp. 279, 280).—The author describes the clinical symptoms and appearances by opaque meal examination of a case of hernia into the duodenal fossa.
R. W. A. S.

The X-ray Treatment of Tubercular Epididymitis and Orchitis.—A. Hyman (*Urologic and Cutan. Review*, May, 1919, pp. 275-277). —It is in the later stages of the disease, with unilateral or bilateral involvement of the testes, that deep X-ray treatment is specially indicated. Even in early cases Hyman advocates its use, provided the question of sterility has been definitely determined. If azoospermia is present no harm can be done; if spermatozoa are present the rays should not be used.

The great advantage of X-ray therapy is due to the fact that the rays, while destroying the spermatogenetic function, have no injurious effects upon the interstitial cells which furnish the internal secretion.

Two cases are reported showing very good results under this treatment (full erythema doses with a spark gap of 9½ inches).
R. W. A. S.

The Sympathetic Nervous System and Diseases of Digestion.—W. Langdon Brown

(*Lancet*, May 24th, 1919, pp. 873-879).—This author reviews the physiology of the alimentary tract. When the bolus has passed the constrictors of the pharynx, voluntary control over the movements of the alimentary canal is lost. The para-sympathetic takes over control, and a slow peristaltic wave, started by the vagus, passes along the œsophagus. With liquids, however, the œsophagus remains dilated and passive. The passage of fluid to the stomach takes four to eight seconds, half of which time is occupied in passing through the cardiac sphincter. Solids take eight to eighteen seconds if well lubricated, but a dry bolus may remain above the cardia for many minutes. After food enters the stomach, it passes rapidly and without the aid of peristaltic waves to the pyloric portion. Active waves soon sweep it towards the pyloric sphincter about three times a minute, gaining force as they go. As the stomach empties it is pulled up until the pyloric orifice becomes the lowest part, which assists the completion of the process. In duodenal ulcer, this pulling up of the stomach can be seen from the beginning.

When it passes into the small intestine, movements of two kinds are seen :—

(1) Pendulum movements, which travel at the rate of 2 to 5 cm. per second, and depend on muscle tone. They serve to mix the contents.

(2) Peristaltic movements, which drive the contents along.

The large intestine can be divided into three portions, which do not correspond exactly to the anatomical divisions :—

(1) The proximal part, characterised by the presence of anti-peristaltic waves.

(2) An intermediate part, with the type of movement seen in the small intestine.

(3) A distal portion, the rectum, where the central nervous system again assumes control.

" Anti-peristalsis," it is stated, is rather a misnomer, for it is really a rhythmical series of reversed segmentation movements, depending largely on the degree of tension present.

Keith's conception of the movements of the alimentary tract is described.

The clinical and radiological aspects of œsophageal and gastric spasm is next dealt with, and it is pointed out that the spasmodic element in many forms of dyspepsia is not sufficiently recognised.

Pancreatitis as a cause of severe abdominal pain is discussed and four interesting cases described.

Reflex dyspepsias from appendix and transverse colon are next touched upon, and the general conclusion that hyperchlorhydria is usually due to some reflex cause—an irritable focus somewhere lower down in the alimentary canal.

Atonic dilatation of the stomach, gastroptosis, and intestinal stasis are finally dealt with.   R. W. A. S.

Radiography by Aeroplane.—Foveau de Courmelles (*Arch. d' Électric. Méd.*, June, 1919).—Both in peace and war there are occasions when very early arrival of medical and surgical personnel and equipment may diminish suffering and save life. To achieve this end an aeroplane equipment has been devised by the Engineer Némirovsky and Dr. Tilmant, and its arrangements and the principles of its use are described by the author. Closed carriers are fitted under the lower plane, one on each side, and contain X-ray, surgical and sterilisation equipment and light stretchers. The X-ray system comprises a small dynamo and accumulators, transformer and interrupter made light and compact, and all capable of being carried some distance from the aeroplane if necessary ; a table of sheet and tube aluminium, which also serves as an operation table; two tubes carried in a fixed box, well padded, and similar to those used on hospital ships and cruisers, which have stood the firing of all the guns without harm to the tubes, a screen and localisation apparatus. The surgical outfit consists of four sealed aluminium boxes of sterilised instruments, for minor emergency surgery, for major surgery of abdomen and thorax, for amputations and for cranial surgery. Eight other boxes carry dressings, gowns, gloves, etc. A last box holds the materials for sterilising skin and hands of patient and operators, anæsthetics and hypodermics. All these boxes are packed in the electric steriliser and autoclave. The crew of the aeroplane is three ; a pilot who takes charge of the mechanical work of the apparatus, a surgeon, and a radiologist who also acts as assistant to the latter. The device enables an injured patient to be carried back on his stretcher to the hospital. The total weight of the load carried is 750 kilos, including petrol for three

hours flying. It is evident that this device has possibilities of usefulness after railway and other accidents in desolate spots, where help has to come from a distance and time is all-important.   N. B.

PUBLICATIONS RECEIVED.

Journals.

Archives d'Électricite Médicale et de Physiotherapie, Nov., 1919.

Bulletin of the Johns Hopkins Hospital, Nov., 1919.

Bulletins et Mémoirs de la Société de Radiologie Médicale de France, Nov., 1919.

Gaceta Médica Catalana, Nov. 15th, 1919.

Good Health, Dec., 1919.

International Journal of Orthodontia and Oral Surgery, Nov., 1919.

Il Policlinico, Nov. 1st, 15th, 1919.

La Radiologia Medica, Nov.-Dec., 1919.

Le Radium, Sept.-Oct., 1919.

Journals—*continued.*

Medical Journal of Australia, Sept. 20th; Oct. 11th, 18th, 25th, 1919.

Medical Science Abstracts and Reviews, Dec., 1919.

New York Medical Journal, Oct. 11th; Nov. 1st, 8th, 15th, 22nd; Dec. 6th, 1919.

New York State Journal of Medicine, Oct., Nov., 1919.

Norsk Mag. for Lægevidenskaben, Dec., 1919.

Rivista Italiana di Neuropatologia, Psichiatria ed Elettroterapia, Nov.-Dec., 1919.

Surgery, Gynæcology, and Obstetrics, Dec., 1919.

Ugeskrift for Læger, Oct. 30th; Nov. 27th; Dec. 4th, 11th, 18th, 25th, 1919.

NOTICES.

ARCHIVES OF RADIOLOGY AND ELECTROTHERAPY is published monthly.

The index for each volume, which ends with the May number, is supplied with the June number of each year.

Communications to the Editors should be addressed to "ROBERT KNOX, M.D., 38, Harley Street, W. 1."

Communications and illustrations from American contributors may be sent to Messrs. REBMAN COMPANY, 141-145, West Thirty-sixth Street, New York City.

All radiographs and photographs must be originals, and must not have been previously published. Drawings should be supplied on separate paper.

Owing to the scarcity of paper the Publishers are reluctantly compelled—as a temporary war measure—to reduce the number of free reprints of Papers to twenty-five.

Annual Subscriptions, payable in advance, 30/- including postage. Single copies, 3/- (postage 2d.) Single numbers and back numbers can be supplied on application.

Vol. XXIV—No. 9   FEBRUARY, 1920   No. 235

ARCHIVES OF RADIOLOGY AND ELECTROTHERAPY

THE OFFICIAL ORGAN OF THE
BRITISH ASSOCIATION OF RADIOLOGY AND PHYSIOTHERAPY

Editors.

ROBERT KNOX, M.D., Hon. Radiologist, King's College Hospital.
E. P. CUMBERBATCH, B.M., M.R.C.P., Medical Officer in Charge, Electrical Department, St. Bartholomew's Hospital.
SIDNEY RUSS, D.Sc., Physicist to the Middlesex Hospital.

IN COLLABORATION WITH

A. E. BARCLAY *(Manchester)*; BELOT *(Paris)*; H. MARTIN BERRY *(London)*; W. H. BRAGG *(London)*; N. BURKE *(Woodhall Spa)*; J. BURNET *(Edinburgh)*; W. J. S. BYTHELL *(Manchester)*; J. T. CASE *(Battle Creek, U.S.A.)*; A. ST. GEORGE CAULFEILD *(London)*; H. A. COLWELL *(London)*; FOVEAU DE COURMELLES *(Paris)*; GUNZBURG *(Antwerp)*; HALL-EDWARDS *(Birmingham)*; HARET *(Paris)*; HAUCHAMPS *(Brussels)*; F. HERNAMAN-JOHNSON *(London)*; W. F. HIGGINS *(Teddington)*; THURSTAN HOLLAND *(Liverpool)*; HURST *(London)*; KLYNENS *(Antwerp)*; LAQUERRIERE *(Paris)*; LAZARUS-BARLOW *(London)*; LEDUC *(Nantes)*; ALEXANDER MACKAY *(Edinburgh)*; REGINALD MORTON *(London)*; HARRISON ORTON *(London)*; W. OVEREND *(St. Leonards-on-Sea)*; PFAHLER *(Philadelphia)*; C. E. S. PHILLIPS *(London)*; GEORGE PIRIE *(Dundee)*; HOWARD PIRIE *(Montreal)*; A. W. PORTER *(London)*; R. W. A. SALMOND *(London)*; WERTHEIM SALOMONSON *(Amsterdam)*; S. SLOAN *(Glasgow)*; SOMERVILLE *(Glasgow)*; W. C. STEVENSON *(Dublin)*; W. J. TURRELL *(Oxford)*; HUGH WALSHAM *(London)*.

Obituary.

WE record with the deepest regret the death of Mr. C. R. C. Lyster, M.R.C.S., which occurred on January 26th, at the age of 60 years. Dr. Lyster, until within a few months of his death, was in charge of the X-ray and Electro-therapeutic Departments at the Middlesex Hospital, a post which he had held for the last 17 years.

Dr. Lyster received his medical education at Charing Cross Hospital, and subsequently became Medical Superintendent at Bolingbroke Hospital. He was largely instrumental in placing Bolingbroke on a stable footing, both financially and from the administrative aspect ; this was, in fact, the first opportunity on a big scale he had of showing one of his outstanding qualities, namely, the faculty of understanding people, especially their troubles.

When Dr. Lyster was appointed in charge of the electrical department at Middlesex Hospital, the department consisted of a temporary structure at the entrance of the hospital, the "old tin house" as it was familiarly called.

X-ray and electrical applications in medicine, however, were a growing necessity, and under his administration a new department came into being. In his opinion it was very desirable that the medical officer in charge of this work should be thoroughly acquainted, not only with radiology but also with electrotherapeutics, and he continued to direct the work of the two sections until within a few months of his death.

No adequate guide to the value of Dr. Lyster's services to medical radiology and electrotherapy is to be found in his publications, which were few ;

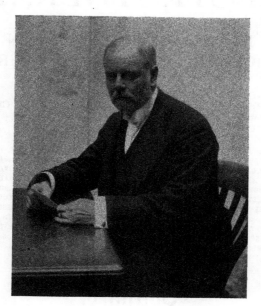

he was never happy with the pen. He served his subject in many other ways. He was President of the Electrotherapeutic Section of the Royal Society of Medicine for the year 1918-19, and served on its council for several years, doing similar service for the Röntgen Society, a society to which he was an excellent friend. His broad outlook on questions and his utter unselfishness of intention always commanded the greatest respect among his colleagues for any views to which he gave expression. It was a matter of much concern to him that advances in his subjects should be continually supplementing routine procedure, and he was always keen to try new methods of treatment which had as a basis for their use the results of laboratory investigation, so the research worker found in him a constant stimulus. He made many efforts to raise the status of the position occupied by medical men in his own field of work. It was largely due to him in the first instance that the Diploma in Radiology and Electrology, now in existence, became an accomplished thing, and it was a great happiness to him that the seal of the University of Cambridge was fixed upon this initiation.

The years of the war entailed fresh burdens upon him at a time when he could least bear them, but they were always cheerfully met. He undertook the direction of the X-ray and Electrotherapeutic Departments at Queen Alexandra's Hospital, at Millbank, and devoted a great deal of time and energy in such administration.

It was during the early part of Dr. Lyster's work at the Middlesex Hospital that he suffered damage from X rays. Those were days in which the potentiality of the rays for good in the treatment of disease was little known, still less indeed of their harmful effects. The damage became aggravated in the course of time ; but although he was fully aware of the extra risks which he incurred, he declined to be set aside from his purpose, and continued to be actively employed in alleviating the distress of others right up to within a few months of his death. It is for this reason that the work of a good many of his later years must be looked upon in the light of a sacrifice. Indeed, it is this viewpoint that gives us the true perspective upon his life, for it was essentially upon the human side that one found Dr. Lyster's qualities developed to the highest pitch. He was a rare friend, a man who thoroughly understood his fellow man, especially if he happened to be a sufferer. We looked upon him as one of the great warm-hearted men whose serenity of outlook no passing clouds could dim, whose spirit no suffering could daunt.

His last public wish was characteristic of him—the flowers that might be brought, and indeed were brought in great numbers as tributes to his memory, were all to be taken to the wards of the hospital he served so well. He leaves a memory that will serve to remind a large circle of a great and lovable man.

THE DIPLOMA IN MEDICAL RADIOLOGY AND ELECTROLOGY.
The Inaugural Lecture.

THE London course of study in preparation for the examination next summer, at Cambridge, for the Diploma in Medical Radiology and Electrology, has now commenced. Clinical instruction of intending candidates is proceeding at various hospitals, and lectures on Electrotherapeutics and Physics are in progress.

The first lecture of the course was delivered on February 4th, at the house of the Royal Society of Medicine, by Dr. Turrell, Physician to the Electrical Department of the Radcliffe Infirmary, Oxford. The subject was, "The History of Electrotherapeutics." The lecture constituted an inaugural address, marking the commencement of a complete and inclusive course of instruction in the medical uses of X rays, electricity, radium and ultra-violet light, and in the necessary preliminary subjects, such as physics and electrotechnics.

The lecture was of much interest, especially to students of electrotherapeutics. Dr. Turrell showed that the foundation of the science of electricity was laid by a medical man, Dr. Gilbert, of Colchester, at the beginning of the 17th century, but that more than 100 years elapsed before it was used in the treatment of disease. Even then, in this country, its medical uses long remained chiefly in the hands of non-professional men, although John Freke, F.R.S., Surgeon to St. Bartholomew's Hospital, wrote on it in 1702.

Dr. Turrell showed a copy of a work by the Rev. John Wesley, entitled, "The Desideratum ; or, Electricity made Plain and Useful." This was published in 1759, and contained accounts of most of the recorded cases in which electricity had been used. John Freke is mentioned in this work.

Dr. Turrell also showed copies of two rare engravings illustrating Galvani's experiments on frog's muscles, which led to the discovery of electric currents. A copy of the *Morning Chronicle*, of the year 1783, was shown. This contained an amusing advertisement by a charlatan, who offered cures of sterility by a form of alleged electrical treatment which he called the "Celestial Bed."

Dr. Turrell's lecture was the most complete that has yet been delivered on the history of electrotherapeutics, and his scholarly address formed a fitting inauguration of a course of study which may certainly be regarded as forming the commencement of an epoch in the medical uses of X rays and electricity.

THE HISTORY OF ELECTROTHERAPY.

By W. J. TURRELL, M.A., M.D.,

Physician in charge of Electrotherapeutic Department, Radcliffe Infirmary, Oxford.

LADIES AND GENTLEMEN,

Before I deal with the subject of my lecture, perhaps I ought to say a few words on the origin of the course which we inaugurate to-day. So far as I am aware, this great advance in the development of our science is due, in the first place, to the inspiration of Dr. Barclay, of Manchester, to the organisation of Dr. Robert Knox, to the hard and disinterested work of Dr. Cumberbatch, Dr. Sidney Russ, Dr. Shillington Scales and others, and to the scientific enterprise of Cambridge University.

In consequence of the priority which the subject of my lecture naturally and automatically assumes, it has fallen to my lot to deliver the inaugural lecture of the course, and I can assure you that this is an honour, accidental though it may be, that I very deeply appreciate.

THE HISTORY OF ELECTROTHERAPY.

It is probable that, even in prehistoric times, the physiological effects of electricity were unpleasantly experienced by unwary bathers and fishermen in the Mediterranean seas from contact with the electric ray, or torpedo fish, three or four varieties of which are met with in those waters.

Aristotle (B.C. 341) states that these fish have the power of benumbing men, and Pliny (A.D. 79) relates that "this fish, if touched by a rod or spear, even at a distance, paralyses the strongest muscles, and binds and arrests the feet however swift" (1) ; he also prophetically hints that considerable therapeutic benefit may be reasonably expected from creatures endowed with such natural powers.

Anthero, a freedman in the time of the Emperor Tiberius, is said by Scribonius Largus (A.D. 50) (cap. 4, XLI) to have been cured of an attack of gout by placing his feet on the back of a torpedo fish. Dioscorides (2) recommends shocks from torpedo fish for the cure of obstinate headache. Galen (A.D. 144) (3) and Paulus Ægineta (4) recommend a similar form of treatment.

The electric ray, or torpedo fish, belongs to the elasmobranch family ; its electric organ consists of about 800 to 1,000 cells connected with large bundles of nerves. It grows to a width of three to four feet, and, when fully grown, is said to be able to give a shock of sufficient strength to stun a man. The dorsal surface of the fish is positive, and its under surface negative.

According to the writer on animal electricity in Todd's "Cyclopædia of Anatomy and Physiology," 1839, the torpedo fish was still used as a therapeutic agent by the Arabians at the beginning of the 19th century. The

---

(1) "Historia Naturalis," XXXII, Chap. I.
(2) "Dioscorides," Lib. II, Art. "Torpedo."
(3) Galen "Simp. Med." Lib. XI.
(4) "Paulus Ægineta," Lib. VII.

method of administering the shocks is thus described: " The patient is placed on a table, and the fish applied to all the members of the body in succession, so that each should receive at least one shock. The treatment causes rather severe suffering, but enjoys the reputation of being febrifuge."

Muschenbroeck, about 1750, was the first to infer that these shocks were electrical in origin; he drew this inference from their resemblance to the shocks received from a Leyden jar.

The gymnotus, or electrical eel, is another fish capable of giving very powerful electrical shocks.

Since the electrical nature of these shocks was not recognised until about 1750, electricity may be said to have been first discovered when Thales, of Miletus (B.C. 600), one of the Wise Men of Greece, discovered that amber, when rubbed, attracted light bodies. This phenomenon induced Thales to believe that amber was endowed with life, and that it derived nourishment from the objects it attracted. From the Greek name for amber, *elektron*, the word electricity has been derived.

About B.C. 300 Theophrastus, in his book on " Precious Stones " (1) states that this property of amber is also possessed by lyncurium (tourmalin). He found that tourmalin, when rubbed, attracted light bodies, such as straw, and small particles of iron and copper.

For nearly two thousand years no further advance was made in electrical knowledge. In 1600 there appeared a book entitled, " De Magnete, Magneticisque Corporibus," etc., by the President of the College of Physicians of that year, Dr. William Gilbert (1540-1603), a native of Colchester, and physician to Queen Elizabeth.

Gilbert found that there were many bodies, such as precious stones, sulphur, imitation stones, glass, crystal, etc., which when rubbed attracted light bodies. He defined electrics as: " Electrica; quæ attrahunt eadem ratione ut electrum."

Gilbert noticed that the electrics were much more readily electrified when the atmosphere was dry than when it was wet; when the wind was in the north or east than when it was in the south. He also found that warming the bodies to be excited favoured electrification.

To the inventive genius of Otto von Guericke (1602-1686), Burgomaster of Magdeburg, and discoverer of the air pump, we owe the first frictional machine for the production of electricity. Guericke constructed his machine by filling a glass globe with melted sulphur, then, not being aware that the glass globe would itself serve for an efficient machine, he broke the glass, and mounted the sphere of sulphur on a wooden frame. With this machine, by holding his hand against the rapidly rotated sphere, he was able to produce sufficient electricity to enable him both to hear and see the spark.

Guericke was the first to discover that bodies bearing electrical charges of a similar character repelled one another. Hawksbee, who wrote about 1709, substituted a glass globe for the sulphur sphere, and performed some important experiments in connection with electrical attraction and repulsion. About

(1) Theophrastus, " De Lapid.," p. 134. Hill's Ed.

1742 Winkler, a professor of languages at Leipsic, introduced a cushion or rubber, in place of the hand, which had previously been used to excite the machines. This improvement shortly afterwards led to the construction of machines with multiple glass globes. According to Dr. Priestley, from whose book, "History of Electricity," most of our information in regard to the development of electricity at this period is derived, "such a prodigious quantity of electricity could they excite from these globes, whirled by a large wheel and rubbed with woollen cloth . . . that, if we may credit their own accounts, the blood could be drawn from the finger by an electric spark, the skin would burst, and a wound appear as if made by caustic."

In 1745 electrical research was still further facilitated by the discovery of the Leyden jar. This advance was due, not to Muschenbroeck, as Wesley and others erroneously state, but to von Kleist, Dean of the Cathedral at Camin, who, on November 4th, 1745, sent the following account of his discovery to Dr. Lieberkuhm, at Berlin: "When a nail or a piece of thin brass wire, etc., is put into a small apothecary's phial and electrified, remarkable effects follow; but the phial must be very dry and warm." This may not seem to be a very clear description of the Leyden jar, but R. Lovett, in his "Philosophical Essays," 1766, describes a method of construction which differs little, if at all, from that employed at the present day: "But the most commodious way is to line the inside of the phial with gold leaf, etc., and to coat it with tin-foil, thin lead, or the like, and to fasten some tinsel fringe or fine wires to the lower end of the cork wire within the phial, so as to reach to the gold lining, by which means the electrical fire is conveyed to it from the revolving rubbed glass."

Von Kleist, in his letter to Lieberkuhm, after describing his jar, gives an account of the powerful spark which he obtained by its means. His arms and shoulders were benumbed by its effects, and he expresses the opinion that Mr. Boze would not have desired a second kiss from the jar. Priestley quotes many instances of the terror inspired by shocks from the jar in Germany and France.

Muschenbroeck, in a letter to Reaumur, states that it took him two days to recover from the shock, and that he would not repeat the experiment for the kingdom of France. Priestley, however, presumably in a sarcastic vein, for Mr. Boze was known to him as a charlatan, differs from the opinion expressed by von Kleist in reference to Mr. Boze, and states that the sentiments of the magnanimous Mr. Boze were far different, "who with a truly philosophical heroism, worthy of the renowned Empedocles, said he wished he might die by the electric shock, that the memoir of his death might furnish an article for the memoirs of the French Academy of Science."

Among many other experiments made with the Leyden jar about this time, the Abbé Nollet tried how many patients he could shock at the same time. He first gave a simultaneous shock, in the presence of the King of France, to 180 of his guards. Afterwards, in the grounds of the Grand Convent of Carthusians, at Paris, the whole community being lined up in a row 1,800 yards long, a shock was administered which elicited a simultaneous spring from them all.

About 1760 a glass plate friction machine was independently introduced by Dr. Ingenhousz, of Vienna, and Mr. Ramsden, of the Haymarket, London. It consisted of a circular plate of glass furnished with four rubbers. Priestley comments on this machine as being ingenious, but states that there was a difficulty in insulating the rubbers, and that the machine was more fragile than those with glass globes. We have now arrived at a period of great activity in electrical research, and it is not surprising to find that medical men and others, now furnished with an electrical machine of considerable power, and also provided with the Leyden jar, which was capable of enormously increasing the output from these machines, turned their attention to the curative effects of electricity. Before, however, electricity was applied to the treatment of disease, the Abbé Nollet had made several experiments in reference to its effects on animals.

Priestley states that the first account which he had "met with of the application of electricity to medical purposes is that of Mr. C. Kratzenstein, professor of medicine at Halle, who, in the year 1744, cured a woman of a contracted finger in a quarter of an hour."

Most of the early cures resembled Kratzenstein's case; we should probably now regard such cases as functional, and transfer them to the psychotherapist, though it is very doubtful whether, even at the present day, many of these functional cases would not be more speedily and effectually cured by the static spark than by suggestion. The torpillage, or torpedo treatment of Dr. Vincent, utilising intensive galvanic currents, yielded most excellent results during the late war, according to the French journals, and this treatment is, in principle, the same as the "commotiones fortiores" of the static spark.

Jallabert, professor of philosophy in Geneva, secured, in 1747 and 1748, results very similar to the one reported by Kratzenstein.

From this date electrotherapy owes its progress chiefly to French workers. The treatment appears not only to have appealed to the imagination of the French, but also from the first they approached the subject in a more scientific spirit than did the workers in other countries. About 1750, an official commission was held at the Hotel Royal des Invalides, Paris, and experiments were performed before it by Dr. Lassonne, physician to the king, Morand, surgeon to the Hospital des Invalides, and the Abbé Nollet. These experiments were not successful.

Sauvages, of the Montpellier Academy, was induced by the reported success of Jallabert to attempt the cure of paralytics, and he met with such success that "the concourse of patients of all kinds which the report of the cures brought together was prodigious." In fact, the success of the treatment was so great that the priests had to be called in to convince the neighbouring people that the cures had not been wrought by witchcraft. Moreover, as the outcome of Sauvage's success, a medico-electrical hospital was founded at the Convent des Celestius, under the authority of the French Government, for the treatment of epilepsy, catalepsy, and nervous diseases of all kinds. This hospital treatment does not appear to have realised the hopes of its founders. Marat attributed its failure to empiricism and a blind routine.

The first treatise published on electricity, of which any record exists, was " De Hemiplegia per electricitatem curanda," written by Deshais, and published at Montpellier, 1749. This work was followed two years later by Bohadatsch's pamphlet, " De utilitate electrisationis in arte medica," published at Prague, 1751.

In England electrical treatment appears to have been first practised by the clerical profession. In 1756 a book entitled, " The Subtile Medium: or, that Wonderful Power of Nature, . . . showing its various uses in the animal œconomy, particularly when applied to maladies and disorders of the human body, . . ." was published at Worcester.

This book was written by Richard Lovett (1692-1780), a native of Chalfont St. Giles, Bucks, and a lay clerk at Worcester Cathedral. Lovett treated a large number of diseases, including St. Anthony's fire, bronchocele, contractions, epilepsy, feet violently disordered, gout, headache, mortification, palsy, rheumatism, sciatica, sore throat, and fistula lachrymalis. His treatment appears to have been very thorough; in reference to hysteria and similar cases he writes: " In these complaints it is not to be done by halves ; not for a few minutes only (which is sufficient in some others), particularly if it has taken deep root ; but the person ought to stand or sit on the electrical stool for an hour in the morning and another in the evening each day; or, if two hours a day cannot be complied with, let it be for two half hours. This may be practised with sometimes simply drawing off sparks ; afterwards with some slight shocks, and then if the disorder requires it, to be increased with more. Such proceeding I seldom found to fail of the desired effects."

In 1780, John Wesley, the great divine, anonymously published a most interesting book, entitled, " The Desideratum; or, Electricity made Plain and Useful. By a Lover of Mankind, and of Common Sense." Wesley follows very closely the practice of Lovett, to whom he frequently refers. The most remarkable feature of the book is the fervour with which he appeals for a trial of the curative effects of electricity. Wesley, to judge from his writings, held a very poor opinion of the ideals of the medical men of his day. In a book, which he wrote on the treatment of disease by drugs, entitled, " Primitive Physic," he thus expresses his opinion of the doctors: " Physicians now began to be had in admiration as persons who were something more than human. And profit attended their employ as well as honour, so that they had now two weighty reasons for keeping the bulk of mankind at a distance that they might not pry into the mysteries of the profession. To this end they increased those difficulties by design, which began in a manner by accident. They filled their writings with abundance of technical terms, utterly unintelligible to plain men. They affected to deliver their rules and to reason upon them in an abstruse and philosophical manner. They represented the critical knowledge of anatomy, natural philosophy (and what not? Some of them insisting on that of astronomy and astrology too) as necessary previous to the understanding of the art of healing. Those who understood only how to restore the sick to health they branded with the name of Empiricks." In the preface to the " Desideratum " Wesley has another tilt at the doctors: " Mr. Lovett is of opinion 'the electrical method of treating disorders cannot be expected to arrive at any degree of perfection till administer'd and applied by the Gentlemen of the Faculty.' Nay, then, quanta de spe decidi! All my hopes are at an end. For when will it be administered and applied by them? Truly, ad Græcas Calendas. Not till the Gentlemen of the Faculty have more regard to the interest of their neighbours than their own. At least not till there are no apothecaries in the land, or till physicians are independent of them."

Wesley concludes his book with the following sarcastic and impassioned, but thoroughly rational, appeal to the medical profession : "Before I conclude, I would beg one thing (if it be not too great a favour) from the Gentlemen of the Faculty, and indeed from all who desire health and freedom from pain, either for themselves or their neighbours. It is, that none of them would condemn they know not what ; that they would hear the cause before they pass sentence ; that they would not peremptorily pronounce against electricity, while they know little or nothing about it. Rather let every candid man take a little pains to understand the question before he determines it. Let him for two or three weeks (at least) try it himself in the above named disorders. And then his own senses will show him whether it is a mere plaything or the noblest medicine yet known in the world."

Time does not permit of an analysis of Wesley's alleged cures, but there are one or two passages in his book which are deserving of special attention. The experience of most electrotherapists would lead them to assent to the following statement : "And yet there is something peculiarly unaccountable, with regard to its operation. In some cases, where there was no hope of help, it will succeed beyond all expectation. In others, where we had the greatest hope, it will have no effect at all. Again, in some experiments, it helps at the very first, and promises a speedy cure ; but presently the good effect ceases, and the patient is as he was before. On the contrary, in others it has no effect at first ; it does no good, perhaps seems to hurt. Yet all the time it is striking at the root of the disease, which in a while it totally removes." Among the 42 electrical experiments which Wesley quotes from Martin's " Essay on Electricity," the following is of special interest as it foreshadows the experiments of Geissler and Crookes with vacuum tubes : " If the globe be exhausted of air, and then turn'd, the electric fire will act wholly within the globe, where it will appear (in a dark room) as a reddish or purple flame, filling the whole globe. But this, as the air is readmitted into it, will gradually disappear."

Though unqualified practitioners, both Wesley and Lovett had a very real and genuine belief in the efficacy of electrical treatment, and their zeal and enthusiasm did a great deal for the early development of this science ; moreover, their work and their writings survived them for many years, and were frequently quoted by their qualified successors. Priestley thus comments on the work of Lovett and Wesley : "This account of the medical use of electricity by Mr. Lovett and Mr. Wesley is certainly liable to an objection, which will always lie against the accounts of those persons who, not being of the faculty, cannot be supposed capable of distinguishing with accuracy, either the nature of the disorders, or the consequences of a seeming cure. But, on the other hand, this very circumstance of their ignorance of the nature of disorders, and consequently of the best method of applying electricity to them, supplies the strongest argument in favour of its innocence, at least. If in such unskilful hands it produced so much good, and so little harm, how much more good, and how much less harm would it possibly have produced in more skilful hands : "

The first treatise on electrical treatment, written in this country by a medical man, was the thesis on paralysis, which J. Smyth Carmichael presented, on October 29th, 1764, for the degree of Doctor of Medicine at the University of Edinburgh. In this "Testamen Medicum Inaugurale de Paralysi," Carmichael describes very clearly the method of administering the electrical treatment of his time. Before entering into the details of the treatment, he first quotes the Abbé Nollet (Memoires de l'Academie de Sciences, 1748) to show the effect of electricity in hastening the passage of water through capillary tubes, and its accelerating action on the germination and the vegetation of plants. Carmichael then states that Verratti, of Bologna, and other Italians were the first to utilise electricity in medicine. The method at first adopted was to insulate the patient, charge him with the electrical current and draw sparks from different parts of his body. Subsequently the introduction of the Leyden jar led to the administration of strong shocks (commotiones fortiores).

The results of treatment showed an increase in the flow of urine (Linnæus, Zetzel, and Verratti) ; the onset of diarrhœa (Jallabert) ; increased secretion of cerumen (Linnæus) ; an increase in the amount and a prolongation of the menstrual flow (De Haen).

The treatment of paralysis by the sparks relieved pain and excited involuntary contraction (Verratti and Jallabert). The parts from which the sparks were drawn off became hot and red. Nollett in his experiments caused blisters by his sparks, but Carmichael was of opinion that this could not occur in man, because the thinness of the human skin readily allowed the sparks to escape. Sparking of the parotid increased the flow of saliva (Boissier, 1744-1740). Strong sparks gave great pain to the sick, greater in the affected than in the healthy parts (Nollet and Morand). The shocks excited contraction in the most insensitive muscles.

Electrisation was found to increase the strength, to restore the pristine bloom to the atrophied parts, to render the veins more manifest, and to bring back the natural colour to the skin.

De Haen stated that the electrical force never hurt anyone. Carmichael, however, remarks that "this ought not to be accepted as the general rule, for Verratti has shown that one ought always to guard against the use of electricity when there is any suspicion of latent venereal disease."

Carmichael concludes the electrical portion of his thesis by quoting two cases of paralysis cured by electricity.

A careful survey of the history of any subject invariably reveals the forgotten existence of many facts and fallacies which, many years later, are rediscovered and heralded forth as new and original observations.   For the past few years no form of electrical treatment has been so extensively practised as that known as "Ionic Medication." It is only within the last year or so that the absurdity of the claim that drugs can be introduced into the deeper tissues of the body and there exercise their specific action has been definitely exposed.   It is very interesting, therefore, to find that Priestley vehemently inveighs against a somewhat similar theory that was in vogue in his time.   "In the course of history," writes Priestley (1775), "we have seen frequent instances of self-deception, for want of persons attending to all the essential circumstances of facts ; but nothing that we have seen equals what was exhibited in the years 1747 and 1748.   Mr. Grey's deception was chiefly due to his mistaking the cause of real appearances ; but in this case we can hardly help thinking that not only the imagination and judgment, but even all the external senses of philosophers must have been imposed upon.   It was asserted by Signor Privati, of Venice (who has all the merit of these extraordinary discoveries), and, after him, by Mr. Veratti at Bologna, Mr. Bianchi at Turin, and Mr. Winckler at Leipsick, that if odorous substances were confined in glass vessels, and the vessels excited, the odours and the other medicinal virtues would transpire through the glass, infect the atmosphere of the conductor, and communicate the virtue to all persons in contact with it ; also that those substances, held in the hands of persons electrified, would communicate their virtues to them ; so that medicines might be made to operate without being taken into the stomach."

They even pretended to have wrought many cures by the help of electricity applied in this way.   Priestley goes on to relate that a man with a pain in his side had hyssop applied to it by the advice of a physician, he then approached the cylinder and was electrified.   " The consequence was that he went home and fell asleep, he sweated, and the power of the balsam was so dispersed, that even his cloathes, his bed, and chamber all smelled of it.   When he had refreshed himself by his sleep, he combed his head, and found the balsam to have penetrated his hair, so that the very comb was perfumed." (1)

Another patient, treated in this way by Privati, was no less a person than Signor Donadoni, Bishop of Sebenco.   He came to the seance attended by his physician and friends.   His lordship was 75 years of age, and had experienced pains in his hands and feet for many years.   Owing to gout, he could not move his fingers or bend his knees.   " In this deplorable condition, the poor old bishop implored Privati to treat him by electricity.   Privati filled a glass cylinder with discutient medicines, and managed it so that the electric virtue

(1) Priestley's " History of Electricity," and Phil. Trans. Abridg., Vol. X, p. 400.

might enter into the patient, who presently felt some unusual commotion in his fingers. After two minutes treatment, his lordship opened and shut both his hands, gave a hearty squeeze to one of his attendants, got up, walked, smote his hands together, helped himself to a chair and sat down wondering at his own strength, and hardly knowing whether it was not a dream. At length he walked out of the chamber, down stairs, without any assistance, and with the alacrity of a young man." (1)

Privati and his followers were probably examples of investigators whose enthusiasm had outrun their discretion ; but an undoubted charlatan of this period was a certain Professor Boze, who practised a sort of Maskelyne and Cook *role*. He initiated a new form of electrical treatment which he termed " Beatification." The patient was seated on a large cake of pitch and electrified ; in a short time he was surrounded by flames and smoke, and a halo of electrical breeze adorned his head. Dr. Watson, who had already disproved the extraordinary claims of Privati, exposed the fraud in this case by showing that the professor, before his experiments, clothed himself in a suit of armour provided with a number of points and bosses.

It was not long, after Lovett and Wesley started their electrical treatment, before quackery made its appearance in this country. James Graham (1745-1794), of Edinburgh, affords a striking example of an electrical quack, a class which still flourishes in this country, tolerated by an indifferent or indulgent Government and largely patronised by a gullible public. Graham was the son of a sadler at Edinburgh, and is said to have studied medicine under Munro, Cullen, and Whytt at that university. There appears to be some doubt whether he took his degree in medicine. His pamphlets are signed, " James Graham, M.D.," but the " Dictionary National of Biography " states : "It is doubtful whether he qualified at Edinburgh, where, in 1783, he was described as the person calling himself Dr. Graham." Graham practised as an aurist and oculist in America, and, perhaps, during a two years stay at Philadelphia, 1772-74, he may have acquired his electrical knowledge from a study of Benjamin Franklin's work. But though he may have learned some electricity from the experiments of Franklin, he certainly did not learn his quackery from that great man, for Franklin was most cautious and reserved in his references to medical electricity.

In a letter to Sir J. Pringle, read at the Royal Society, January 12th, 1758, Franklin writes, " he never knew any permanent advantage from electricity in palsies," and goes on to say that, " perhaps some permanent advantage might be obtained if the electric shocks had been accompanied with proper medicine and regimen, under the direction of a skilled physician." On his return to England Graham practised electrical treatment at Bath, Bristol and London. 1779, we find him at Aix la Chapelle, where he treated Georgina, Duchess of Devonshire. The patronage of this lady appears to have been very useful to him, and in the autumn of the same year he established himself at the Temple of Health, Adelphi House, London. He

(1) Priestley's " History of Electricity," and Phil. Trans. Abridg., Vol. X, p. 403.

fitted up this establishment with most elaborate electrical machines, including an electrical throne, insulated upon glass pillars. He claimed to have spent £10,000 upon the installation. This palace did not for long satisfy his ambitions, and he soon opened the Temple of Health and Hymen, at Schomberg House, Pall Mall. It was here that he acquired his chief claim to fame by becoming associated with the notorious Emma Lyon, afterwards the celebrated Lady Hamilton, the companion of Lord Nelson. Graham is said to have exhibited the "frail Emma" as the Goddess of Beauty, and to have utilised her as a nude model for his lectures on health.

Horace Walpole, in his letters, writes of Graham, "The most impudent puppet show I ever saw, and the mountebank himself the dullest of his profession, except that he makes the spectators pay a crown apiece." Southey describes him as "half enthusiast, half knave."

Graham's method of electrical treatment consisted in placing his patients either in baths, or on a magnetic throne, through which electrical currents were passed. His chief speciality was the treatment of sterility ; its cure was effected by sleeping in the Celestial Bed, at the modest fee of £50.

A copy of the *Morning Chronicle*, Thursday, April 24th, 1783, contains the following advertisement of Graham's establishment:—

"Temple of Health and Hymen, Pall Mall. Dr. Graham begs respectfully to inform the Public that this evening, and every evening this week, he will, at the very earnest request of many Gentlemen of the Navy and Army, lately arrived from abroad, deliver his very celebrated Lecture on Generation, etc. . . . Admittance two shillings. A valuable pamphlet will be given gratis to every Lady and Gentleman as they enter the Temple. Patients are electrified and Dr. Graham may be consulted as usual."

Graham was an early exponent of the virtue of the mud bath, a form of treatment of which he showed his personal appreciation by burying himself in the earth for hours at a time. On one occasion he carried out this treatment in company with a young lady from Newcastle. Having first powdered their heads, they were buried in the earth up to their chins, and were likened by a spectator to two blooming cauliflowers. He decried flesh eating and alcoholic excess; he states that he never ate more than sixpennyworth of food a day. He advocated cold bathing, open windows, and sleeping on hard mattresses. He asserted that all diseases were caused by wearing too many clothes. He appears to have carried this idea to extremes, for Southey records that "he would madden himself with opium, rush into the streets, and strip himself to clothe the first beggar he met."

Towards the end of his career he suffered from religious mania, and at Edinburgh was confined to his house as a lunatic. Had Graham lived at the present time he would doubtless have been a leading Christian Scientist, for in one of his pamphlets he describes himself as "formerly a Physician, but now a Christian Philosopher."

In 1778, Dr. Robert Steavenson, of Edinburgh, presented his thesis, "De Electricitate et Operatione ejus in Morbis Curandis." This dissertation is little more than a *resumé* of the work of earlier writers, and its chief interest lies in the fact that a descendant of the author, Dr. W. E. Steavenson, of St. Bartholomew's Hospital, the first medical electrician of that institution, wrote a thesis on the same subject and under the same title for the M.D. degree of the University of Cambridge, 1884.

Jean Paul Marat (1743-1793), scientist, revolutionist, oculist, pulmonary specialist, and electrotherapist, forms one of the most interesting figures in the history of electrotherapy. This man of many parts spent ten years in London, practising part of the time in Conduit Street, Soho. He frequently attended the meetings of the London scientific societies, and on June 30th, 1775, was admitted to the degree of M.D., St. Andrew's. It was during his stay in London that he published his well known paper, "An enquiry into the Nature, Cause, and Cure of a Singular Disease of the Eye." Marat does not appear to have practised electrotherapy during his stay in England, but shortly after his return to France he took part in a disputation, held by the Academy of Lyon, on the value of electricity in medicine. This disputation appears to have been rather acrimonious, for the judges, in awarding the prize to the Abbé Bertholon, for his paper, entitled, "The Influence of the Electricity of the Atmosphere on Diseases," expressed their regret that the Abbé had not been more courteous to his distinguished opponent, Marat. Bertholon made extravagant claims for the use of electricity in all diseases, basing his theories upon pure empiricism rather than upon actual experience. He contended that all diseases were due either to a deficiency or to an excess of the electric fluid. The former cases he treated by the electric bath, the latter by drawing off the excess from the back of the hand of the electrically charged patient. A somewhat similar theory to that of Bertholon, and one but little less absurd, was recently advanced in this country by an electrical engineer, and, like the absurdities of the past, it was not lacking in followers, even among medical men. Marat would have nothing to do with such nonsense; he showed definitely in what diseases electricity should be used, he determined the method of its administration, and defined the efficiency of its action. Marat, indeed, made no small claims for his book on electrotherapy: "One will not find in this publication any hypothesis, any uncertain experiment, any doubtful principle, any hazardous conclusion ; it is upon facts alone, but upon simple and constant facts that all my reasoning is based." Marat, to some extent, at any rate, justified these ambitious claims, for his work was certainly on far more scientific lines than the writings of any of his predecessors, or even, one may add with equal truth, than the publications of many of his successors.

Marat, in his book, yields appreciative testimony to the work of Franklin, but he rejects the idea that the atmospheric electricity has any effect on the human economy. He states that artificial, as opposed to atmospheric electricity, can alone be of any use. From the electric bath he only obtained moderate results. He studied the effects of sparks and shocks, applied in accordance with the practice of his time. He conducted experiments on animals to study the effects of the sparks. As the result of his experiments he concluded that the urine was the best conductor of electricity in the human body; next in order came the bile, the blood, the lymph, and the synovial fluid.

Marat held that electricity was justified in the treatment of external indolent tumours, œdematous engorgement of the limbs, cutaneous eruptions, paralysis, hemiplegia, rheumatism, sciatica, the colic of painters, founders and enamellers. He insisted that the duration of a treatment should be definitely fixed, that there should be a dosage of electricity as well as of other medicines. A séance should last for twenty minutes or more ; it should be repeated three or four times a day. Strong shocks should not be used at all; they should be weak at first and should be gradually increased in strength.

Up to the period which we have now reached, the only form of electricity known was that obtained by means of friction. According to popular tradition, a certain Madame Galvani, the wife of Aloysius Galvani, Professor of Anatomy at Bologna, was in ill health ; and she was consequently ordered by her physician to undergo a diet of frog soup, a delicacy of which she is said to have been very fond. It so happened that in the neighbourhood of the frogs, laid out on the table in preparation for the meal, one of the Professor's assistants was turning a frictional machine. Madame Galvani, to her great surprise, noticed that when a spark was elicited from the apparatus the frogs' legs became contracted, distorted, and apparently endowed with life. The Professor was immediately summoned to witness the phenomenon, which so impressed him, that he immediately proceeded to perform a series of experiments, which are said to have had as much influence on the advancement of science as the discoveries of Galileo and Newton. Unfortunately for the credit of this story, but fortunately for the reputation of Galvani, who has been said by some writers to have been ignorant of electricity at the time he made his discovery, his manuscripts were collected after his death by M. Gherardi, and were published by the Academy of Science of Bologna. Among these papers was a draft in the handwriting of Galvani, dated November 6th, 1780, in which electricity is dealt with in relation to the excitation of contractions in the legs of frogs. In another paper, dated September 20th, 1786, entitled, " Electricity of Metals," Galvani described the contractions which occurred in the legs of a recently killed frog when the muscles and nerves were touched by an arc formed by two dissimilar metals.

It appears, according to Matteucci, in his " Treatise on the Electro-physiological Phenomena of Animals," that the celebrated entomologist, Swammerdam, showed an experiment of a similar character to the Grand Duke of Tuscany, in 1678. This experiment is thus described : " Into a cylindrical tube of glass was placed a muscle, the nerve of which was enveloped with a small silver V wire, in such a manner that it could be raised without injury. The first wire was passed through a ring, bored in the extremity of a small copper support, soldered to a sort of piston or partition ; but this small silver wire was disposed in such a manner that, on passing between the glass and the piston, the nerve could be drawn by the hand so as to touch the copper, the muscle immediately contracted."

Swammerdam's experiment was apparently lost sight of and was unknown to Galvani.

Galvani's great work, " De viribus electricitatis in motu musculari commentarius, 1791," is divided into three parts, dealing respectively with the influence of (1) artificial, (2) atmospheric, and (3) animal electricity in exciting muscular contractions.

It is evident that the author foresaw the application of his discovery to the treatment of disease ; for, in the opening paragraph, he states that he has undertaken his arduous task and has performed a large number of experiments with a view to its practical application, and also to make its use safer in the treatment of diseases.

Galvani at first maintained that the electricity came directly from the muscles and nerves themselves, and, in the flush of his initial success, he is stated to have believed that he had discovered the origin of life. At this period, Alessandro Volta (1745—1827), professor of Natural Philosophy at Pavia, opportunely came on the scene, and was able to show that the current originated from the contact of two dissimilar metals.

As the result of this conclusion, Volta was led to construct his celebrated Voltaic Pile, consisting of alternate discs of copper and zinc, separated by wet pieces of cloth. The announcement of this discovery was made by Volta m a letter to Sir Joseph Banks, in 1800 ; in the following year he visited Paris and showed his instrument to Napoleon at the French Academy of Science. Napoleon, on seeing Volta's pile in action, is related by Chaptal to have exclaimed: " Voila, l'image de la vie : la colonne vertebral est le pile, la vessie le pole positif, et le foie le pole negatif." Volta subsequently discarded his pile for the " Couronne de Tasses," which he designed in its place. This instrument consisted of a number of glass cups, filled with salt and water, or diluted sulphuric acid, in each of which was placed a zinc and a copper rod, the zinc rod (—) in one vessel was connected with the copper rod (+) in the next ; in this way a battery of cells, in series, was obtained, practically of the same character as those used at the present day.

These discoveries of Galvani and Volta rendered possible the far-reaching experiments of Sir Humphrey Davy in electro-chemistry ; they also enabled Oersted, of Copenhagen, in 1820, to demonstrate the deflection of the magnetic needle by the galvanic current, an experiment which in turn led to the discovery of the induction coil and the dynamo, to which instruments the origin of all the modern theories and applications of electricity may be traced ; but the steps by which these developments have been arrived at is beyond the scope of the present lecture.

When we trace the development of electrotherapy from Galvani's discovery, we find that the apparent restoration of function in frogs' legs, which occurred under the influence of the galvanic current, naturally led to the current being first applied to the apparently dead or drowned ; and, as early as 1792, galvanism was recommended as a means of distinguishing real from apparent death. Valli, about this time, claimed to have restored to life, by means of galvanism, fowls which had apparently been drowned ; therapeutical experiments were also at this period performed on patients at the University of Jena by Professor Loder, and Drs. Bischoff and Leickenstein recorded the cure of two cases of amaurosis, and improvement in a case of hemiplegia.

In 1801 Dr. Grapengeisser, of Berlin, published a treatise on the therapeutical effects of galvanism, and recommended its use in weak sight, amaurosis, deafness, rheumatism, and sciatica. Aldini, of Bologna, the nephew of Galvani, published in 1804 his " Essai theorique et experimental sur le galvanisme," Paris, in which he recommended the use of galvanism for disorders of the mind, neuroses, and the diseases of the organs of special sense.

Partly owing to defective apparatus, but chiefly on account of its failure to fulfil the preposterous claims of its too enthusiastic advocates, galvanism declined for a time into disuse. A revival of its use in the form of electrical acupuncture took place about 1825. In that year Sarlandiere published his " Memoires sur l'electropuncture considérée comme moyen noveau de traiter efficacement la goutte, le rheumatismes, et les affections nerveuses, et sur l'emploi du moxa Japonais en France." Paris, 1825. A work by Majendie appeared a year later, entitled, " On Galvanism, with Observations on its Chymical Properties and Medical Efficacy in Chronic Diseases." London 1826. Sarlandiere used two steel or platinum needles, introducing them as in acupuncture, or as it was then called, acupuncturation, and connecting them respectively with the opposite poles of the battery. Majendie was a bold operator, and his practice was to introduce the needles directly through the eyeball on to the orbital nerves and then apply the current ; it is said that in this way he accomplished some remarkable cures, but, as sometimes happens, even now, in the relation of modern surgical marvels, nothing is said of the occasional disastrous failures resulting from so drastic a procedure.

The discovery of the induction coil by Faraday, in 1831, was attended by less sensational, but by far more valuable clinical results than those which immediately ensued on the publication of Galvani's work. Five years later, in the autumn of 1836, an electrical department was established at Guy's Hospital. A room was set apart for the administration of electricity, under the charge of Dr. Golding Bird, and clinical clerks were appointed to record the cases. Dr. Golding Bird remained in charge of the department for eight years, when he was succeeded by Dr., afterwards Sir William, Gull. Though this was the first electrical department established in this country, electrical treatment had been practised in the Royal Infirmary, Edinburgh, many years previously ; for Dr. Whytt, in his book, " The Cause of Nervous Disorders," published in 1764, records the case of a patient in that institution, " who felt a remarkable uneasiness through his whole body, when it was charged with the electrical fluid by means of a wire held in the hand, although there was no other shock given him."

Dr. Golding Bird's lectures " On Electricity and Galvanism in relation to Physiology and Therapeutics," delivered to the Royal College of Physicians in the spring of 1847, mark a distinct advance in the recognition accorded to electrotherapy by the medical profession. These lectures were published in book form in 1849. This charmingly written book commences with a philosophical discussion on the electrical methods in use in his day, and concludes with a summary of the personal experience of the author of the results of electrical treatment, chiefly in connection with the work at Guy's Hospital. Dr. Bird complains of the position of electrotherapy in his time in much the same terms as we frequently hear used to-day : " Electricity has by no means been fairly treated as a therapeutical agent ; for it has either been exclusively referred to, when all other remedies have failed—in fact, often exclusively, or nearly so, in helpless cases—or its administration has been carelessly directed, and the mandate, ' Let the patient be electrified,' merely given, without reference to the manner, form, or mode of the remedy being for an instant taken into consideration. Conscientiously convinced that the agent in question is a no less energetic than valuable remedy in the treatment of disease, I feel most anxious to press its employment upon the practical physician, and to urge him to have recourse to it as a rational but fallible remedy, and not to regard it as one capable of effecting impossibilities."

Dr. Bird mentions the success which attended the use of faradism by a skilled obstetrician in cases of uterine inertia; he alludes to the scepticism expressed by the famous obstetrician, Dr. Simpson, of Edinburgh, in regard to this treatment ; but Dr. Bird prefers to pin his faith to the facts recorded by Drs. Lever and Radford rather than to the theories of Dr. Simpson. Faradism is also mentioned as having been successful in the control of postpartum hæmorrhage.

This treatment is referred to on the testimony of others as having benefited incontinence of urine and atony of the bladder. Dr. Bird mentions that he had never seen electrical treatment successful in cases of paralysis attended with permanent contraction. He advocated the use of static sparks in lead palsy, and various forms of electricity in the treatment of hysteria, chorea, amenorrhœa, tonsillitis, catalepsy, etc. " In the treatment of amaurosis," he says, " I have seen it employed in the hospital under all forms of this disease, and regret that I have never been able to observe the slightest benefit in whatever way it has been employed. In deafness, also, it has been greatly lauded, but I have seen little which can bear out the commendations accorded to it by some writers."

Dr. Bird is most enthusiastic over the treatment of disease by what he terms the " electric moxa " ; this consisted of a zinc plate and silver plate, connected by a wire, for the treatment of indolent wounds, etc. Under the zinc plate electrolytic action occurred with the formation of zinc oxychloride, and resulted in the formation of a deep slough. When a wound did not already exist, blisters were first induced to overcome the skin resistance. In the case of the silver plate, well moistening the skin with salt and water was usually all the preparation required. In the appendix of the book there are some interesting notes from Mr., afterwards Sir Thomas, Spencer Wells, the celebrated surgeon, at that time a surgeon in the navy, on the treatment of about sixty cases of ulcer, fistula, etc., by this method of electric moxæ. Probably as the result of Dr. Bird's lectures, the Pulvermacher, and later the Harness electrical belts were foisted upon a credulous public during the latter half of the 19th century, and became a most successful and remunerative form of quackery. These belts consisted of metal discs on the plan of Dr. Bird's moxæ, but as the preliminary production of blisters would not have conduced to the speedy sale of the apparatus, the electrical resistance of the skin was ignored, with the result that a credulous public suffered in pocket only, and no sores or moxæ were produced. A large number of medical men of the time, including Sir Richard Quain and Sir Andrew Clark, testified to the efficacy of these electric belts, and, in consequence of their ignorance of electricity, supported the imposture.

It was the discovery of Faraday that led to the electrical work of the most famous and illustrious of medical electricians, Duchenne, of Boulogne : "The man who has played a preponderating part in the researches and the discoveries upon which the edifice of neuropathology has been erected."

In 1849, Duchenne made his first, and in 1852 his second communication to the French Academy of Science : "A Critical Examination of the Instruments of Induction, from the point of view of their application to Physiology, Pathology, and Therapeutics." In 1855 he published his book of 926 pages, "De L'Electrisation Localisée." Duchenne chiefly relied on faradism : "Of the three forms of electricity, induced electricity is the best for muscular electrisation, especially as it can be practised frequently and for a long time. . . . In its application to physiology, pathology, and to treatment, this method of electrisation has surpassed my expectations in yielding scientific and practical results of the highest importance."

Duchenne was of opinion that there was a difference in the physiological action of the primary and the secondary current, but Becquerel (1) pointed out that the variations in the physiological effects of the two currents was entirely due to the difference which existed in their voltage. It was subsequently demonstrated by a special wiring of the coils, which permitted the wiring of the primary and secondary coils to be modified, that the effects which Duchenne attributed respectively to the primary and the secondary currents could be reversed at will.

Dr. Neef, of Berlin, and Masson, of Paris, are said to have been the first to apply faradism to the treatment of disease ; but it is certainly to A. Tripier, of Paris, who began writing on the treatment of the diseases of women by faradism in 1859, that we owe the modern type of faradic coil. In fact, it may be said that, with the exception of the condenser introduced by Fizeau, no definite improvement in this instrument has been made since 1865, when Tripier showed to the French Academy of Science a series of coils with different windings, both in their primaries and their secondaries, and fitted with an interrupter, the rate of vibration of which could be varied at will.

(1) "Traite des applications de L'électricité," Paris, 1857.

Tripier, moreover, shares with Apostoli the credit of being the first to successfully apply electricity in a rational and methodical manner to the treatment of the diseases of women, especially in reference to the treatment of fibroids, Tripier relying in such cases on the faradic current, and Apostoli preferring galvanism.

We have now reached a period where the history of the past merges into the history of the modern development of electrotherapy ; the recent history of light, Roentgen rays, high frequency and diathermy will be more appropriately dealt with by the lecturers on these subjects. There is still, however, to be considered the origin of the introduction of drugs by the galvanic current.

It is generally thought that this treatment was first practised and advocated by Leduc, of Nantes, and that it was introduced into this country by Dr. Lewis Jones. Historical research shows us that the method was used in this country by Dr. Benjamin Ward Richardson, in the year 1858, under the name of " Voltaic Narcotism."

In October, 1858, Dr. Benjamin Ward Richardson produced a local anæsthesia as the result of applying a solution of morphia under the positive pole of the current ; and he published his results in the *Medical Times and Gazette,* of February 12th and June 25th, 1859. Richardson subsequently substituted the following preparation for the solution of morphia.

> Tinct. Aconiti ʒiii
> Extr : Aconiti gr.xx
> Chloroformi ʒiii

Applying this solution under the positive pole, and passing a continuous current for eleven minutes, he obtained local anæsthesia in a dog's leg, enabling it to be amputated with no evidence of pain except when the bone was sawn through. A nævus in a child was painlessly removed, teeth were extracted, and a hernia operated on by the use of the same technique.

It is probably due to the exclusive use of the positive pole, at this time, as the active electrode, that the term " Cataphoresis " was applied, and is still used at such places as hydros and electrical institutes, as synonymous with the term " Ionic Medication." It is remarkable that such drugs as chloroform, etc., were used, as they contain no ions, and are consequently non-conductors.

The chloroform and similar agents were probably absorbed through the skin, which had become inflamed owing to the high voltage required to force a current through it, after its electrical resistance had been enormously increased by the application of these non-conducting fluids. Wagner, at the time, pointed out the non-conducting properties of chloroform, and Waller also showed that the insensibility induced was due merely to the absorption of the chloroform, that the procedure was painful, and resulted in inflammation and destruction of the skin. Richardson subsequently withdrew the claims he had made for the practical value of this treatment.

In taking a general survey of the development of electrotherapy from the earliest times, we cannot fail to be struck by the extremely undulating character of its progress, although on the whole the general tendency may be satisfactory ; yet in almost every instance the sudden advance or boom, consequent upon a new discovery, is followed by a nearly corresponding set back or slump. These failures to realise our earliest hopes are clearly, to some extent, due to the exaggerated zeal of too enthusiastic investigators ; but a careful study of the history will prove that they are mainly due to the immediate exploitation of any new discovery by unqualified and unprincipled quacks. In a paper on the history of electrotherapy in Great Britain, which I contributed two years ago to the *American Journal of Electrotherapeutics*, I wrote as follows : " The science and practice of electrotherapeutics can never develop to their full efficiency until they receive their due recognition as an important branch of the healing art, until they are efficiently taught in our universities and schools of medicine, and are placed in the schedules of the examining boards." Both the past and the present show us that no sooner is a new form of electrical treatment introduced to the notice of the medical profession, than it falls into the hands of ignorant and blatantly advertising quacks, who by using it in an unsuitable manner, and in unsuitable cases, and especially by their preposterous claims unsupported by the testimony of results, immediately bring the method to discredit.

It is manifestly absurd to suppose that such a highly specialised science and art as electrotherapy, comprising as it does, or at any rate should do, an intimate knowledge of anatomy, physiology, electricity and pathology, can be practised by any electrician or masseuse. As Aristotle wrote, more than two thousand years ago : " But nevertheless, I venture to say that if a man wishes to master any art or gain a scientific knowledge of it, he must advance to its general principles, and make himself acquainted with them in the proper method ; for, as we have said, it is with universal proposition that the sciences deal." (1)

By the institution of a diploma in Radiology and Electrology by the University of Cambridge, 1920, an opportunity is afforded to all qualified medical men to become acquainted, in the manner indicated by Aristotle, with the general principles of physiology, pathology, and electricity relating to the practice of Radiology and Electrology, and medical men are thereby enabled to master these arts and to gain a scientific knowledge of them.

(1) Aristotle's " Ethics," Book X, 9-16, Peter's Trans., p. 351.

RADIO TECHNIQUE.

THE EXAMINATION OF AIRCRAFT TIMBER BY X RAYS.

By Captain R. KNOX, M.D., R.A.M.C., and Major G. W. C. KAYE, O.B.E., M.A., D.Sc., R.A.F.

A Contribution to a "General Discussion on The Examination of Materials by X rays," held jointly by the Faraday Society and the Röntgen Society on Tuesday, April 29th, 1919.

(Abstracted from the *Transactions of the Faraday Society*, Vol. XV, Part 1, 1919.)

ABOUT the middle of 1918 the Aeronautical Inspection Department decided to ascertain what measure of practical assistance the X rays would afford to its timber inspecting staff in their efforts to ensure that high standard of quality and workmanship which experience has shown to be so essential. The idea was put to the test, using the equipment of the Cancer Hospital (by kind permission of the Governors). The results were very encouraging, but owing to the severe pressure of other matters progress was somewhat delayed, and at the time of the Armistice the method had not reached the stage of commercial application. But sufficient examples had been obtained to demonstrate the value of X rays in this connection, and the only questions remaining were those arising out of equipment—portability, convenience, and the like.

We would like here to acknowledge our great indebtedness to Lieut. Hudson-Davies, who throughout has shown the keenest practical interest. Mr. G. F. Westlake is responsible for most of the radiographic work.

It was realised from the start that for the method to be worth while, it must permit the rapid visual examination of the part under inspection. This naturally implies fluorescent screen examination, photography being reserved purely for permanently recording such cases which the screen shows to be of interest.

All woods are particularly transparent to X rays, and soft X-ray tubes were necessary, the alternative spark gap being usually from 1 to 2 inches between point electrodes. It may be remembered that the efficiency of both the output of an X-ray bulb and the excitation of a fluorescent screen are much less with soft than with hard rays, and it is therefore expedient to use rays as hard as are feasible for the work in hand. A high tension transformer and Coolidge tube were mostly employed, the latter being adjusted to give an abundance of rays of long wave length, some 15 milliamperes being passed through.

As already remarked, in the construction of all parts of aircraft the best workmanship and material of the highest quality are essential, owing to the low factor of safety. X rays may thus be resorted to at two periods:—

(1) While the material is in the rough unfinished condition, and

(2) When the part is assembled and ready for employment.

It will be convenient to consider these stages separately.

1. *Examination of Raw Material.*

The chief defects that had to be looked for in aeronautical timber during the war were spiral grain (in spruce and spruce substitutes), large hidden knots, large resin pockets, compression shakes, incipient decay (including dote), grub holes, very light wood, etc.

It was realised that the method of X-ray diagnosis could only be helpful in revealing differences of density; and, as was anticipated, no difficulty whatever was experienced in detecting hidden knots and resin pockets, grub holes, and the like. "Localising" depth as well as position was attained by radiographing both a front and a side view.

Localising by stereoscopy can also be employed, and actual measurements of depth obtained.

If the specimens are not too thick, it is possible, though only with difficulty, to detect compression shakes, incipient rot, and spiral grain. The chief feature, however, that the X rays bring out is the difference between the light spring and the denser summer growths, *i.e.*, the annual rings of the tree. From a practical standpoint this is only useful in detecting the presence of localised hard grain—an objectionable feature for aircraft purposes. Six radiographs show different aeroplane woods, all of high quality. The chief feature in those photographs taken tangentially to the annual rings is the "grain" produced by the annual rings. The true grain or fibre is not shown in most of the photographs.

It might be remarked that the method of inspection by X rays is still in its infancy, and that with increasing experience in technique and improvements in plates and photographic methods better results will follow.

The vigilance of the inspectors during the process of construction prevented very many accidents. It must, of course, be realised under what high pressure the various aircraft builders were working during the war, and the fact speaks for itself, that in spite of grave difficulties of both labour and material, British aeroplanes were superior both in quality and numbers to those of any other nation. But there is the tendency which is known to exist in some natures to try to conceal a mistake due to a slip, especially when, from a lack of knowledge of design, the importance of the mistake might be underrated. During the war the various aircraft factories, with this in mind, displayed large notices reminding the staff that "A concealed mistake may cost a brave man his life."

It goes without saying that certain members of an aeroplane structure are more important than others, and that in minor parts departure from highest quality material or workmanship may not be attended with serious consequences. But it is imperative in the case of vital parts that nothing should be tolerated which will imperil or reduce the factor of safety of the machine.

Of these important items, the most vital are :—

    (*a*) Main-plane wing spars—which pass from end to end of each wing.

    (*b*) Compression struts—which separate the spars in each wing.

    (*c*) Interplane struts—which separate the upper and lower planes.

    (*d*) Longerons, cross struts and engine bearers — which make up the fuselage.

In most of these instances the composite, laminated, or hollow "box" method of construction is permissible. In some examples the strut or spar is completely covered with fabric, veneer, or plywood; and ordinary visual inspection of the final part is just as ineffective as with hollow spars or struts of the "box" type. An inspector cannot "stand over" the job all the time, and in many cases has to be content with examination of the part in question when it is put up for final approval. But he now receives a powerful ally in the X rays, which clearly reveal the

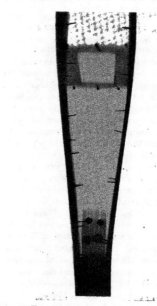

Fig. 1.—X-ray photograph showing the interior of the end of a hollow "Box" aeroplane strut. The internal strengthening block at the end is seen to be badly fitted, and each of the screws has split the block.

quality of workmanship and material of the internal structure of the aeroplane part.

The following examples are selected as illustrating some of the directions in which the method has been developed :—

Fig. 1 shows the front and side view of the end of a hollow box strut. The internal strengthening block is seen to be badly fitted and each of the screws has split the wood, making altogether insecure and poor work.

Fig. 2 is the front and side view of a hollow main-wing spar. In this poor workmanship is shown in the cutting to shape of the internal block. The block is also split across the centre, facilitating the breaking of the spar under sheer stresses.

Fig. 3. This shows the side view of a hollow aileron spar. The spar consists of two halves fitted together by glued joints down centre. It is important that both sides of the outer skin should be of the same thickness; but in reducing the glued-up spar to correct finished dimensions,

construction, and the paper describes a method of examining aeroplane timber parts by X rays which the Aeronautical Inspection Department, with the co-operation of the Staff of the X-ray Department of the Cancer Hospital, investigated during the war.

No difficulty is experienced in detecting concealed knots, resin pockets and grub holes. Excess or deficiency of glue in glued joints is readily revealed. Workmanship and material in the interior of completed laminated or

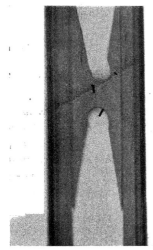

FIG. 2.—X-ray photograph of hollow main-wing spar. Poor workmanship in internal strengthening block.

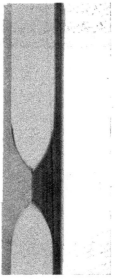

FIG 3.—X-ray photograph showing side view of hollow aileron spar consisting of two halves glued together, after sides have been spindled out. The two halves of the central block should register accurately, and the sides should be equally thick.

workmen are apt to plane away more wood from one side than from the other, occasionally reducing the strength to a critical degree. The use of X rays affords an immediate indication if this is the case. Sometimes the internal block is misplaced or omitted from one of the halves and its absence cannot be determined by external examination. In the present case the block is correctly placed.

SUMMARY.

The best workmanship and the highest quality of material are essential in aircraft

box spars and struts cannot be scrutinised by ordinary methods of inspection, but every detail is shown up by the X rays. The centre veneers of plywood (which enters into the structural design of many aeroplanes) can be examined by the same means.

In almost all instances · fluorescent screen examination suffices.

The original paper gives particulars of some twenty or thirty actual examples collected during the war.

REPORTS OF SOCIETY.

SOCIÉTÉ DE RADIOLOGIE MÉDICALE DE FRANCE.

Séance du 11 Novembre, 1919.

Radiographie d'un volvulus de l'estomac, par les Drs. JAULIN, LIMOUZY, et MARNE. Ces A. présentent deux cas de volvulus de l'estomac, l'un à 90°, l'autre à 180°, avec calques et radiographies. Les deux cas se rapportent à des volvulus partiels n'intéressant que la partie inférieure de l'estomac et à évolution chronique. Ce sont les premiers qui, à leur connaissance aient été révélés par la radiographie. Dans le volvulus à 180° le pylore et le duodénum sont nettement visible sur le bord gauche de l'estomac.

Un cas de calcification artérielle, par les Drs. BRODIER et HADENGUE. Les clichés présentés concernent un homme de 40 ans, atteint de coxalgie. Le réseau artériel est parfaitement visible au niveau des deux membres inférieurs. L'examen des membres supérieurs est négatif.

Constation d'un niveau variable de liquide dans le colon transverse dilaté en amont d'une stricture néoplastique, par les Drs. PIERRE DUVAL, GARNIER, et HARET. Les A. communiquent ce cas pour la rareté de l'image ; à l'examen radioscopique en position debout, le colon transverse apparaissait dilaté à tel point que l'on voyait, de l'angle splénique à l'angle hépatique un niveau liquide horizontal avec une chambre à air. De temps en temps une contraction intestinale refoulait dans le colon ascendant une certaine quantité du liquide opaque qui remontait ensuite dans le transverse.

Calculs du cholédoque, par les Drs. PIERRE DUVAL et H. BÉCLÈRE. Il s'agit d'une femme de 55 ans, soignée pour une lithiase biliaire ancienne compliquée depuis plusieurs mois d'ictère intermittent par rétention avec poussées fébriles. La radiographie faite dans la position ventrale avec rayons très peu pénétrants et ampoule Coolidge - Baby, montre deux groupes de calculs. L'un est constitué par e calculs (vésicule biliaire) et l'autre par l'ombre étagée de sept calculs. La position de ce dernier groupement fait porter le diagnostic de calculs du cholédoque. L'intervention chirurgicale confirma le diagnostic radiologique.

Sur un cas de diverticule de l'œsophage, par le Dr. LAGARENNE. Présentation de clichés montrant un diverticule de la partie tout-à-fait supérieure de l'œsophage, diverticulum très volumineux, situé en arriere de l'œsophage et communiquant avec lui par un canal très rétrèci.

Le Sécretaire Général : Dr. HARET.

Séance du 9 Décembre, 1919.

Incontinence pylorique, par le Dr. AUBOURG. L'A. présente une nouvelle obs. d'incontinence pylorique vraie, caractérisée, au point de vue radiologique par le passage immédiate du liquide opaque, de l'estomac dans le grêle, sans contractions stomachales apparentes, le pylore fonctionnant comme un cardia normal. L'intervention montra une tumeur de la région pylorique ; l'incontinence dans ce cas avait pour cause une lésion pariétale de la région pylorique. A coté de ces formes de lésion du pylore avec signes classiques de sténose et signes radiologiques de stase stomachale dans l'examen tardif de l'estomac, il existe des formes rares de lésions du pylore, caractérisées au contraire par l'absence de vomissements et d'hématemeses au point de vue clinique, par l'incontinence pylorique au point de vue radiologique. Ces faits sont d'autant plus intéressants à connaître que dans ces cas les signes radiologiques précedent les signes cliniques peu accusés. Mais l'incontinence pylorique n'a pas pour seule cause une lésion pariétale de la région pylorique. L'A. rapporte l'obs. d'une malade à laquelle on fit pour lésion pariétale du bord gauche une large résection mediogastrique ; un examen rad. pratiqué ensuite montra une incontinence pylorique bien que cette région minutieusement explorée au cours de l'opération ne présentait aucune lésion ; la raison du non fonctionnement du pylore était du a la section des nerfs de la petite courbure, au cou de la résection déterminant une paralysie du pylore.

Sténose incomplète du pylore, par le Dr. AIMARD. Le sujet présentait les signes cliniques et radiologiques d'une sténose pylorique. L'opération montra un pylore normal, mais il existait un semis de noyaux cancéreux siégeant a la partie sup. de la grande courbure ; il s'agissait donc d'une sténose pylorique réflexe.

Lithiase pancréatique multiple, par les Drs. AIMARD et LAFFOND. Les A. rapportent l'histoire d'une malade qui présenta des crises tres douloureuses avec meloena qui furent attribuées a un ulcus du duodénum. A l'autopsie on trouva une lithiase pancréatique ayant déterminé une hémorragie a travers l'ampoule de Vater ; ces calculs radiographiés a travers l'abdomen d'un sujet sain étaient tres nettement visibles. Les. A. insistent sur la nécéssité de faire non seulement une radioscopie mais une radiographie quand il y a douleur de la région pancréatico-duodénale.

Un cas d'osteome de l'humérus, par les Drs. BAUMGARTNER et MAHAR. Il s'agissait d'une volumineuse exostose ostéogénique.

Un cas de tuberculose du carpe guérie par la radiothérapie, par le Dr. MAHAR. Les radiographies successives montrent l'apparition beaucoup plus précoce en le développement extremement rapide des points d'ossification des osselets du carpedu coté malade irradié. Cette précocité pourrait être due à l'action excitante des Rayons X employés à faible dose.

A propos d'une lésion du carpe, par les Drs. TRIBOUT et AUBOURG. Présentation d'un cliché du carpe montrant la différence de forme d'un scaphoide par rapport à celui du coté opposé, sans que l'exploration au cours d'une intervention chirurgicale ait pu permettre d'affirmer une lésion de cet os.

Le Sécretaire Général: Dr. HARET.

REVIEW.

Roentgen Interpretation: A Manual for Students and Practitioners. By GEORGE W. HOLMES, M.D. and HOWARD E. RUGGLES, M.D. (Philadelphia and New York: Lea and Febiger. London : Henry Kimpton). 15s. net.

This little book comprises a great deal of information within its 208 pages. Works dealing solely with interpretation have hitherto been few and far between. Till recently, it was scarcely possible to purchase a book on radiology in which less than half of its pages were taken up with descriptions of apparatus and technique. But those who have once settled for themselves, at least for a time, what machinery they will use, and how they will use it, are apt to skip all these descriptions ; whereas it is difficult to imagine anyone who is not interested in the question of interpretation. For it is here that we come to grips with the truly medical aspect of radio-diagnosis. All else can, if necessary, be done by the skilled layman.

The book under review deals with bones and joints, the chest, the gastro-intestinal tract, and the genito-urinary system. As regards the bones, the letterpress is excellent, but the reproductions leave much to be desired. The bones are for the most part shown so dark that detail is obscured, and, in some cases at least, the prints have evidently been made from under-exposed negatives.

There is a section of 39 pages dealing with the chest, and the illustrations here are as good, or better, than those shown in most text books.

About the same space is devoted to a consideration of the alimentary tract. This subject being wider from a radio-diagnostic point of view than that of the chest, the account here suffers by compression. The information appears to be sound so far as it goes, but the question of enema interpretation is scarcely touched on, and the recently so much discussed subject of *diverticulitis* does not seem to be mentioned.

The account of the urinary system is compressed into 15 pages. It is pretty complete as regards the ordinary examinations, but

naturally the subject of pyelography is no more than mentioned.

On the whole, this small volume may be described as an experiment in which some degree of success has been attained. It will, no doubt, prove the forerunner of much more complete works dealing with the subject of interpretation.

NOTES AND ABSTRACTS

Electrical Changes Produced by Light.— H. S. ALLEN (*Jour. of the Rönt. Soc.*, April, 1919, pp. 33-44).—The theory of photoluminescence, developed by Stark and by Lenard, is briefly this: the exciting light produces photo-electric separation of the electrons. These in some cases return almost at once to the parent atom, and in their return bring about the emission of light of a somewhat longer wave-length. That is fluorescence. In other cases—as in phosphorescence—the electrons do not at once return to the parent atom, but are, as it were, caught and held by the surrounding molecules, so that it is only after a certain delay that they return to the starting point.

It is well known that certain chemical changes are produced by the action of light. These actions, according to Allen, involve a separation of electrons, which may be complete or partial. At the present time it is not possible to trace out all the stages in the photo-chemical changes, but the author believes that the first step is the production of ionized molecules which are then in a condition suitable for recombination in a different fashion. In the formation of the latent image in photography, the theory of Joly and developed by the author is that the change is purely a physical one, and that in the latent image we have a collection of ionized molecules. Joly has also tried to apply the same conception in radiotherapy. In the case of the living cell, the radiation falling upon it may, if carefully modulated,

stimulate and, if too intense, retard the growth, and ultimately destroy the molecular structure required for mytosis. Joly points out that the growth of the cell is highly sensitive to ionic concentration, so that when radiation falls on the material there may be a change taking place in the number of ionized molecules in consequence of this photo-electric action.

As to the phenomenon of vision, Allen thinks that photo-electric action occurs in the chemical substances of the rods or cones, so that there is a separation of electrons resulting in electrification of the nerve cells which set up the impulse to the sensorium. If this view be correct, the changes in the retina are identical with those which take place in phosphorescence or in the formation of a latent image on the photographic plate.

R. W. A. S.

Köhler's Disease of the Tarsal Scaphoid in Children.—F. W. O'BRIEN (*Boston Med. and Surg. Jour.*, April 17th, 1919, pp. 445-447, with 2 radiograms).—O'Brien adds another case to the literature of this rare condition. The radiographic appearance in the scaphoid is characteristic :—

(a) One half to one-quarter smaller than normal.

(b) Form entirely regular.

(c) Impossible to differentiate between the cortex and spongy portion.

(d) Density increased two to four fold.

R. W. A. S.

The Cardiothoracic Ratio: an Index of Cardiac Enlargement.— C. S. DANZER (*Amer. Jour. of the Med. Sciences*, April, 1919, pp. 513-521, with 10 Figs.).—This method is based on the fact that the heart bears an almost constant relationship to its surrounding framework the chest. This is seen in the narrow vertical type of heart associated with the long asthenic chest and the wide emphysematous chest with a heart of corresponding breadth, and one which is more transverse and at a higher level than in the previous type.

. For practical purposes it may be said that the ratio between the size of the heart and the chest is constant, except when pathological processes set in.

The technique adopted is as follows:— X-ray tube at six feet or more from the patient, who is in the upright position, and the exposure should be made at midinspiration.

- The thoracic measurement is taken at its greatest diameter and the cardiac measurements also at their widest points; for the latter it is usually at the fifth space on the left side and the fourth on the right.

Under these conditions, the ratio is—

$$\frac{\text{Heart (transverse diameter)}}{\text{Thorax (transverse diameter)}}\ \ \begin{array}{l}\text{39 to 50 per}\\ \text{cent.}\end{array}$$

Values of 53 per cent. and over are considered definitely pathological, while below 45 per cent. in the presence of suspicious lung signs is in favour of tuberculosis.

R. W. A. S.

General Discussion on "The Examination of Materials by X rays."—Joint Meeting of the Faraday Society and the Rontgen Society, April 29, 1919.

The Chairman (Sir R. Hadfield) introduced the discussion by making comments on some of the more important recent papers on this subject by workers in the different countries of the world.

The following were delivered :—

"Radiometallography," an address on, by W. H. Bragg.

Short abstracts by A. W. Porter from the following papers :—(a) "Investigation of Metals by means of X rays," F. Janus (Munich) and M. Reppchen (Cologne), in which a description of the Lilienfeld tube is given; (b) "The Principles Governing the Penetration of Metals by X rays," G. Respondek (Halensee), in which the X-ray examination of the metal framework of concrete slabs is described.

" Apparatus used for Radiometallography," a brief description of, by H. Pilon and G. Pearce.

" The Examination of Timber by X rays," a paper on, by R. Knox and G. W. C. Kaye, in which the great value of X-ray Examination of the materials in aeroplane construction was shown.

" Radiographic Examination of Carbon Electrodes used in Electric Steel-making Furnaces," a paper on, by Sir R. Hadfield and S. A. Main.

" A Method of Testing an X-ray Tube for Definition," a paper on, by J. Brooksbank. By means of two fine needles at varying distances from the tube and the sharpness of the resulting shadows, tubes can be classified as to their definition. C. E. S. Phillips demonstrated the actual apparatus for this testing which is used, under his direction, at the War Office X-ray Laboratory.

" The Detection of Hair Cracks in Steel by means of X rays," a note on, by C. F. Jenkin.

" The Behaviour of Photographic Plates to X rays considered in relation to the Radiography of Metals," a paper on, by F. F. Renwick.

"Contrasts in X-ray Photographs," a paper on, by R. E. Slade, in which was discussed at length the quality of X rays which gave the maximum contrast in photographs through metals.

" Researches into the Industrial X-ray Examination of Metals at the Laboratories of Messrs. Schneider, Le Creusot," a paper on, by E. Schneider, in which it is stated that X rays enable an examination to be made of ordinary steels, provided their thickness does not exceed 40 to 45 mm.

The discussion was also taken part in by several well known electrical engineers and physicists. An exhibition and demonstration of apparatus and materials connected with radiometallography was given during the evening. R. W. A. S.

Œsophago-Tracheal Fistula.—I. GERBER (*Amer. Jour. of Roent.*, April, 1919, pp. 191-194).—Gerber records and illustrates a case of the above associated with the presence of a pressure diverticulum of the œsophagus and, in all probability, of syphilitic etiology.

R. W. A. S.

Roentgen Ray Treatment of Tinea Tonsurans.

—H. H. HAZON (*Journal of Cutaneous Diseases*, May, 1919).—Less than one per cent. of ringworm cases can be cured by medicine or local antiseptic applications. Ninety-nine per cent. can be cured by the proper use of the Roentgen rays, and with no harmful results if the technique is right. The object is not to kill the organisms, but to produce a defluvium. This removes most of the spores, and reduces the food supply of the parasites so that the remainder can be killed by antiparasitic remedies, which can penetrate the now empty follicles. The author follows the Kienbock method, as modified by Adamson. The hair is cut short, and along the vertical line from brow to occiput three points are marked at five-inch intervals. Two lateral points are marked at the same distance. The tube is centred carefully over each spot in turn, so that each exposure is at right angles to the others. With the Coolidge tube and interrupterless transformer a standard technique is adopted, and needs no measurement of doses. The author's technique is:—

Focal skin distance, 9 in.; spark gap $7\frac{3}{4}$ in.; ma. 4; time $1\frac{1}{4}$ minutes. This represents a little over 4 Holzknecht units. A mild antiseptic ointment is used until the scalp is clean, yellow oxide or salicylic acid; if erythema is caused there may be a permanent baldness. Once the hair has fallen, full strength ointments may be used to clear up any patches. Out of 225 cases of tinea tonsurans treated by this method only one recurred, and there were only two mishaps. In one the timing clock stopped and an overdose produced permanent baldness, in the other the child moved, so that where the exposures overlapped there was a slightly excessive dose with thinning of the new hair.   N. B.

The Treatment of Guinea-worm by Total Extirpation.

—G. HUDELLET (*Arch. d'Élect. Méd.*, April, 1919).—The difficulty of accurately localising the guinea-worm preparatory to its excision has been partly met by the X-ray method, as shown by Bergonié and

Dimier, but the work is delicate and the parasite not always easy to distinguish. By making use of its capability of penetration by liquids it can be shown up clearly. On finding evidence of the worm, by its pointing on the skin, or on opening an abscess caused by it, a ten per cent. solution of collargol is injected. The whole parasite is then clearly visible under X rays, and is also shown up against the surrounding tissues when operation is performed.

N. B.

Apparent Partial R.D.

—H. BORDIER (*Arch. d'Élect. Méd.*, Feb., 1919).—A series of cases of functional contractures or flaccid paralyses of the arm were examined in the winter of 1915-16, and the dorsal interossei and hypothenar muscles were found to show, almost invariably, a partial R.D. The condition in detail was: Slowed galvanic response, with alteration of the polar formula, and some hypoexcitability and faradic hypoexcitability. In the definite absence of organic lesions the author was at a loss to explain the state of affairs until, on examining several of the men again at the end of April, he found normal reactions, although the functional condition had not cleared up. He then realised that the winter cold, combined with the lack of movement in the part, had caused the whole condition of depression or hypoexcitability. He was able to reproduce the same type of partial R.D. (reaction of hypothermia) by immersing the hand of a normal man in cold water for 15 minutes, and to find it during another winter in a number of nurses who suffered from cold hands. The condition should be taken into account in examining any patient in cold weather.   N, B.

Reconstitution of Muscles, Singly or in Groups, by Rhythmic Intensive Faradisation.

—J. BERGONIÉ (*Arch. d'Élect. Méd.*, Feb., 1919).—The majority of wounds leave one or more muscles in need of rehabilitation. The best method is useful work, professional or preferably agricultural, every day and all day, which brings into play the affected muscle. But there are conditions in which such work is not possible, and then the effective treatment is rhythmic intensive faradisation. The induced waves should be sharp, purely oscillographic, of a frequency of 50 to 55 per second to just produce tetanisation, from a coil with well regulated trembler and without spark, or a special machine giving pointed waves. About 15 of these waves, attaining 12 to 14 volts at their height, form a suitable series to be delivered by a metronome with equal alternations of exercise and rest. The current should be applied longitudinally and over very large surfaces.

N. B.

An Observation on the Movements of the Colon.—CARLO GUARINI (*La Radiol. Med.*, 1919, Vol. VI, p. 99).—It is generally admitted that there are continual movements of the large intestine. They are described as of two kinds, lesser undulatory movements, which cannot be observed in radioscopic examination, but can be made out by a series of plates exposed at short intervals, and the greater pendular movements, described by Ludwig, which are caused by contraction of a length of several centimetres of the tract of the colon. It has been suggested that this big movement is excited by the taking of food or by defæcation. The author shows illustrations of a case in which he was able to observe this large movement taking place spontaneously and without any of these exciting causes. The cæcum and lower part of ascending colon were seen to be distended with the opaque meal, and showed the usual segmental appearance. Suddenly the walls seemed to squeeze themselves together, and assumed a tubular aspect, and the whole mass advanced to fill the angle of the hepatic flexure. The transverse segmentation returned, and the cycle of movements was then repeated once. All happened within the space of three or four seconds.

N. B.

CORRESPONDENCE.

MANCHESTER ROYAL INFIRMARY. X-RAY AND ELECTRICAL DEPARTMENT.

To the Editors of ARCHIVES OF RADIOLOGY AND ELECTROTHERAPY.

DEAR SIRS,

In view of the increased price of silver at the present day I thought it was worth while investigating the waste that was taking place in the X-ray department of this hospital.

I therefore took a sample of the used "hypo," and sent it to my friend Mr. Thomson, who very kindly undertook the investigation, and whose report I enclose, with his permission, for publication. 1 am certain that it will be of great interest and use to other X-ray departments.

I am, yours faithfully,

A. E. BARCLAY.

Honorary Medical Officer in charge, X-ray and Electrical Department.

DEAR DR. BARCLAY,

I have estimated the amount of silver contained in the hypo washings which you sent to me and find them to contain 0·52 per cent. of metallic silver, equal to 415·9 grains per gallon.

RECOVERY OF SILVER.

The old fixing baths should be thrown into a tub containing a solution of sodium sulphide. The silver is thus precipitated as the sulphide. When the tub is nearly full, a sample is taken in a test tube and a few drops of the sodium sulphide solution added; if no precipitate forms, all the silver has been deposited; if the liquid becomes brown more sodium sulphide solution should be added to the liquid in the tub, and the whole stirred and the sediment allowed to settle. A tap should be fitted about 10 in. or 12 in. from the base of the tub, and when the deposited silver reaches this level, or as soon as the tub is full of liquor, the clear liquid above is run off. The sludge is now emptied into a second tub or vessel, and when sufficient is obtained it should be labelled "Silver Sulphide" and sent to the refinery to be reduced.

At the rate of 415·9 grains per gallon, 2½ gallons would contain 1039·8 grains of metallic silver. This is equivalent to 2·38 ozs. avoir. per week, or = 2·17 ozs. troy per week.

Note from British Drug Houses, Ltd., January 1st, 1920: "Silver foil or wire, 9s. 6d. per oz. troy weight."

I remain, yours very truly,

WILLIAM THOMSON.

P.S.—The specific gravity of the solution was 1·1326 at 60° Fah. = 26½° Twaddell,— W. T.

PUBLICATIONS RECEIVED.

Journals.

American Journal of Electrology and Radiology, Oct., 1919.

American Journal of Röentgenology, Oct., Nov., 1919.

Archives d'Électricite Médicale et de Physiotherapie, Dec., 1919.

Archivio Italiano di Chirurgia, Dec. 5th, 1919.

British Journal of Surgery, Jan., 1920.

Bulletin of the Johns Hopkins Hospital, Dec., 1919.

Bulletin et Mémoirs de la Société de Radiologie Médicale de France, Dec., 1919.

Hospitalstidende, Jan.7th, 14th, 21st, 1920.

Il Policlinico, Dec. 1st, 15th, 1919.

International Journal of Orthodontia and Oral Surgery, Dec., 1919.

Journals—*continued.*

Journal de Radiologie et d'Electrologie, Dec., 1919.

Medical Journal of Australia, Nov. 1st, 8th, 15th, 22nd, 29th; Dec. 6th, 13th, 1919.

Medical Science, Jan., 1920,

Modern Medicine, Dec., 1919.

New York Medical Journal, Dec. 13th, 20th, 27th, 1919; Jan. 3rd, 1920.

New York State Journal of Medicine, Dec., 1919.

Norsk Mag. for Lægevidenskaben, Jan., 1920.

Revista Espanola de Electrologia y Radiologia Medicas, July, 1918; Nov., 1919.

Surgery, Gynæcology, and Obstetrics, Jan., 1920.

Ugeskrift for Læger, Jan. 8th, 22nd, 1920.

NOTICES.

ARCHIVES OF RADIOLOGY AND ELECTROTHERAPY is published monthly.

The index for each volume, which ends with the May number, is supplied with the June number of each year.

Communications to the Editors should be addressed to "ROBERT KNOX, M.D., 38, Harley Street, W. 1."

Communications and illustrations from American contributors may be sent to Messrs. REBMAN COMPANY, 141-145, West Thirty-sixth Street, New York City.

All radiographs and photographs must be originals, and must not have been previously published. Drawings should be supplied on separate paper.

Owing to the scarcity of paper the Publishers are reluctantly compelled—as a temporary war measure—to reduce the number of free reprints of Papers to twenty-five.

Annual Subscriptions, payable in advance, 30/- including postage. Single copies, 3/- (postage 2d.) Single numbers and back numbers can be supplied on application.

Vol. XXIV—No. 10   MARCH, 1920   No. 236

ARCHIVES OF RADIOLOGY AND ELECTROTHERAPY

THE OFFICIAL ORGAN OF THE

BRITISH ASSOCIATION OF RADIOLOGY AND PHYSIOTHERAPY

Editors.

ROBERT KNOX, M.D., Hon. Radiologist, King's College Hospital.
E. P. CUMBERBATCH, B.M., M.R.C.P., Medical Officer in Charge, Electrical Department, St. Bartholomew's Hospital.
SIDNEY RUSS, D.Sc., Physicist to the Middlesex Hospital.

IN COLLABORATION WITH

A. E. BARCLAY (Manchester); BELOT (Paris); H. MARTIN BERRY (London); W. H. BRAGG (London); N. BURKE (Woodhall Spa); J. BURNET (Edinburgh); W. J. S. BYTHELL (Manchester); J. T. CASE (Battle Creek, U.S.A.); A. ST. GEORGE CAULFEILD (London); H. A. COLWELL (London); FOVEAU DE COURMELLES (Paris); GUNZBURG (Antwerp); HALL-EDWARDS (Birmingham); HARET (Paris); HAUCHAMPS (Brussels); F. HERNAMAN-JOHNSON (London); W. F. HIGGINS (Teddington); THURSTAN HOLLAND (Liverpool); HURST (London); KLYNENS (Antwerp); LAQUERRIERE (Paris); LAZARUS-BARLOW (London); LEDUC (Nantes); ALEXANDER MACKAY (Edinburgh); REGINALD MORTON (London); HARRISON ORTON (London); W. OVEREND (St. Leonards-on-Sea); PFAHLER (Philadelphia); C. E. S. PHILLIPS (London); GEORGE PIRIE (Dundee); HOWARD PIRIE (Montreal); A. W. PORTER (London); R. W. A. SALMOND (London); WERTHEIM SALOMONSON (Amsterdam); S. SLOAN (Glasgow); SOMERVILLE (Glasgow); W. C. STEVENSON (Dublin); W. J. TURRELL (Oxford); HUGH WALSHAM (London).

EDITORIAL.

IN bringing to the notice of our readers a copy of the first announcement of the proposed memorial to the late Sir James Mackenzie Davidson, we do not think it necessary to dwell at any length upon the various aspects of the proposals embodied in it. Mackenzie Davidson was known personally to a large number of the readers of the ARCHIVES, who deeply deplored his death. The proposed memorial gives them and others the opportunity of paying a tribute to the man and to his work in the domain of radiology. If the two-fold object of the memorial is to be achieved a considerable fund will be necessary, but we have little doubt that the contributions from what we may term the inner circle of radiology will form an appreciable fraction of the sum to be realised from world-wide sources. With this brief introduction we commend the proposals for the consideration of our readers.

THE MACKENZIE DAVIDSON MEMORIAL FUND.

In surveying the devastation of five years of war, the nation is beginning to realise that some compensation may be found in the great stimulus which science has received.

In no branch of science has this been more marked than in the field of radiology. In the diagnosis of disease and in the localization of foreign bodies and bone injuries, radiology has played a vital part in the war and has given invaluable aid to the thousands of medical officers serving in the forces.

Remarkable as has been the development of radiology during the war, there is need for watchfulness lest full advantage be not taken of this stimulus and a period of reaction set in. There is pressing need of unremitting research. For this is required the provision of the best equipment possible and also a more thorough and systematic scheme of teaching.

The University of Cambridge is alive to these requirements, and a Diploma in Radiology and Electrology at the University has been established. It is felt that the success of the step will be greatly assured if similar facilities are provided in London.

The death of Sir James Mackenzie Davidson in the prime of life has deprived radiology of one of its most distinguished exponents, whose name is specially associated with the development of radiographic technique and particularly that of stereoscopic radiography, and with the introduction in this country of the method of the localization of foreign bodies to which so many thousands of wounded men owe a deep debt of gratitude.

Mackenzie Davidson's reputation was international. In this country he was rightly regarded as the head of his profession, and throughout his career he was unsparing in his efforts to raise the status of radiology among the sciences. He was especially insistent on the fundamental value of physics to radiology, particularly in regard to methods of measurement and the designing of equipment, subjects in which he was deeply interested up to the time of his death.

Many in his own branch of the profession and a number of his friends and former patients, wishing to keep his memory green, have suggested that an appeal for funds should be made to found a Mackenzie Davidson Chair of Radiology at some University.

Had Mackenzie Davidson lived he would have been among the first actively and generously to support the foundation of an institute for teaching and research in radiology, of which he was one of the earliest pioneers. If funds permit, it is hoped to found such an institute, to which possibly the chair could be attached, and of which the personnel and equipment would be beyond reproach. The benefit accruing to the British school of radiology would be incalculable.

Till quite recently radiology has been regarded as a purely medical subject, but experimental research has shown that X rays may be profitably employed commercially in a number of industries. A new subject, radio-metallography, has, for example, come into being, which offers great possibilities for examining the internal structure of metals and other materials. In this connection, radiology has already been turned to account by the steel manufacturer, the metallurgist, the engineer, the manufacturer of explosives, the aircraft constructor, the glass manufacturer, etc.

The future of radiology will therefore lie, not only in the fight against disease and suffering, but also in the increase of commercial and industrial efficiency. But these new branches of radiology need much Investigatory work before they can come fully into their own, and a Chair of Radiology associated with an X-ray Institute should play a worthy part in such development.

It is in the belief that the scientific study and teaching of radiology will materially add to the well being of the human race that the Committee venture to put forward this appeal for public support.

A. BONAR LAW.	HARCOURT.
STANLEY BALDWIN.	BERTRAND DAWSON.
J. J. THOMSON.	W. D. COOLIDGE.
CLIFFORD ALLBUT.	W. WATSON CHEYNE.
HUMPHRY D. ROLLESTON.	FREDERICK W. MOTT.
ALEXANDER OGSTON.	ANDERSON CRITCHETT.
ROBERT HADFIELD.	ERNEST RUTHERFORD.
ROBERT JONES.	CHARLES H. WORDINGHAM.
J. Y. W. MACALISTER.	ARCHIBALD D. REID.
A. E. BARCLAY.	C. THURSTAN HOLLAND.
THOMAS J. HORDER.	SIDNEY RUSS.
N. S. FINZI.	W. IRONSIDE BRUCE.
G. HARRISON ORTON.	GILBERT SCOTT.
LENNOX WAINWRIGHT.	G. W. C. KAYE.
CHRISTOPHER ADDISON.	ROBERT KNOX.

Cheques should be made payable to the London Joint City and Midland Bank, crossed "& Co." and marked "The Mackenzie Davidson Memorial Fund," and sent to Dr. Robert Knox, 38, Harley Street, W.1.

MALIGNANCY.

By Morley Roberts.

Before trying to show in what way a general biological principle can assist the investigator of malignancy, I should like to say that it was the special form of it, known as X-ray cancer, which led me to attempt a co-ordination of the many apparently unrelated facts connected with it. To one not unfamiliar with speculation from the time of Durante and Cohnheim, it seemed remarkable that such a new aspect of the problem did not lead the medical profession to discard theories formed before X rays were known. For, in the welter of conflicting opinions as to the causes of cancer, it was at last certain that here were agents which not only might, but, if sufficiently applied, *must* in the end produce it. It seemed to me then, as it seems now, that when such were discovered all arguments as to the part played by "rests," or irritation, or an acquired bad habit of tissues, or some unknown infection, protozoal or bacillary, were partly beside the point. Those martyrs to science, the early radiologists, must have died in vain if no one recognises the high importance of the facts to which their agonies bore witness. That radiologists, so far as I am aware, have not seen the full value of X-ray dermatitis and malignancy in cancer theory is, I can only suppose, due to the immense calls upon their time and the peculiar interest of their daily work. But among them orthodoxy has scarcely had time to rear its head, and those who have seen tissues increase or rarefy almost under their own eyes will probably regard with suspicion a hypothetic unique infection, let us say, which has the remarkable power of causing the proliferation of vigorous invasive tissue. Any theory of malignancy which does not co-ordinate their work with all relevant physiological and pathological facts cannot be a true one. But, by taking their labours into account, and linking them with certain physiological and pathological phenomena, it is, I think, possible to show that a fresh general view may reveal its true nature. If it is then seen that there is no invariable single antecedent to malignancy, it must be admitted that there are many exciting "causes," of which X rays are but one. If such is the case, it follows logically that it is in the tissues concerned, their nature and relationship, that the true cause must be found. Those who have learnt by bitter experience how to upset, and happily more often to restore, somatic equilibrium will be most ready to admit this conclusion. Dynamite may be detonated in many ways, but the scientific cause of the explosion is not the man with the match, or the motive which led to its use, though these may be causes in law or psychology, but its inherent molecular instability. Perhaps the most valuable work done of late is that which shows the means and methods by which an unstable organism is kept in equilibrium, and an explanation of malignancy must take it into account.

It is, however, not common for investigators to work under the influence of general ideas which cannot easily be shown to have strict relevance to their objects. Though this preserves them from the concoction of fantastic views, it is possible that too strong a revulsion against theory tends to atrophy the imagination, which is the most powerful weapon of analysis. If our hypotheses and experiments are always closely related to the particular matter in hand, we learn to distrust unduly the tentative inductions we owe to those who do not fear to put forward provisional results which seem to have no immediate bearing on investigation. Thus we do not commonly speak of an organism as a republic of cells or a federation of organs, and though this seems unprofitable to many, we do so with advantage, since it helps to clarify our ideas on general metabolism. The conception is even more useful when it tends to show that symbiosis is not only found in groups or societies but in those close cell systems to which we commonly restrict the term " individual." The more such ideas are studied the more fruitful they become, though progress has not so far advanced but that it is commonly taken for granted that the essence of symbiotic life is mutual or inter-organic help. We ignore the fact that when two individuals, and definite cell colonies may with advantage be called such, preserve their individuality there is in their relations a certain real, if subdued, hostility. Mutual help, even if indirect, undoubtedly exists, but how easily the relationship may become one of parasite and host all zoologists are aware. There is often a great reluctance to admit that what is true of an organism as commonly conceived is also true of loosely knit human societies, and that the converse is not mere fancy. But when we observe that this fundamental reserve hostility is in fact self-protection in those political federations which help each member of them, while they provide against encroachment on the part of others, or of the federal authorities, and then compare such observations with organic life, it may not, to those with scientific imagination, seem far-fetched to declare that the phenomena of zoological and political symbiosis are intimately related and alike biological. Such a conception helps us to see that, whatever the waste in material, the methods by which life is built up from the apparently simple amœba to the hugest empire are marvellously economical, so economical, indeed, as to suggest that life could only be constructed in one way.

Whether such views are regarded as commonplaces or extravagances every political student will recognise as true the statement of fundamental interstate hostility, while every biologist and physiologist knows that balance between opposing forces in the organism is a *sine qua non* of its existence. To such a degree is this carried in health that every definite organ now appears to rule and to be ruled, to control and to be controlled. The regulators of metabolism are also the regulators of growth, and all alike appear conditioned by the chemical messengers of their environment. This is known to be true of the ductless glands, and as we learn more of their functions we may presently infer that all glands, ductless or not, have several functions, and go on to suspect that every portion of the whole body influences every other part, either for good or evil. What was help may become refusal of aid, and what was due inhibition may exhibit itself as destructive. If we carry these general views with us, and seek for light not only in the lesser laboratory, but in the great laboratory of life all round us in which ceaseless experiment is carried on, we may presently be able to infer from the theory of hostile symbiosis the real nature of malignancy, and to suggest certain paths of enquiry and experiment with a view to discovering a cure.

However much remains to be learnt of the glandular system it is known that the tissues respond, or fail to respond, and that characteristics are moulded in one way or another, in accordance with the presence or absence, the hyper-trophy or atrophy, of these glands. When sex is once determined the genital glands dominate growth ; testes are usually correlated with larger, ovaries with lesser, size. Ovariotomy allows undeveloped male homologues greater oppor-tunities ; early castration by preventing differentiation preserves female characteristics. If growth and size are mainly determined by the pituitary and thyroid, emasculation appears to permit the pituitary to exercise a greater influence on the legs, since the eunuch's are longer than normal. Among the unsolved problems of these organs is the phenomenon known as unilateral acromegaly, but the very fact that it occurs and that perfect symmetry is rare, shows how remarkably a hormone or stimulant can work or be inhibited. It seems that the tissues are moulded according to the stimulation they receive from secretions, of which the chemical constitution may presently be as well known as that of adrenalin, which exercises so powerful an influence on the blood pressure. A bone may be a function of many variables, but one is a gland placed beside the brain. It seems probable that the parathyroids influence the growth of nervous tissue since they control the irregular discharges of motor nerves, and we may yet learn that some forms of epilepsy are due to hypo-parathyroidism. Thus, not only growth, but much normal behaviour, is ruled by what Bland-Sutton well calls a glandular pantheon. That this is obviously so may reasonably lead to the inference that interacting stimulation and regulation is a function of all tissues, and that this is the method of growth and order in every animal whatsoever. All cases of excessive or defective growth must be classed as the result of stimulation, or the want of it, as surely as we see atrophy follow a failure of function or hypertrophy on its excess. But if this is generally true of all the obviously controlled tissues it may easily enough be true of those which are regulated we know not how, and, if that be granted for the sake of discussion, it seems possible not only to class all cases of malignancy but to suggest possible means of combating it by other than surgical means.

That some method should be adopted for clearing up the confusion of theory seems obvious when the battle ground of the cancer authorities and specialists is surveyed without prejudice. Unless there is definite reason for coming to other conclusions, it is usually safest to work on the principle that earnest and able workers are rarely entirely wrong. That the constitutional view of cancer, held by Paget, though undoubtedly "humoral," and therefore suspect, is still advocated by some is not surprising when it takes the form of "pre-disposition," if the word is interpreted in the light of modern physiology and heredity. To go no further than to speak of the cancerous diathesis, after the more ancient manner, is, however, a denial of explanation. The theory of infection may also have something to commend itself, if it is only on the ground that infections may stimulate a latent proclivity, though to declare that malignancy is due to a special pathogenic organism is to ask us to believe that every form of it has its own special bacillus or protozoon, or that a single one can exhibit its potentialities in a thousand shapes, while it is necessary to ignore other very definite phenomena which can with difficulty be brought into line with such views. Moreover, few pathologists will admit that what is seen in cancers has any great likeness to those diseases definitely traced to infection. For such a theory to be a complete explanation it would be necessary to class all inflammatory hyperplasias with malignant overgrowth. It is, of course, impossible to deal with all that has been said in support of the infection theory which at the moment seems the orthodox view, but, so far as I have yet discovered, no exposition of it can be reconciled with the complete pathology and histology of these disorders. All the evidence alleged to support it can be interpreted as conditions tending to upset metabolic balance, and the conclusions drawn from it are not compatible with X-ray cancer or the physiological and pathological phenomena at the base of chorion-epithelioma. Such an explanation will, I feel sure, be found a superfluous luxury, and as such to be dispensed with by the economic philosopher. There are also workers who seem satisfied with the notion that the phenomena in question are due to loss of function in some cells and increase of function in others. This is no doubt true, but again, that is the very thing which needs to be explained. We are often told that irritation is the cause of cancer, and the mere statement seems to be considered an explanation. This is not the case, for, though irritation is often followed by cancer, all that is proved is that in some of the organisms concerned resistance to irritation is weakened, whereas in others it is maintained. Not every clay pipe smoker, even with syphilis, or every burnt kangri-user in Kashmir, or every chimney sweep, or pitch or paraffin worker, gets cancer. We wish to know why these differences exist, and we shall then be able to class malignancy among other phenomena of normal and abnormal growth. The attribution of malignancy to foods is possibly not without value if it leads to a diet which is not irritating to the intestinal canal, and the fact that salmon or trout fry when fed abnormally on hog's liver may, it seems, suffer from an overgrowth of thyroidal tissue which later may become malignant, is of importance, but we are still as far as ever from the knowledge of causes which leads to explanatory classification. It appears that all these views are true, as far as they go. If it can be shown that they all point in one direction we should not be far from the truth.

There are however, other theories to be taken into account which appear of greater value, since they are more than restatement and seek explanation in the nature and functions of the very tissues which become abnormal. Such endeavours take into consideration not only pathology, but physiology as well. If it is said, by the way, that there is no greater hindrance to scientific advance than the separation of physiology and pathology, few who are not specialists in either branch of learning will be found to deny it. The opinions, for they are little more, of Thiersch and Waldeyer have at any rate the advantage of contact with the physiological side of the problem. Thiersch held that with advancing age the connective tissue ceased to be able to hold the epithelium in check. It was a brilliant guess, but it failed to account for carcinomas in the young, nor does it in any way explain sarcomas. Yet how near the truth it was may possibly be shown later, though, according to Bainbridge, the modern view of the function of epithelium during development is that it determines the character of the connective tissue, and that cancer cells mould or determine connective tissue "to their requirements." This may mean much or nothing, for I confess to having seen few such loose statements. Waldeyer's opinion was more complicated than Thiersch's and fuller of assumptions. He held that the epithelium was weakened, and, being pressed on by the connective tissue, was in parts isolated and thereby, in some inexplicable way, liable to transformation into cancer cells. Since this transformation is the problem, we should be no farther advanced if insistence on the material of change were not distinctly useful. Durante and Cohnheim, also, seem to have been in favour of the theory that the epithelium and connective tissue directly influenced each other, but Cohnheim was led away by the sequestration or "cell-rest" theory which is due to him. Modern research seems to support his opinion that tumours are frequently to be attributed to such causes, but the malignity of some and the benignity of others is still to be explained. It is absurd to suppose that embryonic "rests" always occupy the sites of tumours started by irritation, and Cohnheim himself excepted certain cases where that seems the immediate cause of malignancy. Ribbert held that such "rests" can be created post-natally, and that epithelium when cut off from its ordinary physiological control can proliferate malignantly. Implantation tumours by themselves are sufficient disproof of this view. Adami attributes cancer to an acquired "habit of growth." The cells devote themselves to mitosis. After what I have said I need not add that this is merely re-description. It deals with "how?" not with "why?" Green attributes cancer largely to the influence of the combustion products of coal or peat with a high percentage of sulphur, as well as to low-lying valleys. While such may be contributory factors to a loss of symbiotic equilibrium, they certainly do not "explain" malignancy. For it cannot be too frequently insisted on that true explanation is the classification of phenomena under some more inclusive law. Observations, however useful they may prove as regards prevention, are not explanation. For instance, if it be true that atrophy of the thyroid is common, or almost invariable, in cancer, we are not much further advanced in explanation, although in certain cases, say those of familial proneness to malignant disease, such an observation might be useful.

The sole general results which I am able to extract from the argumentative confusio of the subject is that epithelium and connective tissue somehow or other possess the capacity of invasive aberrancy under long-continued irritation. This may be no more than a re-statement, but it suggests that the only hope of explanation lies in the discovery of the reasons for tissue stability or instability. Is there any reason for supposing that instability or invasiveness is in certain conditions a physiological quality in epithelium? That connective tissue cells are capable of reparative work of an invasive order we know already. It seems that the reply to the question about epithelium is ready to hand. Bland-Sutton was, perhaps, on the very verge of a possible explanation of cancer when he declared that in the normal action of the trophoblasts of the fertilised ovum could be seen the physiological type of the invasive action of epithelium. In chorion-epithelioma such a physiological type becomes pathological. This dictum implicitly asserts that where the trophoblastic action becomes malignant there is a loss of balance ; the multinuclear cap of the villus is not inhibited by the normal uterine reactions, which usually prevent such invasion. What is it in the normal uterus which does inhibit it ? We are not going beyond what is known of repair if we say that the reaction tissues are mainly connective. In the normal gravid uterus the erosive action of the trophoblast is thus in all probability stayed by a connective tissue reaction. Yet this erosive action *is* malignancy. Cells in contact with the trophoblast dissolve; are, as it were, digested. As the larva of the blow-fly dissolves dead cells, so the trophoblast cap dissolves live uterine cells by some chemical product, some cytolitic secretion. In normal gestation such action is neutralised sooner or later, and since malignant epithelium when active pierces connective tissues as if they did not exist, the reaction which stays its course in the uterine wall must be more than mere fibrous growth. We seem compelled to assume that some cells can neutralise malignant cytolitic action by their products and thus restore physiological balance. The resumption of pathological action in chorion-epithelioma comes on in the period of involution when all the uterine tissues lose their activity. It seems hardly too much to say that the secretions or cell-products of the active connective tissue are those which inhibit or fail to inhibit the alien epithelium.

If the implications of the argument are clear, it will be seen that the conclusion to be drawn tentatively is that in such reactions lies hidden the mystery of malignancy. It will, perhaps, be objected that the multinuclear cap of the trophoblast is, in a sense, of alien origin, whereas ordinary malignant growths are autochthonous. In this very fact of partial alien origin lies support of the view suggested. It is more than conceivable that the male element in the zygote is here the earliest possible origin of malignant energy. It would not be wholly surprising if future investigation traced such cases to the peculiar energy of some spermatozoa. The ease with which a sperm cell enters the unfertilised ovum might be a measure of the likelihood of chorion-epithelioma, provided that the resistance of the ovum were a measure of the general tissue resistance of the maternal organism. But even granting that the alien, or partially alien, origin of the trophoblast renders malignancy more likely than with ordinary somatic tissues, it may be replied, on the lines adopted at the beginning of this paper, that all such tissues are, in spite of their symbiotic life, fundamentally alien and hostile.   A breakdown in their relations as established by evolution, may, and in many forms of disease, does occur.   By the study of the glandular system the interdependance of all tissues is inferred. There is also, undoubtedly self-protection. "Thus far and no farther," is embryological law. With deficient inhibition we see this law abrogated.   For in a new environment we may see any variation.   Thus, the polymorphism of malignant epithelial cells, described by E. H. Kettle, is just what might be expected on the loss of normal control.   The whole body is a group of organs and tissues which are not always harmonious, and the behaviour of malignant or benign aberrant tissue is by no means a phenomenon standing by itself. Probably all tissues might become malignant if they were as capable of free and rapid proliferation as connective tissue and epithelium.   It is not a loose or wild illustration to point out that in society we are all potential criminals at the mercy of excitation and inhibition, and it may not be otiose to observe that the liability to crime on the part of aliens in this or any country is due to unaccustomed stimulation and the lack of former inhibitions.   Such criminality is an analogue of malignancy.   I owe to Professor Keith the suggestion that the negro in the United States is even a better example.   The negro community there is as much a transplanted tissue as mouse cancer ; it tends to spread, excites violent reactions and might conceivably prove definitely malignant.   I am aware that the remark may excite ridicule, but it can be pointed out that the reaction against the immigrant negro in the north is comparatively slight, and that when trouble occurs it is very frequently due to the presence of a Southerner, who, by his previous contact with the race, has been "sensitised" so as to react violently.   Without desiring to push the analogy to its farthest extreme, it is obvious that a large negrine irruption tends to break up and push apart previous social bonds and regulations.   I do not see how it can be denied that such illustrations help us to understand the more obscure somatic phenomena.

It must be quite obvious by now that the views here advocated link the general theory of malignancy to the doctrine of the endocrine organs, that glandular hierarchy or pantheon which rules growth and metabolism.   When we observe that the absence of a particular secretion limits growth, or that its undue increase make such growth abnormally large, we are assuredly dealing with phenomena closely connected with the existence of epithelial or connective tissue neoplasms.   In both sets of phenomena the root fact is failure of proliferation or its excess.   If we delve deeply enough into causes it will not seem absurd to put cancers and giantism or acromegaly into related sub-classes.   That the latter are due to abnormal glandular activity we know. With normal pituitary influence no overgrowth occurs.   Connective tissue proliferation ceases at a point when the glandular system becomes balanced. This is obviously the case with what we see in repair or normal epithelium and connective tissue.   When the epithelium is stripped away and the underlying structures damaged, the connective tissue cells proliferate rapidly. As the young epithelial cells invade the edges of the wound the underlying cells become fibrous and deep scar tissue. Excessive and unhealthy granulations only arise when the epithelium does not do its work. Histologically there is a great likeness between round-celled sarcoma and granulation tissue, and, after all, granulation is no more than connective tissue cell proliferation growing outwards into a wound where normal tissues are wanting. A sarcoma might almost be called inverted ingrowing granulations. That the varied phenomena of malignancy exceed in variety those attributable to merely defective or hypertrophied glands is only what might be expected. Such a gland is highly specialised epithelium with very definite work. The general epithelium of the body is much less differentiated and nearer the embryonic type. It is found practically everywhere. Connective tissue is the somatic network, in no part is it absent. It exhibits a remarkable capacity for many forms of rapid specialisation, and may be looked on as highly unstable because of these very qualities. But its instability is obviously a function of many variables. From the universal presence of these two tissues we infer that normally there is nothing in the organism which inhibits the existence of either in any part. They can grow anywhere, and if aberrancy occurs at all it is in them we should look for it, if they did not, in some way analogous to the action of the endocrines, inhibit each other's undue growth. The age incidence of sarcoma and carcinoma suggests most forcibly that they do so. Sarcoma is predominantly a disease of youth, though it may be found at any age. It may develop *in utero*. Repair is most active when it is commonest, and epithelium is most delicate. Epithelium reaches its highest state of activity, as shown by its products and conduct, at a later age in which connective tissue activity is lessened and repair slackens. It is a period in which persons of failing metabolism tend to accumulate toxic products in the connective tissue which depress and inhibit its activity. It is the age of cancer. When cancer occurs in the adolescent there is frequently a history of heredity. That the un-balanced should breed unbalanced offspring is not surprising. The cancer house and the cancer valley are unhealthy, mostly low lying. From a defective environment we do not expect tissue health or balance, *i.e.*, the normal influence of one tissue on another in a federated system. It is by no means necessary that such influences must be exerted by definite glands. Every glandular secretion is but a specialised form of some unknown epithelial product. Snake venom arises in a specialised salivary gland ; the secretion of the salivary gland in embryonic epithelial cells. We can hardly go wrong if we say that every cell in the body influences every other cell, and that those which are in an immense majority have much power. Newton's law of gravity might almost be translated into a somatic law.

It is, therefore, by no means mere guess work to assume that the relations of epithelium and connective tissue are the essence of the cancer problem. Quite independent of their cross action in repair, we actually see in atrophic "scirrhus" of the mamma that this slowly developing cancer is surrounded by more or less dense strands of fibrous tissue, and is often known as withering or contracting cancer. Patients may live for twenty years or more with this variety of the disease. In old age the connective tissue appears to give way, and the few imprisoned anarchic epithelial cells may resume their invasive qualities. It was such cancers which showed the older physicians that there were attempts at repair in malignancy, but they attributed its arrest to mere mechanical action, a view not tenable when we consider the great erosive effect of really wild epithelium. Handley has shown that in melanotic cancer, at a later stage of permeation, there is inflammation accompanied by round-celled infiltration and fibrous growths. From the experiments *in vitro* of Champy much can be learnt as to the relations of these tissues. He demonstrated that when renal tissue was grown in a nutritive plasm it showed, after nine hours, new tubules of a primitive order, while still further away from the original section the epithelial cells did not form tubules and were of a simple embryonic type. This can only be attributed to loss of control by normal inhibitions. When the same worker cultivated simpler epithelium and connective tissue together the epithelial cells retained their characteristics, but when they spread and grew apart from the connective tissue they lost their usual order and appearance, and were no longer true epithelium. Only one inference can be made. It is that these tissues are to each other controlling environment. Bayliss says, in commenting on this, "it seems that cells, when they have taken special functions in the organism, are normally prevented by some means from continuing their primitive multiplication, and that when this influence which restrains their growth is removed they start afresh and produce simple embryonic tissue. There is significance in these facts in connection with the formation of malignant tissues." Assuredly nothing could be truer, and, working with the analogy of the endocrines, we are forced to conclude that like effects are produced by like causes. The "influence" at work must be some product of the connective tissue. In an unstable organism any depressing factor inhibiting the activity of that tissue, such as uneliminated katabolic toxins accumulating in the lymphatics and connective tissue generally, may end in allowing the explosive epithelium to break out into embryonic activity. Such instability has many analogues in pathology.

If it be granted that these facts are of importance, it seems that it is by using them and by following the indications afforded us by chorion-epithelioma and X-ray cancer, that we are likely to solve the problem. No doubt it may seem strange to bracket such diseases, but if it be found that two disorders so different in origin point the same way we cannot be far from the truth. In X rays we have an exciting cause of epithelial overgrowth, which not only may, but if sufficiently applied, must produce malignancy. The symptoms of X-ray dermatitis are those of profound irritation, epithelial overgrowth, attempts at repair, which in mild cases succeed, and in severe ones fail disastrously, leaving the skin in epithelial anarchy. It is cracked and fissured in every direction, heaped up in one place and broken down in another, until it becomes a picture of disorder rarely seen even in the domain of dermatology. Such an exhibition of ineffective energy spent at the surface in vain efforts at repair makes it less surprising that what we may call the potential of the deep epithelial layers of the epidermis becomes abnormally kinetic. It may be said that the cells of that layer grow malignant because they find existence impossible in their normal position. It seems certain that the effect of the rays on connective tissue is depressing ; they are, at any rate, totally unable at the last to resist, either by mechanical or chemical means, the push of the escaping epithelium. It is stated by Darier and Wolbarth that in X-ray dermatitis there is hypertrophy of the epidermis and pronounced degeneration of the corium, the most marked result being, as I anticipated before I was aware of the actual facts, the rarefaction of the sub-epidermal portion. I may also mention the work of Lazarus Barlow and his co-workers at the Middlesex Hospital. He points out that in certain conditions the influence of radium rays is one of stimulation. In experiments on rats, which produced what can only be described as squamous-cell cancer, it is especially to be noted that there was degeneration of the subjacent connective tissue, which even extended to bone and cartilage. Obviously radium was here used in time-quantities which carried stimulation into degeneration. These changes are, I may perhaps venture to say, only such as could have been predicted, and I did in fact predict them before being aware of his results. The same can be said of those obtained lately by Russ and his colleagues with regard to lymphocytosis, leucopenia, and immunity. They add immensely to the value of their work by pointing out that a large lymphocyte count is not by itself sufficient to procure or preserve immunity. If the general connective tissue and its catalysts are not active this is to be expected. These catalysts, immune bodies, or anti-bodies, are almost certainly connective tissue cell products. Russ, indeed, says there is some as yet undetermined relationship between the number of lympho-cytes and the occurrence of immunity. But if cancer actually depends on the weakening of connective tissue cells of all kinds, the relationship is no longer undetermined. We have a real explanation why large doses of X rays, which are more or less fatal to lymphocytes, destroy immunity, and get a clue to the reason for small or stimulating doses conferring it on susceptible animals. Hernaman - Johnson states definitely that clinical observation and microscopic research show that carcinoma is favourably influenced as the results of this dual action. Mathematically speaking, the good influence of small doses acts as a " couple," the peccant tissue is inhibited and the limiting or resisting tissue is stimulated to activity. With such phenomena before us there is no need to suppose some unknown cause. In all explanation it is illicit to import the unknown when the known can be made to account for the facts. If radium and X rays, according to their dosage and application, can cause different effects in both tissues, and by restoring or impairing them produce amelioration or further destruction, the case for infection falls to the ground. It is also said by Knox that the curative effect of radium depends in many cases on the Becquerel rays stimulating the connective tissue and producing fibrosis. Under the battery which brings about these results it can hardly be thought that any specific cancer protozoon continues to live. Those who believe in the infection theory must take up the position that the agent is everywhere in the body, or the environment, ready to infect the patient in the so-called pre-cancerous stage of X-ray malignancy. Such a hypothesis is a multiplication of causes. The destructive powers of the X rays on connective tissues in combination with the resistance of the skin are sufficient to account for the results. In what other way can we interpret the conclusions reached by J. B. Murphy and Sturm? These workers found that the entire lymphoid tissue of the body could be destroyed in from seven to twenty-one days by repeated small doses of X rays. In such a condition the theory of this paper would infer that an immense reduction of organic resistance followed. What do we find? First, there is a greatly lessened resistance to all implants; second, a lowered resistance to cancer grafts; third, the destruction of acquired immunity to cancer; and fourth, a lowered resistance to the tubercle bacillus and other infective agents. Murphy, however, remarks that the chief objection to accepting the lymphatics as a great factor of resistance to cancer growth is that the lymph glands are common points for metastatic growths. This appears to be no such objection as he imagines, since the very existence of the primary focus is in all probability due to general loss of tone of all connective tissue cells, stationary or wandering, highly evolved or semi-embryonic. I draw the conclusion with confidence that, as with chorion-epithelioma where infection is negatived by the whole of the phenomena of ovum and uterine interaction, X-ray malignancy and allied phenomena point straight to the conclusion that the explanation of cancer lies in the relations of epithelium and connective tissue, that benignity is a normal reaction and malignity a failure, that irritation is only a means by which the normal reactions of these tissues are destroyed, and that infections are only causes so far as they excite or depress and thereby destroy the balance of tissues which exercise outside control by their mechanical nature and products. I have so far found no theory, but the one here advocated, that reconciles all these phenomena, and the fact that it enabled me to prophesy facts quite unknown to me at one period of investigation form my greatest excuse for supporting it in this journal. Among the multitudinous observations of radiologists I have so far found nothing irreconcilable with these views.

Conclusions of this kind are necessarily as relevant to sarcoma as to carcinoma. The immense activity of connective tissue in youth suggests that it might at any age get out of hand. Fowls seem specially liable to it. Luckily, they mostly die young. An aged fowl, which should be liable to carcinoma, is a rare object. As a domestic animal which, owing to the caprice of breeders, is in a peculiarly fluent condition, it is particularly liable to loss of balance. Uterine or mammary cancer is also rare in bitches, a fact very properly attributed to their commonly dying before involution sets in. It may also be due to their habits, since they are not so much exposed to sexual stimuli as human beings, who only practice continence during the œstrus. It is said that castrated animals are more liable to malignant diseases than others. They have been thrown out of normal balance by operation. The peculiar deadliness of sarcoma seems natural enough if we remember that it is to connective tissue that all repair is due. It is a case of "quis custodiet?" when the guardian tissue becomes anarchic. Whatever influence epithelium may have upon it, epithelial tissue cells cannot surround, or attempt to encapsule, aberrant connective tissue, for as soon as they proliferate freely they are themselves malignant.

That benign tumours should often become malignant is, according to the theory advocated, just what might be expected. With senescence there is in the whole body an increase of static elements as compared with the cytoplasm; a tendency to rigidity, and a loss of the federal unity of the body which we call health. There is less response to regulative stimulation or inhibition and less or more of the normal hormones to respond to. The result should naturally be an increase in the autonomy of separated parts and the increasing dominance of any tissue which is in excess. That the chief tendency of malignancy is towards carcinoma is what we should expect at an age when epithelium in any case tends to become rampant, but that a benign connective tissue tumour in which the epithelial portions are at a minimum should at last break bounds is by no means surprising. When thinking upon such lines and dealing with phenomena of senescence, it is a not uninteresting speculation if we venture to attribute to a temporary rejuvenescence the partial cures or alleviations of symptoms often found when a new empirical remedy is tried in inoperable cases. To inspire hope by whatever means is a function of the physician, and to do so is, in the language of the physicists, to free energy. The hopeless patient, when concentred on his symptoms and his feelings, is doubly the host of a parasite; his energy is bound within a narrow circle, his horizon of life contracted to a mere point. As a result his functions fail; he eliminates less and less toxin, the static elements increase till the cytoplasm of his whole organism is as unable to cope with its work as his cerebral cytoplasm is to face the general situation. If he is afforded hope in any way whatsoever the engine works again; there is at least a temporary rejuvenescence, and the partially freed tissues tend to resume their functions. At such a stage the progress of a tumour may be arrested by the renewed action of connective tissue or epithelium or of the general regulative metabolism of the whole body.

Though cancer "cures" may thus exercise a favourable, if brief, influence on those who suffer, their number and character bear bitter witness to the confusion of the whole subject. In theory I have been unable to find any general principle at work. If it were not that in looking back upon the past of pathology it is seen that most advances have been made rather by trial and error than by any great grasp of the human mind, those who are not wedded to one particular theory might indeed feel hopeless. Amid the din of battle, the confusion and the shouting, it is hard to discover order. Yet to those who are somewhat withdrawn from the arena facts do sometimes emerge which seem of real relevance. The long known occasional cure of cancer due to erysipelas is one of them, and the very failure of Coley's fluid, composed of the toxins of *S. erysipelatosus* and *B. prodigiosus*, to fulfil the hopes of its inventor, may, if considered in a proper light, be of the greatest assistance. That these toxins, without the acute attack, fail of their purpose suggests very forcibly that it is not such toxins which inhibit the growth of the aberrant tissue, but that it is overcome by the immense reactions of the connective tissue which results in the cure of the acute infection. So far as Coley's fluid excites the connective tissue so far it may possibly do good. Such a view is greatly strengthened by the experiments of Ehrlich and Apolant, if they can be regarded as authenticated. This is, I think, thought by many not to be the case, but their results fall in so completely with the views advocated in this paper that I find it impossible to disregard them. That a transplanted mouse carcinoma should in certain cases produce sarcoma seemed to some impossible; and to some a proof that the transplanted tissue was really sarcomatous. Yet, if it is granted for the moment that epithelium and connective tissue live in symbiotic hostility, such a phenomenon is by no means so surprising as it looks. It is but reaction overbalancing itself. On continued transplantation with one strain it is said that the tumour tissue overcame the epithelium till it at last consisted of scattered cells only, so that finally the graft was a pure sarcoma. In another strain this "power to induce sarcoma" was lost, and the tumour remained epithelial in character. The phrase, "power to induce sarcoma" is, to say the least of it, unhappy. By the phenomenon, if correctly reported, we have to understand that the host's connective tissue did not react. No explanation of these observations is to be found in any theory but that of the action and reaction of the two tissues concerned. When their balance is upset one proliferates abnormally. Anything that throws the organism out of gear is a possible factor of malignancy, and that is the reason why, with the increase of wealth, a new and highly varied environment, which tends to produce variation, makes for the increase of such disease.

If the value of a theory depends on the aid it gives in explanation, the one here advocated certainly helps to make it clearer why some forms of malignancy are more deadly and liable to metastasis than others. So far there has been no real explanation of the fact that the forms of it which deviate most widely from the tissue of origin are most rapid and destructive. It has remained an observation, and to say this extreme aberrancy from type renders it more deadly is only to repeat in another form what has been said before. But if it is understood that the immediate and total somatic environment determine cell character, it is obvious that extreme aberrancy implies that the determining tissues generally are weakened to an extreme degree, and that any cancer growth or embolus will nowhere meet with much resistance. That environment has definite results is well known. In speaking of the relatively more deadly femoral sarcoma, as compared with a similar tumour in the tibia, Bland-Sutton says, " this would appear to indicate that the two tumours, though structurally alike, really have different causes, yet these are facts which lead us to suppose that variations in tissue actually constitute a different environment." He adds that echinococcus disease is the only condition which supports this view. Yet surely in studying all diseases we are compelled to come to the conclusion that different reactions in different patients with the same disorder can only be due to their bodies constituting a different environment. Further investigation will almost certainly show that there is some reaction difference in the region of the femur when compared with that of the tibia. The comparative immunity of joints from a burrowing sarcoma supports the view that some tissues have a more powerful resistance than others. It may be that the great resistance of cartilage is due to its lack of channels, but it is far more likely that it is due to the cell products of its closely arranged cells. In studying the various types of malignancy we cannot but be struck by the varying amounts of normal, or fairly normal, connective tissue about them. That the small, round-celled sarcoma should be more deadly than most of the other varieties is what would be expected from the scantiness of the still growing or surviving stroma. Such varieties as are more difficult to distinguish from normal cells seem obviously those in which the whole of the normal inhibition of the environment has not been overcome. These are points in which a considerable knowledge of biology might be of assistance to pathologists.

While it is impossible to deal here in detail with every kind of tumour, something may be said of embryomas and their malignant forms. Obscure and difficult as the subject is, there seems reason to believe that when it is understood many of the basal problems of biology will be solved with it. That they are due to some ovum, or embryonic ovarian tissue, developing parthenogenetically seems more than likely. Shattock's remarkable paper on these tumours supports the view that embryonic ova may be fertilised by errant spermatozoa, but there are many reasons for coming to the conclusion that an embryonic " rest " may develop without such assistance. Such views do not account for infantile, feminine, or testicular embryomas. It is more likely that any epithelium in regions where reproductive processes commence may, under some abnormal stimulation, develop incompletely determined epithelial products or rudimentary organs. The prodigious fertility of embryomas in such products suggests that the imperfect parent tissue is doing its best to be normal, if the phrase is permissible, but that such a result is impossible owing to the necessary lack of normal excitation and inhibition, *i.e.*, of the usual environment. That a simple product of epithelium, such as hair, may be perfect is not surprising. The epithelium from which it grows is practically the only environmental stimulus it requires. That teeth, on the other hand, are rudimentary, mis-shaped, and monstrous, may be regarded as the result of their lacking a normal environment. That embryomas are frequently very deadly is what might be expected from the possibilities of the unspecialised tissues from which they originate. The subject of interaction or environment of the various tissues of the body is one that should include far more than the endocrine organs, since it is more than likely to solve the problems of heredity as well as those of malignant growth. The divisions between physiology, pathology, and biology are responsible in a very large measure for the slowness with which they all advance.

It follows from all these considerations that it must not be supposed that reaction against one kind of overgrowth or the other is due entirely to the tissues principally concerned. Such a view would be a partial denial of the entire independence of the whole organic federation. There is reason to suppose that the blood stream is hostile to intrusive epithelium. Small cancerous emboli excite thrombosis, and are sometimes buried and perhaps destroyed in a blood clot, in which lymphocytes are probably very prominent. The erosive agent of the chorionic villus is in its multinuclear cap, or giant cell, sometimes without warrant called a plasmodium. Properly speaking, a plasmodium consists of fused cells, and there is reason to suppose that a giant cell is one which accumulates nuclear material without normal fission. If we regard the nucleus not as a "director," which is a common psychological fallacy, but as a workshop containing the non-living tools, weapons, or catalysts, by which the cytoplasm works, it is easy to understand that when there is active use and much waste of such tools mitosis does not occur. In normal gestation, when uterine reaction is complete and erosion ceases, there is probably no longer any multi-nucleated cell, for where such are found patho-logical conditions exist. If we knew when such a cell is again formed in fragments of the decidua, we should be able to point to the very moment when chorion-epithelioma starts. It begins when the uterus has involuted and is no longer in its highly developed and vascular form. I say highly vascular because, as said before, it seems that the blood plasm itself exerts a direct inhibitory influence on malignant cells. When considering this aspect of the problem, I came, independently of any suggestion, to the conclusion that I should expect in some carcinomatous conditions to find multinuclear epithelial cells closely resembling the cap of the trophoblast. This inference was con-firmed by Mr. Sampson Handley, who told me, not at all to my surprise, that whereas no such cells are formed at the distal part of a carcinoma while still advancing in the lymphatics, they are to be found as soon as the growth comes in contact with the blood. This implies that there is a new reaction in the growth, and such a reaction seems obviously due to the inhibiting action of the blood stream and the catalysts it carries.

The confusion in theory is more than equalled by that in experimental therapeutics. Leaving aside the cures which are but quackery or empiricism run mad, the attempts to discover a remedy in opotherapy seem in few cases to have been guided by much more than trust in chance. Preparations of every kind of tissue have been injected into patients, and the results have been such as almost to discredit any reasoned series of experiments. Yet if it is agreed that the fundamental principles of organic life are inter-organic stimulation and inhibition, and that want of order is the result of failure in metabolic regulators, such views lead at once to considered experiment. The arguments used to establish this theory may be deemed insufficient as proof, yet if they lead to trial verification may follow. Such trials should be directed to assisting the reaction of all connective tissue in cases of carcinoma, and that of epithelium in those of sarcoma. How this can be achieved is for the physiologist and pathologist to determine, but it may be suggested that after the excision of a carcinoma efforts should be made to irritate or stimulate the connective tissue in the neighbourhood of the removed focus. We know now that this may be done by radiation, while the injection of doses of epithelial juices might assist the process. Moreover, it may be found that the pituitary is a direct or indirect agent both of carcinoma and sarcoma ; of cancer through failure of inhibition by some dystrophy or by hypo-pituitarism, and of sarcoma by over-excitation of repair when the equilibrating reactions of epithelium are wanting. If this be proved the case we might well term such a deadly disease as femoral sarcomas " local explosive osteomegalies." Since we know that many forms of cell proliferation are inhibited by their own products, it is not unlikely that aberrant epithelium may be rendered inactive by injections of healthy epithelial products, or by prepared and filtered cancer juice. With sarcoma similar trials might be made, and, in the meantime, while such experiments are in progress on operated or inoperable cases, it should be the task of the physiologist or bio-chemist to separate from epithelium and connective tissue the chemical compound or complex of compounds by which they exercise their influence. Difficult as such a task may prove the labour might well be worth undertaking when we consider its possible results. In any case much might be learnt by the further study of normal epithelium and connective tissue *in nutrient media* while they are subjected to X rays or radium, or both, or to the influence of endocrine secretions or of various toxins. Malignant tissues *in vitro* should be watched when in similar conditions. We might then learn how and why certain epithelial cells become multinuclear, and whether such can be inhibited by the products of connective tissue or of lymphocytes or lymphoid tissue. Even if little were learnt, a result I refuse to contemplate, the result would be that one field of research had been worked out on scientific lines. Such research, however, would almost certainly suggest that these diseases are indeed diseases of development, and must be combated by rendering the organism stable rather than by seeking any single cure.

If the results provisionally arrived at are summarised, it may be said that—

1. The general biological conception of the organism as a federation of organs and tissues, living in symbiosis and yet fundamentally hostile, or " selfish," is helpful in the study of disease.

2. If atrophy or hypertrophy of the endocrines accounts for certain disorders the failure of normal relations between less specialised tissues may account for others.

3. Order does not exist without control, and the essence of malignancy is lack of control.

4. There is reason to suppose that epithelium and connective tissue influence and control each other, and that their failure to do so is the real cause of malignancy.

5. Irritation, including the effects of infection, acts by destroying such balanced action.

6. The phenomena observed in the chorionic trophoblast, in chorion-epithelioma, in X-ray dermatitis and cancer, as well as the experimental growth of the two tissues liable to malignancy, support the view of this relationship between epithelium and connective tissue, and suggest that a morbid condition of the pituitary may be a fundamental cause of the disease.

7. Malignancy is thus brought into relation with the phenomena of growth and can be classed with developmental diseases such as those due to endocrine atrophy or hypertrophy.

8. Research should be directed to the discovery of the tissue products or secretions by which epithelium and connective tissue preserve their individuality and prevent reversion in each other.

REFERENCES.

Adami, " Medical Sidelights on Evolution," 1919.
Bainbridge, W. S., "Cancer Problem," N.Y., 1914.
Bland-Sutton, Sir John, "Tumours," 1918. Lecture III., *Cham. Jour.*, Vol. XXX, p. 186-08.
Butlin, Sir H., "Unicellula Cancri," 1912.
Darier and Wolbarth, quoted by Hartzell, M.B., "Diseases of the Skin," 1917.
Emery, D'Este, " Pathology of Tumours," 1916.
Green, C. E., " Cancer Problem," 1919.
Handley, Sampson, " Melanotic Sarcoma," Hunt Lect., 1907, *Lancet*, 1905, I, p. 909 ; 1907, I, p. 930.
Hernaman-Johnson, F., "Comparative Values of X Rays and Radium in Malignant Disease," Aberdeen B.M.A.
Kettle, E. H., " Pathology of Tumours," 1916. Path. Sect., R.S.M., 15.4.19.
Knox, Robert, "Radiology," 1918.
Murphy, J. B., Sturn, E., III, *Jour. Exp. Med.*, Jan., 1919.
Russ, Sydney ; H. Chambers, " Exp. Studies with Small Doses of X Rays," *Lancet*, 26.4.09.
Shattock, S. G., "Ovarian Teratomata," *Lancet*, 1918, I, p. 479.
Spencer Herbert B., " Lettsomian Lecture," *Brit. Med. Journal*, 21.2.20.

ON THE VALUE OF COMBINED TREATMENT, WITH SPECIAL REFERENCE TO SURGERY, ELECTRICITY AND X RAYS.*

By Francis Hernaman-Johnson M.D., Radiologist to the French Hospital; Physician to the X-ray Department, the Margaret Street Hospital for Consumption; late Consulting Radiologist, Aldershot Command.

Gentlemen,—

I would recall to your minds for a moment the story of Naaman the Syrian. He was a leper, and went to consult the Prophet Elisha as to what he should do to be healed. The advice given was that he should wash seven times in Jordan. But upon this Naaman fell into a great rage, his indignation focussing itself, as it were, upon two points : he objected to the bathing place as such; but more particularly and strenuously he quarrelled with the simplicity of the prescription. And he turned, and went away in a rage. But his servants, displaying both insight and courage, said to him, "My father, if the prophet had bid thee do some great thing, wouldst thou not have done it ? " And Naaman—so we are told in the fifth chapter of the second book of Kings—took to heart the gentle reproof, washed seven times in Jordan, and was healed.

This story, gentlemen, is not a digression, or in any sense irrelevant to my subject. For this medical generation to which we belong is too apt to seek always to do some great thing, to look for a sign from heaven—which shall not be given unto them—and, incidentally, to stone the prophets. Probably none of us are altogether guiltless in this respect, but it is a pleasant exercise to point out the failings of others, and I venture to say that some surgeons, at least, in the presence of certain serious maladies, spend their time in sighing for serological signs and wonders, instead of utilizing means which, if they do not accomplish results with dramatic suddenness, are at any rate of proved value. The septic wound which persistently remains septic despite thorough surgical cleansing and drainage, and which threatens to kill the patient by exhaustion, is a case in point. Too often one hears the pious hope expressed that in the future a serum will be discovered that will neutralize all wound toxins, or better still, some chemico-therapeutic preparation which, when injected, will kill all pus-forming organisms. The discovery of such agents is a legitimate object of research; but, meanwhile, the aid which can be given by light, X rays and various forms of electricity should not be neglected.

The value of these agents in the treatment of septic wounds can no longer be doubted. The proofs are set forth in numerous monographs published during the past few years; and the whole subject was discussed at length at a meeting of the Electrotherapeutic Section of the Royal Society of Medicine last year. Equally, I shall ask you to take for granted the beneficial effects of

* A Lecture delivered at the House of the Royal Society of Medicine, 1, Wimpole Street, November 25th, 1919, under the auspices of the Fellowship of Medicine and Post-Graduate Association.

X rays in localized tubercular conditions, and in malignant disease; also their power to disperse pathological fibrous tissue. In short, for the purposes of this lecture, it will be assumed on the one hand that most of the statements made by responsible practitioners of electrical medicine are justified; and, on the other, that modern surgery can accomplish all, or nearly all, that its exponents claim for it.

What I want to put before you is that, in many instances, no single method of treatment is adequate to cure a patient—or, at any rate, to cure him with the minimum of risk, pain and delay.

Let us consider first the question of tubercle. Tuberculous affections of the skin are notoriously difficult to deal with. It is but rarely that surgical scraping in itself leads to an ultimately satisfactory result. The operation is performed, an apparently healthy granulating surface is obtained, and all goes well for a few days. Then, too often, the healing process becomes arrested, and, to a greater or less degree, the disease recurs. The outcome of unaided treatment by X rays or light is not seldom equally disappointing. But a combination of surgical and electrical methods, while not infallible, gives much better results. On the surgical side, it is necessary to curette almost as deeply as if one intended to depend on this alone, and also to go at least a quarter of an inch beyond the margins of the diseased patch. The wound will, of course, begin to heal from the edge in the normal way, leaving a healthy granulating surface which decreases in size day by day. The object of post-operative treatment by electricity and radiation is to keep this process going. It is not easy to describe in words the appearance which must be maintained, but anyone familiar with the healing of granulating wounds can tell by daily inspection whether or not healing is proceeding normally.

To secure such orderly progression is not by any means always a simple matter. Sometimes the daily application of a very small dose of X rays is all that is necessary ; more often one finds that after a short time a particular form of stimulus fails to act, and the wound hangs fire ; or, what is worse, shows a tendency to false healing. It is here that skill and experience come in; but it may be said briefly that the secret of success lies in variation of stimuli according to the behaviour of the wound. Short sparks from a high-frequency vacuum electrode, and zinc ionization, suffice as variants in most cases. Sometimes it is good practice to cause a sharp reaction by ultra-violet rays from a tungsten arc; or it may even be necessary to resort to further curettage of a part of the diseased area. An essential point is that not the smallest scab must be left at any point; for if such remain, it is nearly always an indication of unsound closing, and the probability of recurrence is great.

Once genuinely healed, a particular patch is not likely again to become the seat of tubercle; but, of course, the constitutional tendency remains, and should be combated by all known means. Whether or not tuberculin in any of its multitudinous forms should be numbered among those means, may be left to serological experts to determine. But I take the opportunity of emphasizing thus early, that the advocate of true combined treatment cannot concern himself with local measures alone, but is bound to call in the aid of any vaccine, serum or drug which is of *proved* value in combating the morbid condition with which he is dealing. In some cases, for example in the local lesions of syphilis, there is little likelihood of this principle being neglected. But we must always remember that there is a constitutional factor in most local disturbances. When these troubles are the result of bacterial invasion, lip service, at any rate, is paid to this truth; but it is scarcely so well recognized that even in the case of a traumatic lesion of an aseptic nature, one must beware of not seeing the wood because of the trees. For example, a simple fracture may be slow in uniting chiefly because of thyroid deficiency, and will be speeded up by administering the appropriate extract.

Tubercular neck glands offer a useful field for combined surgical and electrical measures. Surgery alone often fails to eradicate the trouble, and its cosmetic results are sometimes far from satisfactory. Recently, for example, I saw a child of twelve who had had fourteen operations on her neck in six years, and I know of many cases where four or five excisions or scrapings have been undertaken within a comparatively short space of time.

This is certainly not a desirable state of affairs, and, in an endeavour to better it, attempts were made years ago to cure tuberculous neck glands by X rays. Some few of these attempts succeeded, and were reported in medical journals ; but mostly what happened was that after some weeks of rapid improvement progress became arrested, and eventually recurrence took place.

X-ray treatment therefore fell into disrepute, but unjustly so. Used for certain definite ends, it is invaluable. The rule to follow may be briefly stated as follows : When there is no detectable softening, X rays should precede surgical treatment by a month or six weeks, small doses being given three times a week. This causes all surrounding inflammation to subside, and the gland itself usually shrinks until it can be detected only by careful palpation. This is the time to operate—only a small incision is required, and the gland can be readily excised. If the surgeon decides to close the wound at once, no further radiative treatment need, as a rule, be given ; but if there is any subsequent discharge, a few post-operative sittings are desirable.

If, on the other hand, softening has already occurred when the case is first seen, no X-ray treatment should be given before operation. The resulting sinus, if left to itself, may discharge for months, but X-ray treatment commenced within a day or two will generally result in healing, with a minimum of scar tissue, after a few weeks. The surgeon, on his part, must, of course, see to the vital matters of free drainage and healing from the depth no less carefully than if X rays were not being employed. *It may be laid down here as a general proposition, that if combined treatment is to succeed, its various component measures must be carried out as fully and as skilfully as each would be were it alone being looked to to effect a cure.*

I come now to the question of malignant disease. X rays are of greater or less value in most neoplastic conditions, but they have their most striking success in cancer of the breast, and to this I purpose confining my remarks. Malignant growths in this region can often be made to disappear by X rays alone, so far as inspection and casual palpation are concerned ; but rarely to such an extent that remains cannot be detected when carefully sought for. Far more important is the fact, long suspected on clinical grounds, but recently—in the opinion of many competent to judge—experimentally proved, that X rays in suitable doses raise the immunity of the body to cancerous invasion. Radiotherapy should therefore be administered before operative removal. Such pre-operative treatment has the dual advantage of depressing the cancer cells locally before any surgical trauma has disturbed them ; and, at the same time, increasing the general powers of resistance to any subsequent migration. In view of what Sampson Handley has shown as to the radiating growth of cancer along the lymphatics, it is obvious that local treatment should embrace a very wide area. The individual doses should be small, and repeated two or three times a week ; it is possible to obtain a quick local effect at the expense of the general resistance. From two to three weeks should be spent in this preparatory treatment.

Post-operative raying is, of course, a well known procedure, and should at this date require no argument in its support. Nevertheless, there are still many surgeons who do not advise it, or do so only when recurrence is already manifest. It is true that excessive radiation may do harm by lowering resistance ; but experience has taught us the limits of safety. No one disputes the value of prophylactic inoculation because of the harmful effects of over-dosage. In my opinion the best form of post-operative raying consists in giving a course of about a dozen sittings spread over a month or six weeks, with periods of rest of two to four months between. This should be continued for at least two years. If this treatment be carried out properly, it can be practically guaranteed that the patient will have no externally visible recurrence.

The case which is, at first sight, surgically inoperable—or, at any rate, incurable—offers much scope for a combination of surgical and electrical treatment. Fortunately, one does not in these days very often see hopelessly advanced cases, but if there is already a fungating mass, it may be destroyed by the diathermic cautery, and the raw surface treated by X rays. By these means one can sometimes bring about surface healing, and reduce in size and render less adherent the main growth, so that all or most of it may be removed surgically, and a satisfactory external appearance results. Of course, in such cases the disease has nearly always reached the chest cavity. But even here X rays are not powerless, and such patients may live in comfort for months, occasionally for years. Only when the cancerous process has reached the spinal bones does the case seem beyond the possibility of any relief—at least so far as our present experience goes.

I have purposely deferred until now to refer to septic wounds, as they are so firmly rooted in the professional mind as almost wholly the products of war. But, so long as industrial accidents occur, it is unlikely that we shall completely banish the septic wound—and its sequela, the septic amputation stump. A seriously infected stump after an amputation, say, below the knee, may mean the loss of the entire limb, if not the death of the patient. In the early stage, characterized by acute inflammation, profuse discharge, and severe pain, there is nothing so useful as the incandescent lamp of 2-3000 c.p. Physicists tell us that ordinary light rays alone are produced in such a lamp ; nevertheless, experience teaches that its glass should be of a kind readily permeable by rays of short wave length. The effect of the combined light and heat rays is to cause the raw surface exposed to them to ooze serum freely, while at the same time pain is relieved. After a few days, when the acute stage has subsided, zinc ionization and X rays should be applied to the stump on alternate days. Surgical drainage and irrigation of dead spaces is likewise necessary, but by a combination of means re-amputation may be avoided in many cases where at first sight it appears inevitable.

The good effects of X rays in causing the absorption of keloid are well known, and electrical departments during the war were overwhelmed with requests to deal with exuberant and unhealthy scar tissue. But the sad part was that in many, if not in most of these cases, the deforming scars need never have been allowed to form. It may be accepted as undeniably true that whenever X rays or other electrical measures can cause more or less absorption of scar tissue, these same agents, properly employed at an early stage, would have minimised its formation. Such treatment involves the use of bedside apparatus, and, to conduct it on a large scale, it is necessary to have a special ward practically duplicating the electrical department.

Various difficulties of a financial and administrative nature prevented this bedside treatment of septic wounds from being given a full trial during the war. My own experience of it at Aldershot—where I directed the electrical service for a considerable time during the progress of hostilities—is limited for the most part to amputation stumps, and to face wounds in the plastic surgery wards at the Cambridge Hospital, where Major Harold Gillies had his cases previous to his taking charge of the special hospital at Sidcup. The results obtained were, however, quite sufficient to show that the proper course to follow is to secure that the progress of a septic wound is normal day by day, rather than to seek to remove the end results of vicious healing. To accomplish this requires daily inspection of the wound, and close co-operation between the surgeon and the electrical expert. It is the business of the latter to prescribe and vary the electrical procedures, but he may from time to time call on his colleague for minor surgical measures—*e.g.*, the removal of a small slough, the curettage of a sclerosed portion of a wound, or the re-opening of a too-rapidly closing sinus.

Plastic surgeons have certainly shown an excellent example in the matter of combined treatment. Not only have they sought the aid of the electro-therapeutist with regard to the bedside treatment of septic wounds, but also in cases of delayed union in simple fracture of the lower jaw. In the absence of sepsis, necrosis, mechanical obstacle or malposition, non-union indicates a failure of the bone to bone to respond normally to the stimulus of fracture. The bone is a living tissue whose functions are as readily modified, for good or evil, by local or constitutional causes, as are those of any other tissue. Properly applied electrical stimuli always tend to jolt a pathological functioning back into a normal functioning, no matter in what direction the variation from the normal has occurred. It is therefore not surprising that applications of the high-frequency vacuum over the site of a fracture, or the passing of a galvanic current in its neighbourhood, should frequently bring about the desired result.

This subject of non-union is obviously of great importance to anyone who is either in general or surgical practice. It rarely happens that treatment by galvanism at any rate cannot be made available, and, as it involves no risk in trained hands, it should always be given a trial.

From a consideration of fracture, one is naturally led to the question of adhesions. In most electrical departments much time is spent in attempting to relieve adhesions about joints. Here again, would it not be better to try to prevent their formation? This is, of course, already attempted by massage and early passive movement, but no one would claim that these measures are wholly successful, especially where a joint is actually involved in the fracture. A preventive measure to which no surgical exception can possibly be taken is the exposure of the joint to X rays while splints and bandages are *in situ*. If this be done, it will be found that, even in complicated fractures about the elbow, there is surprisingly little limitation of movement—apart, of course, from any due to actual displacement of fragments.

As to what I have said so far, I speak from personal experiences. But it is my firm belief that peritoneal adhesions—the bugbear of the abdominal surgeon—could be to a great extent prevented by post-operative raying. Certain it is that symptoms of a kind usually held to be caused by adhesions can often be relieved by radiotherapy ; and prevention is proverbially both easier and better than cure. The proposition that X rays would tend to prevent the formation of abdominal adhesions is obviously a difficult one to prove. A comparatively small percentage of the patients operated on develop serious trouble of this nature, and it would be necessary to treat a large number of cases, and to observe them over a period of months, or even years, before definite conclusions could be arrived at. Nevertheless, the proof should be attempted, as the amount of radiation required could do no harm.

This is a suitable point to enquire what it is that the X rays accomplish when suitably applied. There is a Greek fable about a traveller who sought shelter from a storm in a satyr's cave. His hands were stiff with cold, and the satyr, observing that he blew upon his fingers, asked him why he did so. "To warm my hands," the traveller replied. His host then hospitably busied himself in preparing a hot drink, which, as soon as made, he handed to him. It was, however, too hot and the traveller blew into it as he had done against his fingers. "Why do you blow again?" said the mystified satyr. "To cool the drink," replied his guest. Whereupon, crying out that he could be no honest man, the satyr, in a fury, fell upon the traveller and slew him. Now, the radiotherapist is much in the position of this traveller. He uses X rays to assist the formation of fibrous tissue, as in cancer ; to destroy it, as in keloid ; and there are those who would like to fall upon him as no honest man. Yet the explanation of the seeming paradox is simple : *in both cases the stimulus provided by the X rays gives nature the necessary impetus towards healing in her own way.* In so far as nature herself partially or wholly destroys a malignant growth, she does so by strangling the cancer cells by connective tissue. But in the case of a keloid, the connective tissue has itself taken on a pathological form, and a return to normal requires its absorption. This tendency to restore balance, to soothe or stimulate, augment or repress, according to what is needed, applies to electrical treatment in general, except when a definite suppression or destruction is aimed at—in which case one is really dealing with a form of surgery. For instance, X rays may be used over a considerable period of time to regulate ovarian function where there is excessive bleeding at the menstrual periods ; or, in women over forty, a few massive doses may be given which completely and permanently stop the ovarian function. In this latter case a kind of bloodless ovariotomy is in reality performed, which is not without special risks of its own, and the whole proceeding partakes of the nature of a surgical operation.

A simple analogy may help you to understand the essential difference between radiotherapy and what I may call radio-surgery. A plant which has been suffering from lack of light will benefit in all its functions by exposure to a suitable amount of sun ; but if we concentrate sunlight on a particular leaf or organ, this part will wither and die in a period long or short, according to the excess of light which is allowed to fall upon it.

I have gone into these theoretical questions at some length because some medical men still fear that actual harm may be done by X rays if they are used for the various purposes for which I have advocated their employment. It is of course true that grave injury may result from faulty methods ; but the same may be said of any powerful therapeutic agent. Accompanying the use of radio-surgery—using the term in the sense which I have defined—are certain risks which must be duly weighed against the looked for results— results as definite as those obtainable by the knife. I use the word "results" rather than "benefits" of deliberate purpose. The surgeon may remove a man's appendix : the disappearance of the organ is a definite result from the operation. But the patient is not necessarily cured of his complaint. Similarly, the permanent destruction of ovarian function can always be accomplished in patients in their fifth decade—this is the result of radio-surgery ; but if disturbed ovarian function is not the cause of the patient's symptoms, or only in part the cause, again cure will not result. The risks of radio-surgery are : irritation of the skin, usually trifling, but sometimes serious ; and possible injury to other organs besides those which it is desired to affect. But when the individual doses are small, and the course limited to a few weeks, the patient runs no risk in the hands of a competent physician. If no good is done, at least the patient has had the chance of benefit, and is no worse off than previously. This is so even in cancer—except in certain advanced cases where risks are justifiable. The pre-operative treatment previously advocated does not in any way interfere with subsequent normal healing.

The agents included under the general term " electrical" are X rays, light, high-frequency and static discharges, galvanism, faradism and various modifications thereof. The use of X rays and light in conjunction with surgery I have discussed at some length, and I propose to devote the remainder of my time to a consideration of combined treatment in infantile paralysis, into which treatment X rays do not enter. American writers claim that the high-candle power lamp applied over the spine is of use in the acute phase of the disease ; of this I have no personal experience. As to the more chronic stage, the mild case comes almost wholly into the domain of physical medicine ; the very severe case is largely a surgical problem, but there are few patients who cannot derive some benefit from physical measures. Leaving aside the few instances in which a late relapse is believed to have occurred, we are dealing in this disease with a destructive process which ceases after a few hours, or, at most, a few days. The extent of the initial paralysis is well known to be no guide to prognosis, except in the sense that the worst possible is known, but not the best. A very common result is for a lower limb to be still more or less seriously paralysed when the period of natural recovery seems to be coming to an end. The treatment of a case not requiring surgical interference must first be briefly dealt with, in order that the *rationale* of combined measures may be understood. First, deformities must be prevented by suitable appliances ; secondly, all muscles which can be made to contract by any form of electrical stimulus must be systematically exercised, and, thirdly, the limb as a whole should be stimulated by high-frequency applications both locally and to the spine. If all the cells in the affected region of the cord were either dead or capable of spontaneous recovery, electrical treatment would be useless. But there are, as a matter of experience, always numerous cells which remain, as it were, in a state of suspended animation ; and it is these which the electrical stimulus can call to life. Unfortunately, they often tend to become sluggish again after a few months, and the electrical excitations must be continued at intervals until full adult growth is attained.

There is sometimes a tendency to be concerned too much with the mechanical side of a case. Deformities are corrected, tendons are transplanted from muscles more or less healthy to do the work of those which are paralysed, and apparatus is prescribed to give mechanical support when necessary. But when all is done the limb too often remains blue, cold and shrunken, the transplanted tendons insufficiently energised properly to carry out their new work, and year by year the difference in size between the sound and the affected member becomes increased rather than lessened.

Massage and exercises are always prescribed, it is true ; and the days are gone by when the value of electricity in the treatment of paretic muscles can be questioned. The electrical stimulation of paralysed muscles has, in fact, become orthodox, and already it has been almost forgotten that electro-therapeutists only a few years ago were fighting tooth and nail for its acceptance. The doctrine of the stimulating effect of electricity on the growth of limbs is not yet canonical, but it is nevertheless true. With the exception of a few rare cases in which only a single important muscle is affected, it may be said that any limb sufficiently injured by polio-myelitis to need surgical attention is also in need of electrical stimulation. A six weeks course will often result in a spurt of growth lasting several months ; and if the stimulus be repeated at suitable intervals over a period of years, the development of the injured limb may lag but little behind that of its fellow.

Combined treatment must be carefully distinguished from blunderbus therapy—this latter may be defined as the simultaneous employment of a whole host of drugs or methods, each individually of doubtful utility, in the hope that, in the mass, they may accomplish some useful purpose. In combined treatment we employ agencies, each of which has been separately tested and found to be of definite value, often to the point of actual cure, in the malady to be attacked. And we make use of these various methods in such a manner and in such sequence that they amplify and reinforce each other.

Let us remember that nature recognizes neither the surgeon nor the radiologist, nor the expert in drugs, nor yet the lord of germs. She will put forth her best efforts only when she is assisted without stint. General practice is in reality the only logical form of practice. But no human mind can compass the whole field of medicine. Hence the hope of the future lies in specialism tempered by co-operation.

REPORT OF SOCIETY.

SOCIÉTÉ DE RADIOLOGIE MÉDI-CALE DE FRANCE.

Séance du 13 Janvier, 1920.

Utilisation du meuble d'Arsonval - Gaiffe pour l'alimentation du tube Coolidge- Baby, par le Dr. AUBOURG. L'A. donne les modi-fications très simples a apporter au meuble d'Arsonval pour permettre de se servir du tube Coolidge. Au point de vue radioscopique, le coefficient de visibilité à l'écran lui a paru très nettement supérieur à l'emploi des anciens

tubes ; pour la radiographie, le temps de pose doit être légérement augmenté. Mais d'une façon générale, l'emploi du tube Coolidge réalise un très grand progrès pour tous les actes radiologiques.

La protection du malade et du médecin avec le matériel Coolidge, par le Dr. H. BECLERE. Les nouveaux transformateurs pour l'aliment-ation des tubes " Baby-Coolidge " ont réalisé un immense progrès dans la technique radio-logique, par la simplicité de leur fonctionnement, mais il y a le revers de la médaille. Par le fait qu'ils ne limitent pas le débit, ce sont des instruments qu'il faut manier avec certaines précautions indispensables.   Pour protéger le malade et le radiologiste contre les possibilités d'électrocution, l'A. propose: 1° Utilisation de salles de gran des dimensions, sans appareils inutiles, avec postes multiples de lumière, faciles à reconnaître, même dans l'obscurité ; 2° Mise à la terre de toutes les parties métalliques des appareils ; 3° Commandes à distance ou marche à la pédale avec arrêt instantané ; 4° Plombs de sureté pour la radioscopie, différents de ceux employés pour la radiographie ; 5° Manettes de commandes en matière isolante et non plus en métal ; 6° Fils d'utilisation dans l'axe du tube, toujours tendus et munis de crochets de rappel ; 7° Large filet métallique relié à la terre, placé sous les trolleys en cas de rupture ; 8° Double prise des fils sur les trolleys ; 9° Drap métallique, léger, relié à la terre, placé sur le patient.

Nouvelle méthode pour le repérage des corps étrangers de l'œil par la radiographie stéréoscopique, par le Dr. CHÉRON.   Cette méthode consiste essentiellement à rendre les parois du globe visibles sur deux radiographies stéréoscopiques de l'œil bléssé en superposant aux clichés deux schémas représentant l'aspect droit et gauche d'un globe oculaire normal vu de profil et formés de cercles entrecoisés. Ces schémas, inspirés des anaglyphes des à M. Richard, permettent de voir dans l'examen au stéréoscope, par le simple effet du relief et de la perspective, si le projectile se trouve en dehors de l'œil ou dans l'œil, et, dans ce dernier cas, dans quelle portion du globe il se trouve.

Perforation de l'œsophage et communication avec la bronche droite, par le Dr. HARET. L'A. présente la radiographie d'un malade chez lequel on soupçonnait une tumeur néoplasique de l'œsophage et qui fut envoyé à la radioscopie pour voir la perméabilité de son œsophage.   Dès les premières gorgées de lait bismuthe, on vit apparaitre sur l'écran dans la partie moyenne et inférieure de la plage pulmonaire droite, toute une arborisation opaque due à la pénétration du lait dans la bronche droite.   Il existait une perforation de l'œsophage avec communication dans cette bronche.   Le fait curieux de l'observation est la tolérance parfaite du malade pour ces corps étrangers des voies respiratoires : c'est à peine s'il avait, au début de l'examen une petite toux qui ne durait que quelques secondes, et aucune suite fâcheuse ne se manifesta après cette absorption.

Le Sécrétaire Général : Dr. HARET.

NOTES AND ABSTRACTS

Some Causes of Kidney Pain and their Treatment (Exclusive of Stone, Tuberculosis and Infection).—S. H. HARRIS (*Med. Jour. of Australia*, Jan. 18th, 1919, pp. 41-48 with 16 skiagrams and 14 figs.).—Amongst intrinsic causes of renal pain are stricture of the ureter and renal tumour.   In the early stages of ureteral stricture, before any palpable enlargement of the kidney has taken place, complete cystoscopic and pyelographic examinations will establish the diagnosis. Secondary strictures following the passage of ureteral calculi or their operative removal are by no means uncommon.   When a renal tumour is small or growing upwards from the upper pole of the kidney, especially in a fat person, the diagnosis may be very difficult. Pyelography, by showing characteristic deformities in the outlines of the calices and pelvis, will often establish an otherwise doubtful diagnosis.

Amongst the extrinsic causes, obstruction of the ureter and uretero-pelvic junction by aberrant vessels, fascial bands, etc., is of considerable importance, and vies in frequency with ureteral stricture as a cause of often unrecognised renal pain. Its symptomatology is practically identical with that of ureteral stricture. Differentiation of the two conditions may be made by pyelography, it is stated, in nearly all cases. Another cause of pain is movable kidney. Examination of a large number of cases has convinced the author that true renal pain is rarely present in this condition without evidence of dilatation of the renal pelvis in the affected, as compared with the opposite, side.

In the author's experience, renal pain is due to the presence of calculi in less than one-third of all cases. Exclusive of tuberculosis, stone and gross renal infections, some form of ureteral obstruction is the cause of renal pain in the vast majority of cases. The diagnosis can and should be made in the early stages, when correct treatment results in a practical *restitutio ad integrum.* For the diagnosis, the cystoscope and ureter catheter may suffice, but often pyelography will be necessary. R. W. A. S.

Remarks on Dilatation of the Œsophagus. —S. G. SHATTOCK (*Proc. Roy. Soc. of Med. Sect. of Laryngology,* March, 1919.)—The following abstracts are the results from the study of specimens illustrating the condition of œsophagectasia.

The thickening of the muscular coat varies in degree in different cases ; and even in the same specimen, in different zones, or at different levels of the dilatation. In some, the amount of muscular thickening is not merely proportional to the increased capacity of the tube, but is absolutely above the normal. In none is the muscular wall atrophic. In one there is a well defined and pronounced hypertrophy of the circular fibres around the terminal part of the œsophagus.

As to the part played by the diaphragm, the skiagrams undoubtedly demonstrate the the presence of an undilated segment of the œsophagus above the stomach, the upper limit of which segment corresponds with the superior surface of the diaphragm. This, however, does not prove that the diaphragm is the *cause* of the obstruction. The obstruction, one may still think, is below at the cardia ; the tone of the diaphragm disallowing the dilatation of the included part of the tube. The dilatation in the specimens ends only at

the gastric orifice, and Shattock concludes that one is dealing either with spasm of the cardia or with a form of obstruction due to inco-ordination. R. W. A. S.

Roentgen-Ray Intoxication : Disturbances in Metabolism Produced by Deep Massive Doses of the Hard Roentgen Rays.—C. C. HALL and G. H. WHIPPLE (*Amer. Jour. of the Med. Sciences,* April, 1919, pp. 453-482, with 15 tables and bibliography).—The results of experiments on dogs by these investigators are given in a valuable paper as follows :—

The general constitutional reaction after a lethal dose of hard X rays from a Coolidge tube is remarkably uniform and constant. A double lethal dose does not modify the clinical reaction. A latent period of 24 hours or longer is the rule, and during this time the dog is normal except for an increase in the excreted urinary nitrogen. Vomiting and diarrhœa then dominate the clinical picture until death, which, as a rule, follows on the fourth day.

The blood non-protein nitrogen commonly shows a marked increase (twice normal) on the day before death, and often more than three times normal on the day of death.

The elimination of urinary nitrogen is increased on the day following the X-ray exposure and remains high until death, often an increase of 50 to 100 per cent. above the normal base line.

P.M. findings are : Spleen small and fibrous, a moderate degree of congestion and mottling of the intestinal mucous membrane and strong evidence for *epithelial injury* in the intestinal mucosa. The epithelium lining the intestinal crypts may show actual necrosis and invasion of polymorphonuclear leucocytes. This epithelium also shows a remarkable speed of autolysis and may vanish by autodigestion within a few hours post mortem. The epithelium of the small intestine is apparently sensitive to large doses of X rays, and the injury of these important cells may give the correct explanation of the general intoxication associated with the vomiting and diarrhœa.

The so-called X-ray anaphylaxis or hypersensitiveness to a second proper time exposure found no support in the experiments. In fact, there is some evidence for a slightly increased tolerance to the second dose.

The liver epithelium is not fundamentally involved in the fatal X-ray intoxication, nor is there any evidence of nephritis.

Increased spark gap greatly increases the severity of the constitutional reaction and subsequent intoxication. The fatal dose for a dog is about 500 m.a. minutes with a 6 inch spark gap, but only 210 m.a. minutes with a 9 inch gap.

Burns caused by X rays are not associated with any distinct increase in urinary nitrogen during the long latent period between the exposure and the early dermatitis which precedes the actual ulcer. No satisfactory explanation of this is known.

The X-ray intoxication or general constitutional reaction is a good example of a "non-specific" intoxication. Bacteria and specific toxins and endotoxins or antibodies cannot possibly be concerned.   R. W. A. S.

Radiotherapy and Corneal Opacities.—BONNEFON (*Arch. d'Élect. Méd.*, May, 1919).—To the problem of restoring sight to those blinded by corneal opacities the oculist Sulzer had applied himself from 1906 until the war interrupted his researches. He has since died, and his pupil Chappé has published the results so far obtained by his unfinished work. The author quotes from this to make a plea for active collaboration between radiologists and ophthalmologists. The patient, aged 50, contracted an extensive opaque leucoma, occupying nearly the whole of the left cornea, in 1906. He received 6 séances of phototherapy during 1908 to 1909 at the hands of Dr. Sulzer. There was a very slight improvement at first, and from perception of light the vision increased to counting the fingers. No more result could be obtained. In March, 1911, radiotherapy was begun, and altogether 9 séances of from 7 to 12 minutes, and 3 to 5 H. were given during 15 months. The opacity so cleared up that by July, 1918, the patient could read ordinary newspaper type with a + 3 D lens.   N. B.

Upward Dislocation of the Ilium.—MASMONTEIL (*Gaz. des Hop.*, March, 1919. Abstracted in *Arch. d'Élect. Méd.*, May, 1919). —The author describes a case whose curious gait led to suspicion of malingering. He publishes the radiographic finding, which showed the whole right half of the pelvis raised 3 cm. upwards by dislocation of the sacro-iliac articulation, accompanied by separation of the symphysis.   N. B.

Clinical Types of Lichen Planus.—JOHN A. FORDYCE and GEORGE M. MACKEE (*Journal of Cutaneous Diseases*, May, 1919).—The value of arsenic and mercury in the treatment is open to discussion. The Roentgen ray will arrest the itching, and will in most cases cause involution of the lesions in a few weeks. In acute lichen the ray acts rapidly, with only a mild dose, $\frac{1}{16}$ to $\frac{1}{4}$ H. units, once or twice weekly. Hypertrophic lesions need larger doses and yield more slowly. Radium has the same effect but of course cannot be used for large areas.   N. B.

The Radiological Appearance of the Stomach in Tetanus.—LUIGI SICILIANO (*La Radiol. Med.*, Vol. VI, 1919, p. 97).—The author has seen a few cases of tetanus in which he was able to study the stomach radiologically. The patients were women, in whom the convulsions had ceased for a few days, but in some the hyperexcitability of latent tetanus was still evident. Except for anorexia in a few cases there were no symptoms of gastric disturbance. The result of radiological examination showed that the shape of the stomach was normal in each case, the volume was slightly increased in a few, the tonicity of the walls was well maintained, but there was diminished or absolute loss of peristaltic movements, and this was characteristic of all patients observed. In two girls with well marked Chwostek's symptom, and definite electrical hyperexcitability of the nerves, it was possible to thoroughly examine the motor functions of the stomach. Light and superficial waves of peristalsis began as soon as the meal was introduced; they started simultaneously in different points of the greater curvature, were never more than superficial, some reached the pylorus but many stopped after a very short course. The horizontal position did not increase peristalsis at all. In all but one patient the stomach emptied in normal time, presumably because tonicity was maintained. The author does not agree with the theory of alimentary intoxication as the cause of tetanus; he believes that the diminished peristalsis which he has observed is a collateral phe-nomenon to the disordered nervous condition of the organism.   N. B.

On the Provocation of Latent Malaria.—
TEMPINI (*Proc. of the Lomb. Soc. of Med. and Biol. Science*, 1918, Vol. VII. Abstracted in *La Radiol. Med.*, 1919, VII, 143).—Among various experimental efforts to provoke latent malaria, the author has tried the effect of X rays on the spleen. The questions he has tested are :—

1. If irradiation of the spleen mobilises the malarial parasite.

2. If it stimulates the generative activity of the gametes and provokes the outbreak of a malarial attack.

3. If it has a curative action on the infection.

4. If it reduces the enlarged spleen.

Forty cases were studied, in which the primary infection took place some months or a year previously; during this time relapses had been verified. They were resistant to ordinary cures, had a moderate degree of splenic enlargement, and excluded serious cases and those of long standing where there was probability of re-infection and much splenic change. The technique consisted of three successive daily sittings of fifteen minutes, $6\frac{1}{2}$ to 7 Walter, $1\frac{1}{2}$ to 2 ma., 3 mm. filter, 25 cm. distance from anticathode. Methodical repeated examination of the blood was made during and after the sitting, and a three-hourly temperature chart was kept during the period of test. In the results the author obtained mobilisation of the parasites in 35 per cent. of cases, pathogenesis in one third, and sensible reduction of the tumour in all cases; no therapeutic action. There was no influence on temperature in cases where mobilisation was negative. Of the fourteen positive cases, a typical febrile attack followed the irradiation of four. Of these four cases, three had shown sexual forms in the peripheral blood, while the fourth had crescents, which does not exclude the possibility of sexual forms in deep organs.   N. B.

UNIVERSITY OF CAMBRIDGE.
DIPLOMA IN RADIOLOGY AND ELECTROLOGY.

In connection with the Courses now running in London, at University College and at the Royal Society of Medicine, the Committee for the Diploma propose to announce to the Senate the following dates for the next Examination, which will be held at Cambridge. Part I (A and B), Tuesday, July 27th, 1920, with practical work and *viva voce* examination on July 28th; and Part II (A and B), Thursday, July 29th, with practical work on July 30th.

Candidates desiring to take the Diploma by Thesis next Term, under Regulation 13, should apply to the Secretary, Dr. Shillington Scales, Medical Schools, Cambridge, without delay, for the necessary certificate forms.

The Committee propose to hold Courses of Lectures and Practical Work in Physics and in Electrology during the ensuing Long Vacation in Cambridge, beginning June 22nd and finishing about the middle of August ; in Radiology in the next Michaelmas Term, beginning October 12th, and finishing in time for the Examination at Christmas. The necessary clinical work can be carried out at Addenbrooke's Hospital, Cambridge. The Physics Course will be given by Dr. Crowther, by arrangement with Prof. Sir Ernest Rutherford; the Course in Radiology and Electrology by approximately the same lecturers, all leading workers in these subjects, who have given the Courses now running in London. The holding of these Courses in Cambridge, will, however, be dependent on a sufficient number of students entering for them, and for this reason early application should be made to the Secretary, Dr. Shillington Scales. It is

hoped in future to hold Courses and Examinations twice a year, the Courses in Cambridge alternating with those in London, so that candidates from overseas may have an opportunity of taking the Diploma.

CORRESPONDENCE.

LONDON HOSPITAL RADIOLOGICAL DEPARTMENT.

To the Editors of ARCHIVES OF RADIOLOGY AND ELECTROTHERAPY.

DEAR SIRS,

Dr. Barclay, in his letter in the February issue, draws attention to the value of hypo "waste." It may interest him, and others, to know that the London Hospital has benefited to the extent of close on £100 in the last six years from the sale of hypo "waste," discarded plates, old X-ray tubes, apparatus, etc. The hypo "waste" is collected by the Refining Company, who supply an empty cask to be filled, and even before the present increase in the value of silver, the money return was considerable by the end of the year.

In a large hospital, where radiographs run into many thousands per annum, it is impossible and unnecessary to keep them all,

consequently some method has to be adopted. On their return to the department at the London, they are classified by the radiologist, and those to be discarded are put aside for a minimum period of six months, and are then sold at the market price of glass. During the war this was a substantial amount.

The Jews in the neighbourhood of the hospital are anxious to get hold of these old negatives, consequently I get them to bid against one another. I recommend this plan if there are any Jews handy!

The question of waste should be considered as part of the organisation of a department.

I am, yours faithfully,

S. GILBERT SCOTT,
Radiologist in Charge.

6, Bentinck Street,
Cavendish Square, W. 1,
March 16th, 1920.

NEW TECHNIQUE.

THE COOLIDGE RADIATOR X-RAY TUBE (SPECIAL DENTAL TYPE).

THE Coolidge Radiator X-ray Tube, like the well known Universal type, employs a cathode with a special tungsten filament and an anode having a tungsten target. X rays are produced by the projection from the heated cathode on to the face of the target of continuous streams of electrons.

There is, however, this important difference between the two types, that whereas the universal tube must be used on rectified

current, the radiator tube is self-rectifying, and can be used directly across the terminals of either an induction coil or a high tension transformer, without the necessity for any auxiliary rectifying device.

A special dental type of Coolidge Radiator X-ray Tube has now been developed, which is similar to the ordinary radiator tube, excepting for a few important differences in form and construction, which have been adopted to make it suitable for dental work. The dental radiator tube has been designed for the particular purpose of making radiographs of the teeth and jaw, and is not intended for general radiographic work.

The bulb of the Coolidge dental tube is $3\frac{3}{4}$ inches in diameter, and the cathode arm extends 2 inches from the bulb, at right angles to the anode arm, which measures 9 inches from the bulb to the end of the radiator. For dental work, the advantages of this mode of construction are :—

1. The rays are emitted from the tube in a line with the axis of the anode, making it easy to manipulate to the best advantage.

2. The cathode circuit is grounded so that there is only one high tension wire, which is always connected to that part of the tube farthest from the subject.

3. It is possible to reduce to a minimum the distance between the film and focal spot, and consequently to make satisfactory radiographs of the teeth and jaws with comparatively short exposure.

As the dental type radiator tube is designed to operate only in connection with special machines, and always at a fixed voltage and current, the procedure is limited to closing the switch for the time necessary to produce on the photographic film the desired effect. The factor of time is the only variable in making radiographs with the dental tube, and this factor will be adjusted in accordance with the judgment and experience of the operator.

Since the cathode terminal is earthed and the anode end of the tube is always farthest from the patient, it is possible to bring the tube very close without risk of shock. The short focal spot-film distance reduces the energy expenditure necessary for satisfactory dental radiographs. Using an 8 in. focal spot-film distance the same radiographs may be obtained with one fourth the energy necessary for a distance of 16 in. The dental type radiator tube should be operated with an energy input not exceeding that corresponding to a current of 10 milliamperes, at a "useful" voltage corresponding to a 3 in. parallel spark gap between points.

A glass protective shield has been manufactured for use with the Coolidge radiator tubes of both the ordinary and dental types. This shield is made of glass containing enough lead to give the same degree of protection as a sheet of lead one quarter as thick. The walls of the glass shield are $\frac{1}{4}$ in. thick, and therefore give the same protection against X rays as a lead shield $\frac{1}{16}$ in. thick. The shield is made in two halves, which are identical and interchangeable. The joint is ground, and made at right angles to the axis of the shield. It is evident that even if the joint

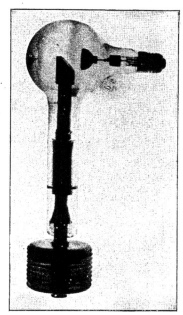

Coolidge Dental Radiator Tube.

does not fit tightly, no X rays can escape unless the focal spot happens to be centred directly in line with the ground surface of the joint.

Coolidge X-ray Tubes of the Universal, Radiator and Radiator Dental Types are supplied in this country by the regular dealers in radiographic apparatus, and also by the patent owners, the British Thomson-Houston Company, Limited, of Rugby, and 77, Upper Thames Street, E.C. 4, to whom application for technical and commercial information should be made.

PUBLICATIONS RECEIVED.

Journals.

American Journal of Electrotherapeutics and Radiology, Nov., Dec., 1919.

American Journal of Roentgenology, Dec., 1919.

Archives d'Électricite Médicale et de Physiotherapie, Aug., 1919 ; Jan., Feb., 1920.

Archivio Italiano di Chirurgia, Jan. 31st, 1920.

British Journal of Dermatology, Jan., Feb., 1920.

Bulletin of the Johns Hopkins Hospital, Jan., 1920.

Bulletin et Mémoirs de la Société de Radiologie Médicale de France, **Jan.,** Feb., 1920.

Gaceta Medica Catalana, **Nov.** 30th, 1919.

Good Health, Feb , 1920.

Hospitalstidende, Nov. 5th, 12th, 19th, 26th ; Dec. 3rd, 10th, 17th, 24th, **31st,** 1919.

Il Policlinico, Jan. 1st, 15th, 1920.

International Journal of Orthodontia and Oral Surgery, Jan., 1920.

Journals—*continued.*

Journal de Medicine de Lyon, Feb. 20th, 1920.

Journal de Radiologie et d'Electrologie, Jan., 1920.

Journal of the Röntgen Society, Jan., 1920.

Le Radium, Nov., Dec., 1919.

Medical Journal of Australia, Dec. 27th, 1919 ; Jan. 3rd, 10th, 17th, 1920.

Medical Science, Abstracts, and Reviews, Feb., Mar., 1920.

Modern Medicine, Jan., Feb., 1920.

New York Medical Journal, Jan. 10th, 17th, 24th, 31st, 1920.

New York State Journal of Medicine, Jan., Feb., 1920.

Norsk Mag. for Lægevidenskaben, Feb. 1920.

Quarterly Journal of Medicine, July, Oct., 1919 ; Jan., 1920.

Surgery, Gynæcology, and Obstetrics, Feb., 1920.

Ugeskrift for Læger, Jan. 15th, 29th ; Feb. 19th, 26th, 1920.

NOTICES.

ARCHIVES OF RADIOLOGY AND ELECTROTHERAPY is published monthly.

The index for each volume, which ends with the May number, is supplied with the June number of each year.

Communications to the Editors should be addressed to " ROBERT KNOX, M.D., 38, Harley Street, W. 1."

Communications and illustrations from American contributors may be sent to Messrs. REBMAN COMPANY, 141-145, West Thirty-sixth Street, New York City.

All radiographs and photographs must be originals, and must not have been previously published. Drawings should be supplied on separate paper.

Owing to the scarcity of paper the Publishers are reluctantly compelled to reduce the number of free reprints of Papers to twenty-five.

Annual Subscriptions, payable in advance, 30/- including postage. Single copies, 3/- (postage 2d.) Single numbers and back numbers can be supplied on application.

Vol. XXIV—No. 11   APRIL, 1920   No. 237

ARCHIVES OF RADIOLOGY AND ELECTROTHERAPY

THE OFFICIAL ORGAN OF THE

BRITISH ASSOCIATION OF RADIOLOGY AND PHYSIOTHERAPY

Editors.

ROBERT KNOX, M.D., Hon. Radiologist, King's College Hospital.
E. P. CUMBERBATCH, B.M., M.R.C.P., Medical Officer in Charge, Electrical Department, St. Bartholomew's Hospital.
SIDNEY RUSS, D.Sc., Physicist to the Middlesex Hospital.

IN COLLABORATION WITH

A. E. BARCLAY (Manchester); BELOT (Paris); H. MARTIN BERRY (London): W. H. BRAGG (London); N. BURKE (Woodhall Spa); J. BURNET (Edinburgh); W. J. S. BYTHELL (Manchester); J. T. CASE (Battle Creek, U.S.A.); A. ST. GEORGE CAULFEILD (London); H. A. COLWELL (London); FOVEAU DE COURMELLES (Paris); GUNZBURG (Antwerp); HALL-EDWARDS (Birmingham): HARET (Paris); HAUCHAMPS (Brussels); F. HERNAMAN-JOHNSON (London): W. F. HIGGINS (Teddington); THURSTAN HOLLAND (Liverpool); HURST (London); KLYNENS (Antwerp); LAQUERRIERE (Paris), LAZARUS-BARLOW (London); LEDUC (Nantes); ALEXANDER MACKAY (Edinburgh); REGINALD MORTON (London): HARRISON ORTON (London); W. OVEREND (St. Leonards-on-Sea); PFAHLER (Philadelphia); C. E. S. PHILLIPS (London); GEORGE PIRIE (Dundee); HOWARD PIRIE (Montreal): A. W. PORTER (London); R. W. A. SALMOND (London); WERTHEIM SALOMONSON (Amsterdam): S. SLOAN (Glasgow): SOMERVILLE (Glasgow); W. C. STEVENSON (Dublin): W. J. TURRELL (Oxford): HUGH WALSHAM (London).

EDITORIAL.

THE paper by Dr. Mottram and Mr. Clarke, reproduced from the Proceedings of the Royal Society of Medicine (Electrotherapeutic Section), Vol. 13, calls attention to the blood changes produced in man by the gamma rays from radium. The problem of adequate protection from these very penetrating rays is perhaps the most difficult with which the radiologist has to contend. The growing recognition of the necessity for protective measures in all X-ray work is partly the outcome of the war and partly the result of the wider knowledge of the harmful effects which result from inadequate protection.

In the case of radium, the use of which in medical procedures is limited to therapy, the question is likely to become more and more pressing as larger and larger quantities are handled. With quantities of the order of a gram the gamma radiation is considerable, and though very much less active as regards photographic or electrical action than the X rays emitted by a Coolidge tube, we can look upon the act of handling such a quantity as that of handling an

X-ray tube in operation, and, in fact, a tube that is continuously in operation. That is the nature of the problem with radium, and any protective measures to meet the case must be thought out at each step, from the moment the radium is taken, say from its safe, to the time when it is applied to the patient, how to protect the operators. It is not an easy matter and will doubtless receive different treatment in different centres of radium therapy.

The paper in question shows that remarkable changes occur in the blood of people exposed daily to small doses of such radiation ; changes in fact of an undesirable nature. The authors have, no doubt, used the most appropriate indicator under the circumstances, for it is now a well established fact that in the X-ray and gamma ray portion of the spectrum, the skin is less sensitive to the rays of very short wave-lengths than it is to those of longer wave-lengths, *i.e.*, to " softer " rays ; the blood changes however are found to occur with hard X rays as well as with soft X rays, and, it so happens, also with gamma rays.

The importance of Dr. Mottram's paper will not be lost upon those who are vitally interested in seeing the whole of radiological work freed from the dangers which have attended it in the past.

A UNIVERSITY CHAIR OF RADIOLOGY AT MIDDLESEX HOSPITAL.

On the tragic death of Mr. C. R. C. Lyster, the authorities of Middlesex Hospital and Medical School were faced with the immediate necessity of appointing a Medical Officer in Charge of the X-ray and Electrotherapeutic Department. It had been felt for some time that if real progress was to be made in radiology in this country it was necessary to ensure that an expert in this branch of medicine should be able to devote his whole time to the charge of this department of the hospital and to the work of education and research. With this object in view the hospital authorities approached the University of London to secure co-operation in achieving their object by giving high academic position to any whole-time officer appointed.

At the last meeting of the Senate (Feb. 25th), a resolution was passed instituting a University Chair of Radiology tenable at the Middlesex Hospital Medical School.

At this hospital there are unique opportunities for the investigation of the possibilities of radiotherapy. Over one hundred beds are constantly occupied with cases of cancer ; in the Physics Department there are special laboratories for the investigation of physical and other problems (also a large supply of radium is available).

Intimate connection will be maintained between the new department and that of physics, which has now been placed in an unique position through the endowment of a University Chair by Messrs. S. B. and J. B. Joel, and it is from this association that the hospital authorities hope for great progress to be made in the treatment and cure of cancer, and for the development of a department which will be of special service to men proposing to specialise in radiology, a branch of medicine which has lately been recognised by Cambridge University as requiring specialist training and worthy of a diploma.

The maintenance of this professorship will be a financial strain for the institution to bear, but it is hoped that some assistance may be obtained by gifts for the purpose of endowment.

HENRI DOMINICI AND HIS WORK (1867-1919).

By Dr. J. Barcat.

The year 1919 (21st May) saw the last of Henri Dominici, who was pre-eminently the leading man in the French School of Radiumtherapy between 1906 and 1919. We are indebted to him in particular for the very important method which he has described as the method of ultra-penetrating radiation, a method which has notably extended the horizon of radium-therapy, and which radiotherapy also had a tendency to realise with the progressive improvement of the apparatus used, the most perfect type of which is at the present time Coolidge's tube.

Although M. Dominici held no official titles, he made for himself a world-wide reputation in scientific circles. This was due to his far reaching work, denoting the stamp of a truth loving intellect, as capable of minute analysis as of general ideas. His courtesy, his absolute straightforwardness, his innate distinction and good breeding caused all those with whom he came into contact to love and respect him.

Of Corsican origin, H. Dominici was born in England, of French parents. He was educated in France, at the College of Vaugirard ; licentiate of science in 1888, he began the study of medicine in 1889, was appointed "interne" in 1893, and from that time applied himself to morbid anatomy and experimental physiology, as well as his ordinary clinical work.

After a three years course at the College of France, under the direction of M.M. Suchard and Malassez, H. Dominici began the publication of a series of original works on the normal and pathological histology of the blood and of the hæmatopoietic organs, which made him the undisputed expert of French hæmatology (formation of nucleated corpuscles in the bone marrow, under the influence of toxins — myeloid reaction of the lymphoid organs in the course of certain morbid states—connective origin of certain lymphatic cells [lympho-connective cells].)

In 1902 he continued his work in Dr. Sabouraud's laboratory, at the Hospital Saint-Louis, and it is there that I had the honour of knowing him and becoming his pupil and friend.

In 1903 he was offered the management of a sanatorium at the "Mont des Oiseaux"; he accepted the post, but not finding there the facilities for study which he had hoped for, he returned to Saint-Louis, to take up once more his work on the morbid reactions of the connective tissue and of the hæmatopoietic organs.

In 1906 radiumtherapy, which had just been brought before the medical profession by Drs. Daulos, Rehns, Salmon, Soupault, A. Daries, etc., and had fallen into unjustifiable neglect, revived again under the auspices of M. Armet de Lisle, who established a centre of studies and therapeutic applications. H. Dominici was invited to study the biological action of radium. He accepted, and asked us to collaborate in his researches, in which later on our excellent friends, H. Rubens-Duval and Faure Beaulieu, took part.

It is in this laboratory that H. Dominici, whose attention was awakened by the process of evolution without necrosis, which histology showed us to take place in the deeper tissues exposed to radiation, noticed, in collaboration with the distinguished and regretted physician, Beaudoin, the homogeneity of the radiation after it had undergone filtration by ·4 millimetre of a dense metal such as lead. Eliminating secondary radiation by another filter of very slightly dense matter he noted that the rays thus selected presented remarkable properties, characterised by a relatively marked innocuousness for healthy tissues, whereas, on the other hand, they preserved all their special action on neoplastic tissues. He thus established the method of *ultra-penetrating radiation* at a time when official opinion maintained that filtration removed from radium its essential properties.

Thanks to this method, large and deep seated cancers, and in particular cancer of the uterus (Chéron et Rubens-Duval), uterine fibroma (Chéron), were treated with success.

In the same laboratory we also studied together the action of the radiation on the connective tissue, an action which is characterised by the momentary return of this tissue to an embryonic state, and later, to a fibro-cicatricial state, which explains the retrogression of angiomata, the fibrous transformation of tubercles and the softening of scar tissue.

With Rubens-Duval and ourselves he studied the comparative susceptibilty of the different tissues, a susceptibility governed by the two great laws of age and species. *Of age*, in the sense that the nearer the cellular elements of a tumour are to the embryonic state, the more sensitive they are to radiation. *Of species*, in the sense that normal epithelial cells are more sensitive than those of the connective tissue. Of the *variety*, in this respect, that the basic cells of the skin are less sensitive than those of the hair bulbs, and also that the cells of the connective tissue are less so than those of the lymphoid tissue.

He also discovered the very remarkable curative action of radium in gonorrheal rheumatism.

With Faure-Beaulieu and the Pr. Petit of Alfort he showed that it was possible to inject into the organism radium salts, and in particular sulphate of radium salts in fine suspension in saline solution (Jaboins' preparation).

He showed that sulphate of radium thus injected persists during many weeks, sometimes more than a year, in the neighbouring lymphatic interstices, if it has been introduced by subcutaneous injections ; in the lymphatic interstices of the lung, if it has been injected in the trachea; in the capillaries of the lung, the liver, the kidneys, and spleen, if it has been introduced intravenously, and that these salts produce therapeutic effects : stimulation of hæmatopoiesis, regulation of the digestive functions, and also those of the nutrition and of the nervous system (results which had been corroborated almost at the same time by Chevrier).

In 1912, H. Dominici left the radium laboratory for a private one of his own, and devoted himself to the study of tuberculosis toxins. The result of these studies was the remarkable work published, together with Ostrowsky, at "Masson's," in 1914. At the same time he attended to the practice of medicine with the help of Rubens-Duval and of Oppert, and was carrying on, with Faivre and Bader, very interesting research work on serums and vaccines when the war broke out. From that time, unhappily, owing no doubt to the anxieties of the war and to the dispersion of his friends, his health, which had ever been frail, began to give way, and, in spite of giving up all work, his malady made steady progress, and shortly after the great victory of the Allies he was carried off, this causing irreparable loss both to his friends and to French science.

THE LEUCOCYTIC BLOOD-CONTENT OF THOSE HANDLING RADIUM FOR THERAPEUTIC PURPOSES[1].

By J. C. MOTTRAM, M.B., and J. R. CLARKE.

(From the Research Department, Radium Institute, London).

[Reprinted from the *Proceedings of the Royal Society of Medicine*, 1920, Vol. XIII. (Section of Electro-Therapeutics, pp. 25-30.]

THESE radium workers are subject to widely different amounts of irradiation according as to whether their employment necessitates their being near to or distant from the radium, and whether for long or short periods of time. Among the workers under observation two classes were especially subject to exposure : (A) Laboratory workers who prepare and measure

[1] At a meeting of the Section. held December 19, 1919.

applicators containing emanation and radium ; and (B) clinical workers who attach various screens to the radium applicators and subsequently apply them to patients. The remaining workers receive less exposure, down to the servants of the institution, who are only subject to very small quantities of the γ-radiation which prevades the whole building.

The leucocytic blood content of all these individuals (twenty in number) is shown diagrammatically in Fig. 1, in which a comparison is made with thirty-eight normal individuals. (The normal figures were obtained from a paper on the effect of solar dermatitis on the leucocytes of the blood [1].) The diagram shows that the polymorphonuclear leucccytic and the

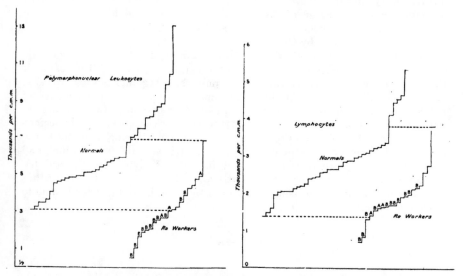

FIG. 1.—Each step in the diagram repesents a single individual. *A*, laboratory worker ; *B*, clinical worker.

lymphocytic blood content of the radium workers is decidedly lower than than that of the normals. In the case of the polymorphonuclear leucocytes, there are eleven individuals below the lowest normal, and in the case of the lymphocytes three below the lowest normal. The lowest figures are : For polymorphs, 522 and 1,035 per cubic millimetre, and for lymphocytes, 706 and 855 per cubic millimetre. The classes A and B are indicated in the diagram, and are seen to form the large majority of the more affected workers. The exceptionally high A in the polymorph chart showed subsequently much lower readings of 2,048 and 2,343. Similar, but less marked, blood changes have been described in X-ray workers [2], and a leucopænia has been produced experimentally in animals with X-rays by a number of observers [3], [4].

Attention is drawn to the absence of any evidence of a leucocytosis even among the less irradiated workers, the highest counts falling near the middle of the normal series. This indicates that a daily dose of irradiation, even when very small, will not produce a leucocytosis; whereas it is known that in small animals alternate periods of X-radiation and freedom from irradiation will, under certain conditions, produce a profound leucocytosis [5], and that the leucopænia following a single dose · of X-rays is often followed by a leucocytosis [6].

The leucopænia of radium workers, classes A and B, manifests itself after a few weeks' exposure—for instance, a class A individual showed a fall from 7,283 to 3,077 polymorphs, and from 4,544 to 1,612 lymphocytes after one month; the corresponding figures for a class B worker were 4,448 to 2,398 and 1,824 to 1,690 after two weeks. The effect of a holiday of two months is well seen in the following case :—

	Before holiday	After holiday	25 days later
Polymorphonuclears ...	522 ...	1,909 ...	1,063
Lymphocytes	885 ...	2,158 ...	857

On the other hand in several cases a holiday of two months was followed by a fall instead of a rise. It is thus clear that the onset of the fall is rapid, and the recovery by comparison slow.

No association between this leucopænia and · any condition of illhealth has been definitely recorded. Whitlows of the fingers and other infective conditions of the hands are of common occurrence in radium workers; this is, however, probably due to local changes.

An attempt has been made to estimate the daily amount of irradiation which workers of class B receive. Electroscopic measurements were found to be impracticable, as the leak was so great that the instrument could not be charged in the room where the attachment of the screens to the radium applicators was carried out. A photographic plate was, therefore, made to occupy the place of a worker. It was screened with varying thicknesses of aluminium from 0·2 mm. to 2 mm. The shadows which resulted on development were of nearly equal density, showing that γ-radiation was chiefly affecting the plate. A control plate was exposed to the γ-radiation (3 mm. lead and 0·2 mm. aluminium screens) from an aplicator having 9 mgr. of $RaBr_2 2H_2O$ per square centimetre for varying lengths of time. The two plates were developed together, and it was found that one minute exposure to the applicator produced a shadow similar to that on the experimental plate. This may be conveniently expressed in biological X-ray units, Rads [7].

This unit is an exposure to the β- and γ-rays from 2·75 mgr. of $RaBr_2 2H_2O$ per square centimetre for one hour; this dose is just sufficient to prevent the growth of rat sarcoma and to produce an erythema when applied to the human skin [8]. Assuming that the radiant energy of β-plus γ-rays is to γ-rays as 50 to 1, then class B workers receive $\frac{1}{500}$ of a rad daily per square centimetre. This small amount is, however, incident

over the entire front surface of the body, and, as a generalized condition
is under consideration, an attempt is made to estimate the total amount of
incident radiation and to compare this with the amount received by a patient
undergoing treatment for cancer of the breast.

The intensity, of the γ-radiation from a radium applicator at a distance
r therefrom is proportional to $\frac{e^{-\lambda r}}{r^2}$ where λ is the coefficient of absorption
of the medium traversed by the rays. In the case of a patient undergoing
treatment the radium is concentrated over a small area (of the order of
2 sq. cm.) situated about 2 mm. from the skin. The radiation received
by a small area δA, distance r from the centre of the applicator or
group of applicators, is thus equal to $I_o e^{\frac{-\lambda r}{r_2}} \delta A$; I_o being the intensity of
the radiation at a point on a circle unit distance from the centre, and λ the
coefficient for absorption of the γ-rays by air.

The integration of this quantity over the irregular surface of the

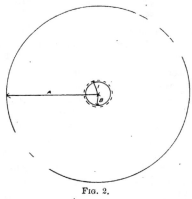

FIG. 2.

body of the patient is very difficult. It was found, however, that a full
strength applicator, 2 sq. cm. in area, prepared as for a carcinoma case,
when laid at one end of a photographic film for twelve hours, had no
effect 1 ft. away. A case of this type usually receives about thirty hours'
treatment, and hence the radiation received by the remote parts of the
body can be neglected. The integration, therefore, was simplified by
considering the body to be a cylinder with its axis horizontal, the front
elevation being a circle.

It is assumed that the applicator is placed at the centre of this circle,
which is of radius a, Fig. 2, and that it is itself circular, of radius b, Fig. 2 ;
b being small compared with a. Measure a and b in such units that
$a > b$, but b is very nearly equal to unity. Then the intensity of radiation,
received by the body at unit distance from the centre, is equal to the
strength of the applicator, to a degree of approximation sufficient for our
purposes. Let this be I_o

The radiation received by annulus, thickness δr at a distance r from the centre, is—

$$I_o, \frac{e^{-\lambda r}}{r^2}, 2\pi r, \delta r.$$

Thus the total radiation received is—

$$R = \int_1^a I_o, \frac{e^{-\lambda r}}{r^2}, 2\pi r, \delta r,$$

+ the radiation received by the circle of unit radius.

But, we have supposed the intensity of the radiation over a circle of unit radius to be constant and equal to I_o.

$$\therefore R = 2\pi I_o \int_1^a \frac{e^{-\lambda r}}{r} \delta r + \pi I_o.$$

$$\text{Let P} = \int_1^a \frac{e^{-\lambda r}}{r} \delta r = \int_1^a \frac{1}{r} \left[1 - \lambda r + \frac{\lambda^2 r^2}{2!} - \frac{\lambda^3 r^3}{3!} + \dots \right] \delta r$$

$$= \int_1^a \left[\frac{1}{r} - \lambda + \frac{\lambda^2}{2!} r - \frac{\lambda^3}{3!} r^2 + \dots \right] \delta r$$

$$= \left[\log a - \lambda r + \frac{\lambda^2 r^2}{2, 2!} - \frac{\lambda^3}{3!} \frac{r^3}{3} + \dots \right]_1^a$$

$$= \log a - \lambda (a - 1) + \frac{\lambda^2}{2, 2!} (a^2 - 1) - \dots$$

Now $\lambda = 6 \times 10^{-5}$ (cm.)$^{-1}$ (9); so λr is of the order 10^{-3}, and powers higher than the first can be neglected.

$\therefore$ P $= \log a - \lambda (a-1)$,

Hence R $= 2\pi I_o [\log a - \lambda (a-1)] + \pi I_o$.

Taking now, as the case of a typical radium treatment for cancer of the breast, a set of applicators grouped over a circle of 3 cm. radius, totalling 200 mgr., and left on for thirty hours, screened by 2 mm. of lead. In this case the "dose" is 6,000 milligram-hours.

Measure a and b in units of 3 cm.

then $b = 1$, $a = 10$,

λ in this case = about 1.8×10^{-4} (cm.)$^{-1}$

$I_o = 200$,

$\therefore$ R $= 2\pi \, 200 \left(\log_e 10 - 9 \times 1.8 \times 10^{-4} \right) + 200\pi$,

$= \pi \, 200 \, (4.6050 - 0.0032 + 1)$.

$= 3413.5$.

$\therefore$ = Total radiation is measurable as 102400.

The area exposed by a class B worker, assuming the body cylindrical as before, of the same radius, and 20 cm. thick, is 3,000 sq. cm. From the results given above a total radiation measurable as 1,413·72 would be received per day. In other words class B workers receive daily about 1·4 per cent. of the total radiation received by a patient during a course of treatment for carcinoma. It follows, therefore, that every ten weeks a class B worker receives the same quantity of radiation as a patient undergoing treatment for cancer of the breast. It is clear, however, that whereas in the case of the patient the radiation is concentrated over a small area, in the case of the class B worker the radiation is spread over the whole body surface.

REFERENCES.

1. TAYLOR. *Journ. Exper. Med.*, 1919, xxix, p. 1.
2. AUBERTIN. *Comptes-rend. Soc. de Biol.*, 1912, p. 84.
3. AUBERTIN and BEAUJARD. *Arch. d. Méd. exp. et d'Anat. path.*, 1908, xx, p. 273.
4. MOTTRAM and RUSS. *Proc. Roy. Soc.*, 1917, B, xc, pp. 1-38.
5. RUSS, CHAMBERS, SCOTT and MOTTRAM. *Lancet*, 1919, i, p. 692.
6. TAYLOR, WITHERBEE and MURPHY. *Journ. Exper. Med.*, 1919, xxix, p. 53.
7. RUSS. *Arch. Radio-Electrotherapy*, 1918-19, xxiii, p. 226.
8. MOTTRAM and RUSS. *Pro. Roy. Soc. Med*, 1917, x, (Sect. Electr.-Therap.), pp. 121-135.
9. RUTHERFORD, E. " Radio-active Substances," 1913, p. 266.

REPORT ON A METHOD OF FLUOROSCOPIC EXAMINATION WITH THE ARMY BEDSIDE UNIT.

By Capt. FRANCIS F. BORZELL, A.E.F.

(Authorised for publication by the Surgeon-General's Office in Washington, D.C., U.S.A)

THERE has been, perhaps, no one phase of war radiology which has attained such a field of usefulness as has bedside radiology, with the possible exception of localizations of foreign bodies. Even the refinement and simplification of localization and removal of foreign bodies, as developed by war necessities, has to a great extent fulfilled its usefulness when the war has ended, but the development of bedside examination has opened a vast field for radiology, hitherto a closed book. It is largely as an expression of appreciation of the value of the Army bedside unit that I am presenting this report.

During the last three months, which represents the actual time this hospital has been doing active service, we have examined a few more than 150 cases at the bedside.

The examinations have been radiographic, with and without the intensifying screen and fluoroscopic, for fractures, foreign bodies, and pulmonary conditions of those patients who could not be transported to the laboratory. One is often called upon to exercise every bit of ingenuity he possesses to secure two views to determine position. Stereoscopic studies have assisted many a time. With the aid of Bowen plate holders, and by marking the horizontal sliding bar on the tube carriage, the required shift can readily be made.

Radioscopic studies with the Dessane bonnet fluoroscope, have been made for fracture position, foreign bodies, and pulmonary conditions.

I have found one method of examination for pulmonary conditions very valuable. We have had a number of patients who required radiologic studies to determine the presence of fluid, empyema, hæmothorax, bronchopneumonia, lobar pneumonia, pericardial effusions, pulmonary abscess, subphrenic abscess, or foreign bodies. Many of these patients were too sick to be moved or even turned upon their side, or else by reason of being splinted and slung in Balkan frames, and other fearfully and wonderfully contrived devices, could not be moved.

By the use of four stilts, which, when placed under the legs of the bed, raise the bed twelve inches, I can drop the tube beneath the bed, and fluoroscoping through the mattress secure very satisfactory information.

The bed springs of the regulation bed do not interfere materially with the study, due to the fact that being some distance from the screen, and a greater distance from the screen than the tissues to be examined, the mesh shadow is very much exaggerated and but few of the lines of the spring intercept vision. I found the average ward bed spring cast a shadow which placed the spring shadows twenty cm. apart on the screen. In the case of a search for foreign bodies a slight shift of the tube will shift the shadows of the spring.

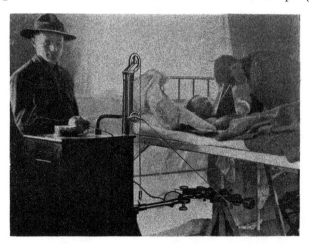

By this method the patient is not at all disturbed, nor is the position of the fractured limb disturbed. Where the Balkan frame is being used, the frame which is lashed to the bed is lifted with the bed and rests with the legs of the bed on the stilts.

Our hospital being of the barrack type, it is necessary to carry the bedside unit from ward to ward. This is readily accomplished by suspending the unit by the handles on a litter made of timbers of sufficient strength and fastened together by two cross pieces. The one we use was made in a few minutes by one of my men. It consists of two timbers, two inches by three inches, five feet long, and set sixteen inches apart, being held together by two cross pieces thirty inches apart.

Conclusion : A bedside examination by this method affords :—

    1. Easy access to entire torso and limbs, fluoroscopically.

    2. Patients can be examined who would otherwise not be available.

    3. No risk to very sick pulmonary cases.

TWO SKIAGRAMS.

Taken by FLORENCE A. STONEY, O.B.E., M.D., B.S.

Case 1.

THE skiagram shows a watch lying in the œsophagus, in the episternal notch. The patient was a lunatic, aged 38, who lost his watch on 23rd November, 1916, 40 hours before the X-ray examination revealed its position.

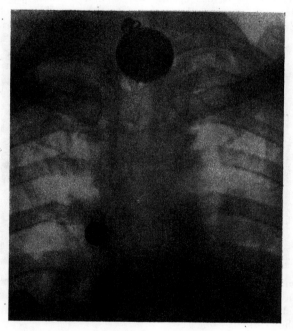

In the interval he had swallowed bread and milk and bread and butter; he made no complaint of his throat, but was much worried at the loss of his watch, continually hunting for it everywhere, and he bothered his attendants so much about it that the orderlies, half in fun, brought him to the X-ray room for examination.

The position of the watch having been disclosed, chloroform was given on the X-ray table, and the watch easily removed by Major J. R. Lee, who passed a long pair of curved forceps through the mouth, and down the throat till they were seen by X rays to have hold of the ring, when forceps and watch were withdrawn.

By this means the foreign body was quickly and easily removed, and without any risk of breaking the glass ; chloroform anæsthesia lasted three minutes. Would it not have taken longer to find and extract the watch with an œsophagoscope, but without X rays during the operation ? (*Cf.* Irwin Moore in *Lancet*, pp. 566 and 609.)

Case 2.

A well built soldier, aged 42, came into hospital December, 1917, with chronic asthma, and also an abscess in his neck of one week's duration.

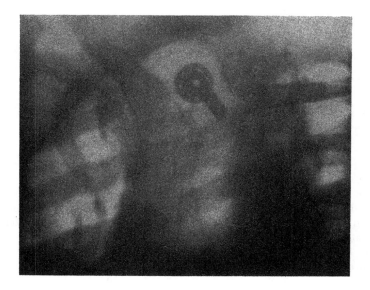

In April, 1915, he had had a slight wound opposite the right thyroid cartilage, which had healed quickly but left him with cough and shortness of breath ever since.

February, 1917, he had been buried.

December, 1917, at Fulham Military Hospital, he complained of rheumatism and asthma, he spoke hoarsely, his neck showed firm swelling below the cricoid, with a small sloughy brawny opening to the right and below the larynx.

X-ray examination revealed no missile of war, but the surprising fact that a tracheotomy tube was present, which by stereoscopic localisation was shown to be a child's size and situated low down in the trachea.

He did not remember ever having had an operation ; but enquiry of his mother elicited the fact that he had suffered from " bronchitic croup " when two years of age, at which time he was dangerously ill and nearly died; he had been nursed at home by his father and mother.

On December 18th, 1917, Mr. Nourse and Major J. R. Lee in operating found the superficial abscess was in the tissues surrounding the trachea, which were much thickened by chronic inflammation. They removed from the trachea a child's tracheotomy tube—a double tube, No. 6, of antique pattern, with no tapes attached. This had been inserted in 1877, the wound had closed over, and it had remained 40 years in the trachea.

He rapidly healed up, and his asthma and hoarseness disappeared within a fortnight.

This is the latest cure for asthma !

A CASE OF TUBERCULOSIS OF THE STOMACH AND ITS SURROUNDINGS.

By the late Dr. H. C. Geuken, Apeldoorn (Netherlands)

The fact that we so seldom meet with radiograms of stomach tuberculose in periodicals induced me to publish the following case.

Both the accompanying radiograms have been taken from a thirty-five years old patient, suffering from several nervous complaints, who a short time ago had suffered from pleurisy, but whose lungs on percussion and auscultation did not show any signs of tuberculose.

Fig. 1 has been taken about ten minutes after a subcutaneous injection of 1 mgm. atropine. The two halves, in which this stomach is divided, are united by a long, narrow tube running in vertical direction and both are filled with bismuth-meal up to about the same level. They both show an air bubble and an intermedial layer ; the upper bubble seems to extend into the œsophagus, the figure of the upper projecture of the air bubble is crossed by the line of the diaphragm. The distinctly visible duodenum shows also a bismuth-accumulation with liquid level.

Fig. 2 has been taken one hour later, and gives a somewhat different image of the communication between the upper and the lower half of the stomach.

Six hours later the stomach was empty. During the operation it appeared that a hard string of tuberculous tissue was compressing the stomach in several places, whilst in the fore-wall of the stomach were to be found tuberculous hearths. Four years afterwards the patient died of general tuberculose.

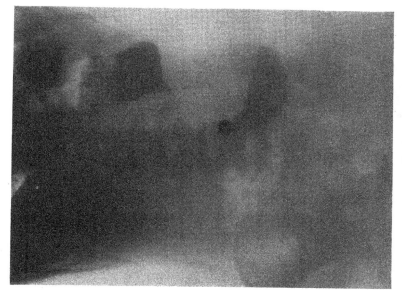

FIG. 2.

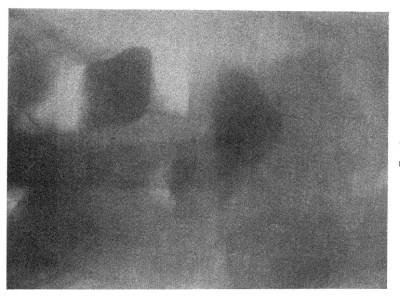

FIG. 1.

A NEW STANDARD CHART FOR RECORDING TRACING OF OPAQUE MEALS.

By C. P. G. WAKELEY

Surgical Registrar and Tutor, King's College Hospital ; late Demonstrator of Anatomy, King's College. London.

THIS figure represents the pelvis, lower part of the vertebral column, and last three ribs of a woman 50 years of age. The soft parts were removed by

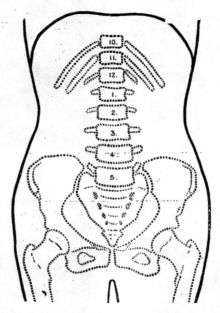

dissection from in front, and a drawing made with the tracing telescope, provided with cross wires, of a pantograph. This drawing was afterwards photographed, and the present drawing was subsequently accurately copied from this. It has the advantage that it is anatomically correct, and by having the last three ribs in position the outline of the kidneys can be shown, or the position of a renal calculus.

By including the upper ends of the femora, fractures of these bones can be demonstrated on the chart.

NOTES OF SOME RECENT CASES OF ELECTROTHERAPY.

By Samuel Sloan, M.D., Glasgow.

Ex-President Electrotherapeutic Section of the Royal Society of Medicine and of the Section of Radiology and Electrology, British Medical Association, etc.

The success of electrotherapeutics during the war has been great, and much experience has been gained in this department of therapeutics. It may therefore seem strange that comparatively little literature on the subject is appearing in the medical journals at the present time. The reason for this is not at once obvious. A possible explanation may be found in the fact that radiology has become so highly specialised that those who engage in it must devote practically all their energies to its pursuit, and they are not doing so in association with ordinary medical practice, but are employing it as valuable aids to the physician or the surgeon in his endeavours to form a correct diagnosis of cases of obscurity. The radiologist is thus thrown out of sympathy and interest in ordinary medical practice. Again, radiology is more of an art than a science, whereas electrotherapy is more of a science than an art. Now technique in any art is more easily acquired in youth, whilst much time is necessary for experience in diagnosis and in ordinary treatment ; knowledge of which is essential to the successful pursuit of electrotherapy. Radiology is, therefore, naturally attractive to the young, whilst those who have had the necessary medical experience to equip them for the practice of electrotherapy are prone to be too conservative to care to take up new methods of treatment. The time necessary is also in their case a drawback. But, if the electro-therapeutist is also a man of wide experience in general medicine, he is more likely to be a successful therapeutist, for he has both general and special knowledge. This will be greatly to the advantage of his patients. He will have more successes and fewer failures in his practice. In his case, however, the special knowledge will be, not the foundation of his skill in the art of healing, but its crown, as the late Dr. Lewis Jones once said.

That there is a large field for electrotherapy when combined with this experience of general therapeutics I am convinced, and an attempt to show how useful this special branch of therapeutics is, alone or in combination with other methods, may not be out of place at the present time. With this object in view I wish to put on record notes of a few of my recent cases ; which, while intractable by ordinary methods of treatment, have in my hands yielded to electrotherapy, alone or in combination with ordinary therapeutic measures. The examples I shall record are more of an illustrative than an exceptional character, and they may prove interesting and encouraging.

Muco-colitis.—It is well known how obstinate and almost incurable cases of this affection may be, but experience has taught me that they may yield to treatment, part of which is electrotherapeutical, when all the ordinary measures have failed. The following is an illustrative case, and, although the result is not all that could be desired, it is yet an encouraging instance of the beneficial influence of the combination of methods I am advocating:—

R. M., male, railway clerk, aged 28, came to me in October, 1919. Since his school days he had had " bilious attacks," generally once a week, consisting of severe abdominal pain, sickness and vomiting of " undigested food and bile " ; was in Edinburgh Royal Infirmary 14 years ago for three weeks for "inflammation of the stomach "; had slightly better health for two months after ; but since then has been much the same as he was before entering the infirmary ; has had chronic diarrhœa since a residence in South Africa from 1911 till 1914. The motions are offensive, contain mucus, sometimes blood, and average two per day; and he has been steadily losing flesh. There is no special abdominal tenderness or local sense of resistance, and no epigastric splashing ; the urine is normal and there are no abnormal eye symptoms. No X-ray abdominal examination was deemed to be necessary, the case being considered one of feeble gastro-intestinal muscular tone with muco-colitis.

He was ordered three dry meals a day, and daily enemata of a dessert spoonful each of Condy's fluid and bicarbonate of soda. Under this treatment the diarrhœa lessened, the motions became less offensive, and he was ordered a dessert spoonful of bynin amara three times a day. A few days later he had an attack of pain and sickness, followed by the discharge from the bowels of large masses of mucus in tape-like pieces of about nine inches long ; but this attack was less severe than previous ones, and the general health was improving. As the progress thereafter was slow he was advised to ask leave of absence from work for four weeks, so that he might obtain the necessary rest during a treatment of dorso-abdominal application of the *rapid* sinusoidal alternating current. After twelve such treatments, which occupied four weeks, he declared himself to be better in health than he had been for fourteen years ; though there were still small pieces of mucus appearing occasionally in the stools, which were otherwise normal. Report one month later: "Appetite good, no pain, still as well, enjoying life now."

The electric treatment was, as is my usual practice, applied by means of a large warm moist clay electrode placed between the shoulder blades, and another, larger one, of the same material, covering the whole of the abdomen. The dose was 7 ma., as measured on the faradimeter. At first the effect was, as I have generally found, a sensation of exhaustion, lasting for several hours, but this diminished in amount and in duration as the treatment progressed, finally giving place to a sensation of well-being, a feeling of having more grit, as he expressed it.*

The vomiting recurred once in this case somewhat severely after a day of special fatigue, beginning at 5.30 a.m., spending five hours on a "fish bank " in the open on a cold, dark, wet morning, and ending with a meeting, late at night, in a close, hot atmosphere. The vomiting was followed by a slight return of the diarrhœa, no mucus being observed.

* For an explanation of these symptoms and for details as to the effects of dorso-abdominal alternating currents in a series of 67 cases so treated, see " The Therapeutic Value of Alternating Currents Applied to the Abdominal Sympathetic Nervous System," by the writer, *The Lancet*, May 30th, 1903,

The patient having become anxious on account of this recurrence, an X-ray examination was kindly made by Dr. Riddell, whose report was as follows: "Tone poor, peristalsis feeble. There is some distortion of duodenum but no delay in emptying of stomach. Five hours after food most of the barium meal is in the cæcum. In this case I don't see that an operation is indicated."

Although this examination afforded little help it was satisfactory to have the diagnosis confirmed. Notwithstanding the recurrence, the patient now reports himself as feeling "splendid," the occasional attacks of sickness are comparatively trifling, and are unaccompanied with pain. Any mucus in the motions is slight and soft in consistence. Although not actually "cured" he is quite fit, he says, to start work at 5.30 in the cold winter mornings. He resumed work three months ago, and has not been one day off work since.

Alopecia.—Mrs. G., aged 40, was sent to me in February, 1919, for my opinion as to the probable effect of electrotherapy. It was a case of absolute alopecia. There was no trace of hair on any part of the body; the whole of the scalp was as devoid of hair as the palm of the hands, and so were the eyebrows, while there was not a single eyelash present. The condition had resisted all kinds of treatment for years. I said that I could not promise any improvement from any kind of electric treatment, but I was willing to try it.

The high-frequency vacuum electrode was applied to the whole of the scalp, to the eyebrows, and to the eyelids. This was followed at each sitting with the effleuve, till the skin was red and slightly tender. A course of twelve treatments was given, and as there was some desquamation, due to the irritation of the current, the patient was ordered to rub hazeline cream into the scalp daily, and to return after an interval of four weeks. At the end of this period there could not be said to be any improvement in the case. A second course of treatment was given, and, on the patient's return three months after, there were several patches of strong dark hairs in the temporal and occipital regions, the hairs being fairly long and the patches about half an inch each in diameter. There was also a crop of fine hairs covering both eyebrows, and on the left eye there were eyelashes over the outer half of the upper lid. All the rest of the scalp was hairless.

Another course of the same treatment was given, and at its close the whole of the scalp was covered with a close crop of fine hairs, the hair on the eyebrows was growing, and both eyes had a complete fringe of normal hairs on each eyelid.

Probable Laceration of the Brain.—Major H., aged 42, applied to me in February, 1919. He had received a gunshot wound in the head, fracturing the skull in the left post parietal region, early in 1917, and he had been afterwards trephined. Present condition: mental confusion, attacks of loss of memory, cerebration slow, slight ataxy, nystagmus, sluggish initial movement of the eyes, pain in back and front of right side of head, and especially in the right eye, knee reflexes greatly exaggerated with slight ankle clonus, blood pressure normal, urine normal.

Asked for an opinion as to treatment by the War Office, I advised rest amid pleasant surroundings and electrotherapeutic treatment three times a week over a period of two months. The treatment consisted of high-frequency applications—effleuve—to the head, occasional couch treatment (auto-condensation) and, when required for special tender spots on the scalp, the vacuum electrode. After two and a half months of such treatment—twenty visits in all—the condition was a general improvement all round, the only persisting complaint being occasional severe attacks of neuralgic headache. After an interval, a second course of treatment was given, after which the headaches soon disappeared. He spent the summer in the country, had a few applications during the autumn, and became so well that four months ago I advised him to resume the business he had followed before the war. The knee jerks had become normal, although there seemed a possible exaggeration in the left knee, and there was no ankle clonus. He has led an active business life since, and has remained "very well" without further treatment.

Locomotor Ataxy.—I have frequently observed that in incurable diseases, such as this, considerable improvement—almost an arrest of the signs and symptoms—may follow electrotherapeutic treatment. The following is an instance of such a case:—

Mr. A., age 54 years, came to see me in April, 1919. His case had been pronounced as advanced locomotor ataxy, and the pains and feeble unsteady gait had been increasing. I advised the stoppage of all drug treatment, and gave him effleuve applications to the spine—five minutes each to the cervical, dorsal, and lumbar regions. At first there was no sensation of the electric impulses. After the second application the legs "felt firmer," but the pain did not yield till the fourth sitting. He had in all twelve applications, during which time he passed through a period of great mental strain, due to a break up of the partnership in his business. Notwithstanding this, he declared himself at the close of the treatment to be greatly improved, said he had much less pain, was eating and sleeping better, and had "a better grip of the ground."

I have been much impressed during the past years with the great benefit to be derived from this form of electrotherapy, and have often wondered what was its mode of operation. I used to compare the effects of the faradic current to microscopic—cellular—massage. Is it not reasonable to conclude that the high-frequency currents employed as above may have an ultra-microscopic—an atomic—massage effect?

This patient remained as well as at the conclusion of the treatment for a period of nearly three months. He then, owing to excessive fatigue in attending to business, took a holiday of two weeks, after which he found himself able to continue at business for some months longer. He visited me again a few weeks ago, saying that he found the pain and difficulty of walking returning. I asked him if he was worse than he had been before the treatment I had given him nine months previously. His answer was, "I was led to understand, before I visited you, that I had about one year to live, whereas I am now very, very much better than I was then."

The result of the present treatment is much as it had previously been. The first impression was on the walking, the pain has begun to diminish, and normal sleep is returning.

Pre-Cancer of the Uterus.—A paper on this subject was read for Dr. F. J. McCann, at the meeting of the Obstetrical and Gynæcological Section of the Royal Society of Medicine, on 9th October last. Dr. McCann's contribution, and the discussion which followed, are both interesting and important; for they reveal a serious difference of opinion amongst gynæcologists as to the existence of a condition, not benign and not yet malignant, which may be found in the uterus.

Dr. McCann has perhaps exaggerated the possible malignancy of some apparently benign affections of the uterus before the menopause. This, however, is an error on the side of subsequent safety. The President of the Section, though he disagreed with Dr. McCann's views as to the gravity of morbid conditions of the uterus, even about the time of the menopause, yet admitted that "when a discharge or a hæmorrhage was present in patients after the menopause, without any apparent cause, hysterectomy was the proper treatment." Granted a pre-cancerous condition, the discussion mostly dealt with the question as to the kind of operation required. No suggestion as to the possibility of a substitute for amputation of the cervix or removal of the womb, in early cases of suspected malignant disease, was made. The following report is, I venture therefore to think, opportune as an illustration of such a condition, and of the treatment which I carried out for it with success. It may throw light on the subject and prove encouraging to those who may happen to come across such a case in the future.

Mrs. F. came to me in November, 1917, complaining of a "red fluid coming from the front passage," this condition having lasted for about two months. She was then 59 years of age, had had four children, and her last menstruation had been nine years previously. On examination I found a slight tear of the cervix, but no undue patency of the os or dilatation of the cervical canal. The anterior lip of the os was, however, red and swollen, compared with the posterior lip. I labelled the case at the time as a possible pre-cancerous condition of the cervix. My diagnosis was based on the clinical aspect and history, and I did not deem it safe or necessary to remove a section of the cervix for laboratory examination. Iodised phenol was freely applied to the parts. The patient returned in four weeks, when the anterior lip was less swollen, but a cotton covered probe gently passed into the cervix caused bleeding, whilst there were two red spots on the anterior lip which looked as if they would readily bleed. Saturated solution of chromic acid was applied to the spots and to the interior of the cervix. Two weeks later there was an ulcer the size of a pea on the right side of the cervix. Formaline was applied on two occasions, but, though there was some improvement, there was still a tendency to bleeding. Frequent applications were made of iodised phenol, and the exterior surface of the cervix became fairly healthy. The os, however, became more open, and the cervical canal more dilated, whilst its walls bled when the cavity was being cleansed. This was the condition six weeks after the patient's first visit to me.

Ionisation with copper was now employed. After seven applications the external surface of the cervix became absolutely normal, and the cavity was contracting. As a precaution the whole of the cavity of the uterus was afterwards treated with the copper. ion, the electrode having been passed three inches into the uterus. It should be noted that at the age of 59 the normal length of the uterine canal is little over two inches.

After two intra-uterine ionic applications the patient was sent home. Two months later my report is, "Os small and practically no bleeding when the cervical cavity is being cleansed." Six weeks later the record states: "Patient very well in every way, cervix externally and internally perfectly normal, no discharge whatever lying around or over the cervix ; only a plug of pure mucus covering the os." Three months later the report is : "No bleeding, no discharge, and no pain during the past three months." Occasional slight relapses occurred during the following six months, but a few antiseptic applications sufficed to keep the parts healthy. Shortly after this, however, there appeared on the anterior lip of the os four small ulcers, and the cervical cavity again bled when gently touched. Copper ionisation was again employed. After five applications the record says : "The ulcers have all disappeared." The cervix continued to be contracted, and the os was so small that the uterine sound could with difficulty be passed into the cervical canal.

The patient's next visit to me was two months ago. The ulceration had not returned, and the os and cervix were as previously noted, but there was some muco-pus around the cervix. It was not thought necessary to ask the patient to remain in town for a further course of ionisation. The last course had been four months previously. Since then there has been no return of ulceration or bleeding or other abnormal discharges, but at times the lips of the cervix become slightly swollen and small nodules appear. There had not, till the time of writing, seemed any need for ionisation, but occasional mild antiseptics have been applied and the parts are being cleansed about once a month.

This case must be set down as one either of cancer or of pre-cancer of the uterus. It is so easy to keep the disease in abeyance that I am inclined to call it the latter, although I strongly suspect that if the case were left to drift an acute malignancy would be the result. I intend, therefore, to ask the patient to report herself, at intervals of not less than two months. This case is exceptional in that, in my experience, a uterine diseased condition once cured by ionic medication practically never requires the treatment to be again resorted to.*

In this patient we have, then, an active pathological condition of the uterus at the age of 61, presumably, therefore, of a malignant nature, and yet

---

* For a list of the cases I have published, which were treated by ionic medication, together with details as to its principles and methods of administration, see "Electrotherapy in Gynæcology," Heinemann, London, 1917.

she is practically free from the disease fully two years after the onset of the malady, whilst her general health is perfect.

Paresis of left Arm and Leg.—Mr. W., aged 40, was sent to me in October last with a history of "shock," following fatigue and excitement during a local trade strike two months previously. He had never lost consciousness nor had any symptoms of aphasia, although the cause of the loss of power was evidently of cerebral origin. I found the left deltoid muscle and the left quadriceps extensor femoris markedly paretic; the rest of the arm and leg less so. His right hand grasp, as measured by the dynamometer, was 70—distinctly under normal for so robust looking a man. The left hand grasp showed distinct paresis of the muscles of the forearm, the dynamometer reading being only 35. The attack was too recent to show the reaction degeneration. As might have been expected, from the cause of the paralysis, there was exaggerated left knee reflex and also left ankle clonus. When walking the left foot came to the ground with a flop. I tried various forms of electric stimulation, placing a well moistened pad, with an area of about 24 square inches, over the interscapular region—the neutral electrode, the active electrode of the same size being placed over the deltoid muscle. To the terminal to which the latter electrode led there was attached a smaller pad for the hand. Thus, the greatest action would be on the deltoid muscle, a lesser degree of stimulation sufficing for the muscles of the forearm and hand. In the case of the leg the arrangement was similar, the neutral electrode being placed on the hypogastrium, and the active electrode on the anterior portion of the thigh and the sole of the foot. The aim was to obtain energetic contractions of the deltoid and the quadriceps extensor femoris, and moderate contractions of the muscles of the forearm and hand, and of the leg and foot where the paresis was less severe, whilst at the same time there should be as little burning or irritation of the skin as possible. The results were completely satisfactory when the *slow* alternating sinusoidal current, with rhythmic surgings, was applied, the quantity of current being, as registered by my faradimeter, $2\frac{1}{2}$ ma. The Leslie Miller clockwork interrupter was employed, the contractions occurring 50 times per minute, the intervals of relaxation occupying about the same time as the duration of the contractions, and the whole of the operations on the arm and leg occupying about one hour. The treatment was given on an average of three times a week, and it was always found that the best results were obtained when the current was of slow periodicity. Altogether eight treatments were given.

After three applications the dynamometer registered in the right hand 80, and in the left 50. After the seventh sitting the right hand grasp was 90, and the left was 70. Thus, while the general muscle tone, as measured by the normal arm, had gained 30 per cent., the paralysed arm had gained 100 per cent.

This patient was unable to remain in Glasgow for further treatment, and I advised him to resume the electric treatment he had been receiving from Dr. Sandison Crabbe, of Birmingham, under whose care he had previously been, and who had kindly referred him to me during his stay in Glasgow.

Trifacial Neuralgia (Tic Douloureux).—This affection is accompanied by so much anguish that it is probably responsible for more temptation to commit suicide than any other disease. Its intractable nature is also evidenced by the variety of drugs proposed for its relief, one of the consequences of which is frequently the formation of the drug habit.

I have treated three cases of tic douloureux which could, owing to their severity, be truly designated as malignant, and yet two of these have yielded to electric treatment and in an amazingly short time.

Case 1.—Mr. S., aged 54, residing in the South of Scotland, was referred to me by a London physician in January, 1916. There was no history of previous illnesses ; the pain was in the ophthalmic and superior maxillary branches of the fifth nerve on the right side, and it had lasted for seven years. It was at first spasmodic in character, but after treatment by hypodermic injections of alcohol, it became less severe though continuous and still desperate, whilst the area supplied by the affected nerves had lost its sensibility to touch. He declared that he would refuse to continue alive if it were not for his wife and children. He had been treated at Duff House for "intestinal stasis," but, although the bowels became more regular, there was no improvement in the face pain. He had also received six applications of the salicylic ion in London, but with no effect.

This patient was treated by me with every form of electric energy I could think of—vacuum electrode, effleuve and mono-polar high-frequency applications, ionisation with cocaine, quinine, and chlorine, and with the rapid sinusoidal alternating currents, which were applied over the face and the abdomen.

Each new form of electrotherapy had some beneficial influence, but the sinusoidal alternating currents in 5 ma. doses, as measured by the faradimeter, seemed to be most helpful. On the whole a fair amount of relief was obtained, so much so indeed that he proposed to take a house in Glasgow and continue similar treatment for as long as might be required. This was his condition when he received a great shock in the sudden death of his wife, to whom he was greatly attached. The result was a recrudescence of the pain, so severe that he went to London and had the gasserian ganglion removed, with what result I have not been informed.

Case 2.—Mrs. M., aged 49, was sent to me in February, 1918, after her physician had decided that if electricity could not help her she must just consider her case incurable. Since the pain was most intense in the ophthalmic branch of the nerve, I advised her medical attendant to send her to an oculist before visiting me.

His treatment having failed to relieve her she begged me to try the effect of electric treatment. With the recollection of almost complete failure in my previous case, I told her that I could not promise relief, whilst I was far from sanguine in being able to cure her. She replied, "All I want is that you will do your best for me, and I shall be most grateful to you if you will take my case in hand."

I at once began with the vacuum electrode from the eighth ring of the high-frequency solenoid, regulating the force of the current by my fingers on the extremity of the cylindrical tube, so as to make the application pleasant, or at least in no degree irritating.

The first application resulted in a diminution of the pain. After the second application the tic pain almost, and finally after six weeks entirely, disappeared.

The drug treatment consisted of iron, arsenic and strychnia ; whilst a dose of five grains of quinine and thirty of bromide of ammonium at bed time, with the application of the vacuum electrode to the scalp, entirely removed a neuralgic pain in the head which had lasted for nearly thirty years.

She remained for a year after the close of the treatment absolutely free from pain, but a slight threatening of pain, then, brought her to me in dread of its return. Her complaint was of "a tingling sensation, as if the pain were not far off." A few similar applications of the vacuum electrode sufficed to free her of this sensation. The pain again threatened three months later, July, 1919, but this time there was decided pain, and as I was then just leaving for a holiday I could give her only a few treatments. On September 2nd the treatment was resumed, but it required six applications to remove the pain. There has been no pain since.

Case 3.—Mrs. C., aged 65, was sent to me in December, 1918, by a relative of the previous patient. This was certainly the severest form of the disease I had met with. The right side of the face was affected, especially in the ophthalmic branch of the nerve, and the pain had lasted for six years. It had been impossible to leave the house, except for a few weeks during the height of the summer season. She could not enter a room unless it had been previously heated, and for weeks at a time she was unable to touch the affected place with water ; whilst, if a hair happened to rest on the cheek, the thought of having to remove it and thus start a spasm of pain was almost more, she said, than she could bear.

A powder of two grains of quiniae and ten grains salicylate of soda was prescribed twice daily, and the vacuum electrode treatment was commenced.

Improvement began at once. After the second application the patient declared that she had not had "so beautiful a night for months and months." I had the greatest difficulty in persuading her to stop the treatment, so great was her dread of the return of the pain.

Six months after the close of the treatment, owing to a slight amount of pain in the mouth and above the right eye, she came to me because of her fear of the return of the old pain. A few treatments were given and the pain passed off. Experimentally I now prescribed thyroid extract, a grain and a half daily, as a possible prophylactic.

Latest report : " Never was better in my life, nor happier."

What, it may be asked, is the explanation of the success of Cases 2 and 3 and the comparative failure of Case 1 ? Is it because in the latter the origin of the disease was central, whereas in the former it was peripheral, or had the hypodermic injections of alcohol anything to do with rendering the electrical application ineffectual ?

A CLINICAL METHOD OF DOSAGE OF ULTRA-VIOLET RAYS.

Unit of Quantity: Chromo-actinometer.

By H. Bordier, Professeur agrégé a la Faculté de Médicine de Lyon.

In the therapeutic application of ultra-violet rays there has been lacking a measure of quantity. Since the bio-chemical reactions depend on the dose absorbed by the tissues this measure is indispensable for obtaining the desired therapeutic results.

I have sought to fill up this gap by establishing a method akin to that which serves to control the dosage of X rays (1), and by creating a unit of quantity based on weights. The latter was necessary to give a numerical equivalent for the quantities of ultra-violet rays capable of producing the colour change in a special reagent when irradiated at the same time and in the same manner as the tissues.

Unit of Quantity.—To establish a unit of quantity I used the property possessed by ultra-violet rays of reducing salts of silver, and I chose the deci-normal solution of the chemical laboratories. It was probable that one could define a unit of quantity of rays by determining the weight of silver reduced, the rays acting along the line of normal incidence on unit area (square cm.) and on unit thickness (cm.) of the standard solution.

I began, by preliminary experiments, to find out the order of weight of silver reduced ; in one I irradiated, for a period of one minute, the standard solution, which was so arranged as to have a thickness of 1 cm. The weight of silver reduced was found to be 1·03 mg. per square cm. (All the silver measurements were, made by Dr. Phillippe, Head of the Laboratory of the Faculty of Medicine.)

After a series of experiments and dosages with varying intensities of current in the lamp, and varying exposures, and with estimation of the bio-chemical effects produced, I saw that the unit of quantity could be defined as follows : The quantity of ultra-violet rays which, acting normally on a deci-normal solution of silver nitrate of 1 cm. thickness, can reduce 1 mg. of silver per square cm.

Chromo - Actinometer.—Having got this unit, it only remained to find a medium with the property of changing colour under the influence of ultra-violet rays, and to translate into units of quantity the different tints acquired by the reagent corresponding to the determined bio-chemical effects.

After many trials (paper impregnated with citrate, santonin, cryogenin), I settled on the choice of a 20 per cent. solution of potassium ferrocyanide (2). On exposing to ultra-violet rays a strip of thick bibulous paper carrying this solution, the colour passes from the initial white to deeper and deeper yellow, through all the intermediate stages of the cream and sulphur shades. I could thus try the changes of tint of the indicator under the influence of different doses of rays reckoned in units of quantity, and could, at the same time, note the cutaneous reactions to these different doses. My chromo-actinometer (3) consists of five tints, which are those taken by the reacting strip, and correspond to the following doses :—

| ·5 unit. | 2 units. | 6 units. | 12 units. | 18 units of quantity. |

The skin effects of each of these doses measured by the chromo-actinometer are as follows :—

$\frac{1}{2}$ unit	.	.	.	Slight erythema.
2 units	.	.	.	Erythema, followed by desquamation.
6 ,,	.	.	.	Photo-epidermatitis.
12 ,,	.	.	.	Intense photo-epidermatitis.
18 ,,	.	.	.	Photo-dermatitis.

These different reactions are utilised for the treatment of several affections, particularly certain dermatoses.

To use the chromo-actinometer in ultra-violet radiotherapy it is sufficient to place a sensitive strip on the same plane as the irradiated tissue, and to carry on the treatment until the strip has assumed the colour of the scale which corresponds to the number of units, and therefore to the bio-chemical effect that is desired. The comparison of the tints should be made in day-light and not in artificial light.

This method of dosage has enabled me to study how the quantity of rays emitted varies with the intensity of current in the lamp in a given time ; this is of great importance in ultra-violet radiotherapy.

Intensity.				*Quantity emitted.*
6·5 amps.	.	.	.	1 unit.
6 ,,	.	.	.	·8 ,,
5 ,,	.	.	.	·5 ,,
4 ,,	.	.	.	·3 ,,

These wide variations in the quantity of rays emitted must obviously lead to gross errors in ultra-violet therapy unless there is measurement of the radiation from the source.

I have also been able to show the influence of the age of the mercury vapour lamp. In working with three lamps of similar character, but of greater or shorter periods of use, I found very different figures for the output. For the same length of irradiation :—

New lamp	.	.	.	.	3 units.
Used lamp	.	.	.	.	1 unit.
Much used lamp	.	.	.	·5 unit.

These results demonstrate clearly the usefulness of dosage in ultra-violet therapy. It may also be hoped that the method of measuring the quantities of rays, and the unit that I have succeeded in establishing, will be an effective help in raising ultra-violet therapy from the condition of empiricism in which it has hitherto lain.

(1) Bordier. "Nouveau Chromoradiomètre." *Arch. d'Elect. Méd.*, 1911, p. 71.

(2) *Arch. d'Elect. Méd.*, 1908, p. 556.

(3) Obtainable from Westinghouse Cooper Hewitt Co., Ltd., 11, Rue du Pont, Suresnes, Seine.

REPORT OF SOCIETY.

SOCIÉTÉ DE RADIOLOGIE MÉDI-CALE DE FRANCE.
Séance du 10 Février, 1920.

La radiothérapie des fibro-myomes utérins et sa technique, par le Dr. A. BÉCLÈRE.—L'A expose que cette technique soumise aux règles générales de la radiothérapie profonde, est en outre subordonnée à l'opinion adoptée sur le mode d'action du traitement. D'après la théorie allemande, il s'agit d'une castration sèche avec regression consécutive des myomes, les ovaires sont la cible unique sur laquelle doivent converger de toutes parts les irradiations, une technique uniforme convient à tous les malades. Au contraire, d'après l'opinion française à l'appui de laquelle M. Béclère a apporté récemment des preuves irréfutables, l'action de la radiothérapie s'exerce simultanément sur les myomes et sur les ovaires, mais se manifeste tout d'abord sur les premiers dont la régression précède de loin la suppression des règles ; elle s'applique aux femmes de tout âge, aux tumeurs de toutes dimensions, avec ou sans exagération des ménorrhagies ; c'est un département de la radiothérapie des néoplasmes et la technique, variable avec le siège et les dimensions des myomes, doit s'adapter aux exigences de chaque cas. M. Béclère fait ressorter tous les avantages de la méthode des doses modérées à intervalles rapprochés, d'une à deux semaines au maximum.

Mécanisme de certaines déformations non lésionnelles de l'estomac ; la distension de l'arrière-fond tubérositaire, par le Dr. BARRET.—Il étudie le mécanisme de certaines biloculations gastriques qui doivent être considérées, sauf exceptions rares, comme purement fonctionelles. L'examen de profil montre en pareil cas que la poche supérieure, située tout-à-fait en arrière, est constituée par une dépression en cuvette de la paroi au niveau de l'arrière-fond de la grosse tubérosité. La formation de cette poche est déterminée essentiellement par la faiblesse de la tunique musculeuse dans cette région ; la dépression se produit dans la zone de moindre résistance lors que la tension intragastrique augmento suffisament ; le seuil qui sépare les deux poches se trouve à la limite de cette zône et répond au renforcement de la tunique musculeuse au niveau du corps de l'estomac.

Modification du porte-ampoule de Drault, par le Dr. BARRET.—L'A présente un pied porte-ampoule Drault dont il a fait modifier l'anneau porte cupule ; la mise en place de l'ampoule se trouve grandement facilitée par cette modification, en particulier dans les applications radiothérapiques.

Présentation d'un chassis radioscopique pour examen vertical, par les M. M. MALAQUIN et DUTERTRE.—M. Dutertre présente un chassis vertical d'examen radioscopique entièrement métallique, à mouvements doux sur galets, et muni d'une plate-forme permettant l'examen du malade sous différents angles mesurables.

Le Secrétaire Général: Dr. HARET.

REVIEW.

Constipation and Allied Intestinal Disorders. By Dr. ARTHUR HURST. London: Oxford University Press. 16s. net.

This book is an exhaustive survey of the important subject of constipation, and its careful study will well repay every practitioner. It is well and clearly written, and full of information; indeed, it may be said that it is so full of information as to be somewhat heavy reading.

The section on the physiology of the intestinal movements is particularly interesting, as is also the section on the constipation of infants, and many valuable hints on treatment may be gained by the practitioner.

The book is characterised by the number and excellence of the diagrams, but it is remarkable that no radiograms are reproduced, and that Dr. Hurst apparently relies entirely on screening in bismuth work. The majority of radiologists will certainly not agree with Dr. Hurst in his statement that "it is quite unnecessary to photograph the shadows.

Examination with the fluorescent screen gives much more information than is obtainable from skiagrams, and the outline of the colon can be traced on a piece of lead glass placed over the screen, from which it can subsequently be copied. . . . Skiagrams produce so much distortion that they are quite useless if measurements are required."

With modern apparatus and proper technique there need be no distortion, and skiagrams have the advantage that their record is independent of the individuality of the observer.

Further, when exact measurements are required, stereoscopic radiograms will give all necessary information with accuracy, including the relative position and depth of the parts. The value of stereoscopic radiograms in gastro-intestinal work is well shown in Dr. J. T. Case's "Atlas of Stereo-Roentgenography of the Alimentary Tract."

The book is well produced, on good paper, with excellent prints and illustrations. The Table of Contents is particularly valuable.

NOTES AND ABSTRACTS

Apparatus Used in Radium Therapy.—A. LABORDE (*Jour. de Radiol. et d'Elect.* March, 1919, pp. 153-163).—In an extensive paper, the author deals with the absorption of the alpha, beta, and gamma rays, the secondary rays given off and the scattering of the rays. He describes the different preparations and apparatus used, the units of activity and how it is measured. Lastly he deals with the recording of the exact conditions of dosage.   R. W. A. S.

On the Importance of De-ionization in the Treatment of Plumbism in Queensland Children.—J. L. GIBSON (*Med. Jour. of Austral.*, April 5th, 1919, pp. 272-274).—The author describes the good results he has obtained with this method of treatment, which consists essentially of foot and hand baths and a galvanic current passed through the body from hands to feet.

On analysis, the negative pole will be found to have lead deposited on it after treatment of such cases.   R. W. A. S.

Geometrical Proof of Sweet's Method of Localizing Foreign Body in the Eye.—(*Med. Jour. of Austral.*, March 8th, 1919, pp. 191, 192).—T. D. SAWKINS shows by means of figures and mathematics the theory of this method of localisation.   R. W. A. S.

Mechanics of the Stomach after Gastro-Enterostomy.—J. T. MURPHY (*Amer. Jour. of Roent.*, March, 1919, pp. 148-150).—From radiological observations upon 25 cases, in which gastro-enterostomy had been performed for ulcer of the stomach or duodenum, Murphy comes to the following conclusions:—

Patients having gastro-enterostomy operations properly performed are uniformly well. A patent pylorus does not interfere with the function of a properly placed gastro-enterostomy opening. The opening must be of sufficient size, placed at the lowest point, and almost directly below the lesser curvature of the stomach. Openings so made remain open permanently.

It is not a necessity but a good surgical procedure to occlude the pylorus, causing the stomach to empty, at least temporarily, by the gastro-enterostomy opening. Gastro-enterostomy is a drainage operation.

Regurgitation of food into the stomach does not seem to make any difference in the results of the operation. Ulcer diet should be used after operation. Liquid food, by preference cool liquids, leave the stomach with the least peristalsis. All gastro-enterostomy patients should eat frequently and a less quantity of food at each meal.   R. W. A. S.

Direct Action of X Rays on Transplantable Cancers of Mice.—E. HILL, J. J. MORTON, and W. D. WITHERBEE (*Jour. of Exper. Med.*, Jan., 1919, pp. 89-96).—The present tendency of workers on X-ray therapy of cancer is to devise methods of increasing the amount of X rays delivered at the seat of the cancer process. From the findings of these observers there is one point which should be taken into consideration; that is, whether or not one is justified in using a procedure which apparently only inhibits the cancer temporarily, while it incidentally lowers the resistance of the individual to the growth. It is well recognised that a proportion of cancers held in check for a time by X-ray treatment will later grow more rapidly. Blood counts on a number of these individuals have been made, and they all showed remarkably low lymphoid counts. These observers feel justified in suggesting that powerful doses of X rays which are only capable of inhibiting cancer growth for a time may bring about eventually a

lowered resistance to a return of the disease process.

Their experiments indicate that the direct action of X rays in more powerful doses than can be applied therapeutically is somewhat injurious to tumour cells, but by no means destroys them. The cancer cells appear to establish a resistance to X rays after repeated doses. This harmonises with the experience of clinicians who have succeeded in checking cancerous growths for some time but reach a point where no response can be effected by repeated doses. Rays of low penetration are apparently more harmful to tumour cells than penetrating rays.   R. W. A. S.

Effect of Exposure to the Sun on the Circulating Lymphocytes in Man.—H. D. TAYLOR (*Jour. of Exper. Med.*, Jan., 1919, pp. 41-52).—Chronic solar dermatitis was accompanied, in 25 of the 38 individuals studied, by an appreciable increase, percentage and absolute, in the number of circulating lymphocytes. Of the 13 with no increase in blood lymphocytes, 6 failed to tan, 3 were so dark originally that to determine an increase was impossible, and 5 had an extremely high lymphocyte count from the first.

Because of the parallelism between the tanning and the blood changes it seems probable that the lymphocytosis observed in the majority of instances, which is similar to the response of the blood of animals to small doses of X rays, is due to the effects of the ultraviolet rays contained in the solar spectrum, though it is impossible to rule out the effect of the infra-red or heat waves in these observations.   R. W. A. S.

Stimulative Action of X Rays on the Lymphocytes.—M. M. THOMAS, H. D. TAYLOR, and W. D. WITHERBEE (*Jour. of Exper. Med.*, Jan., 1919, pp. 75-82).—This study consists of blood counts on 9 rabbits after an exposure of 20 minutes, spark gap $\frac{1}{4}$ in., milliamperage 25, distance from the target 8 in. In 7 of the 9 animals there resulted an increase of the circulating lymphocytes, in 5 the increase was marked, and in 2 definite but not striking. A higher penetrating dose (6 in. spark gap, milliamperage 5) given to two animals produced no appreciable stimulation. This suggests that the effect on the lymphoid organs is not the result of a direct action of the rays, but is secondary to changes brought about either in the circulating blood or in the superficial tissues. The amount of X rays penetrating to the deeper structures with the former dose must be infinitesimal. Another question arises as to the nature of the energy generated by the tube worked on such a small spark gap. This point has not yet been taken up, but it is conceivable that other factors than pure X rays may play a part. R. W. A. S.

Experimental Studies with Small Doses of X Rays.—S. Russ, H. Chambers, G. M. Scott, and J. C. Mottram (*Lancet*, 26th April, 1919, pp. 692-695, with 5 Figs.).—In a series of experiments upon rats, in which the time of exposure varied from two seconds to thirty minutes, these observers found that one hour after the exposure the number of circulating lymphocytes was reduced to about 50 per cent. of the initial count. It was also found that the time elapsing before they return to the normal number is longer the more prolonged is the X-ray exposure. From the results of many experiments it has been concluded that the action is a direct one of the X rays upon the lymphocytes in the circulation.

If a small dose (12 seconds) be repeated a fortnight later a similar drop in the lymphocyte count occurs, the recovery is slightly delayed, but the number of lymphocytes finally reached is generally greater than at the beginning. Repeated applications of such a small dose may result in a high degree of lymphocytosis.

In determining the part played by the lymphocytes in resisting the growth of rat sarcoma, these observers believe that some factor other than mere numbers of lymphocytes in the circulation has to be recognised as playing an essential part in the immune process.

It has been shown that X rays administered to an animal have two actions, apart from their direct effect upon a tumour : (*a*) a large dose by destroying the immune condition will favour the growth of a tumour ; (*b*) a small dose by producing the immune condition will help to control, and may overcome the growth of a tumour.

The bearing of the facts upon the radiological treatment of malignant disease in man appears to these observers to be as follows : Whenever a tumour is exposed to X rays the lymphocytes circulating in the blood vessels of the growth and surrounding tissues will be irradiated, or if the site of operation be treated the lymphocytes in the normal vessels and tissues will be similarly exposed. The radiologist may thus be giving the primary growth the dose of radiation required for its disappearance, but, at the same time, he may be indirectly encouraging the development of secondary growths by lowering the natural powers of resistance of the patient, especially if this comparatively large dose is repeated at fortnightly intervals, as in post-operative treatment.

All possible precautions, therefore, should be taken to prevent the destruction of such cells as the lymphocytes, which, there is good reason to believe, play a defensive *rôle* in many varieties of malignant growth.

As regards the possibility of using X rays to increase the natural powers of resistance against cancer, up to the present it is only resistance against cancer inoculation that has been increased. There is, nevertheless, a distinct analogy between a graft introduced experimentally and a lodgment of cancer cells at a distance from a primary focus. By the use of small doses of X rays, repeated at intervals it may be that the resistance against the development of secondary deposits can be increased in a similar way to that which occurs in the case of an experimental inoculation. R. W. A. S.

Some Effects of Roentgen Rays on Certain Bacteria.—M. W. Perry (*Amer. Jour. of Roent.*, Sept., 1919, pp. 464-466). — As a result of experiments, this author finds that X rays in human dosage do not prevent the development of B. typhosus and staphylococcus aureus on inert media. In twice the human dosage they do not kill cultures of the same.

In human dosage they do not prevent the development of experimental glandular tuberculosis, neither do they destroy the organisms in fully developed glandular tuberculosis.

On the other hand, they seem to definitely increase the susceptibility of B. typhosus and staphylococcus aureus to killing by heat. This, he says, may indicate a method by which therapeutic results are obtained in the X-ray treatment of bacterial conditions. R. W. A. S.

PUBLICATIONS RECEIVED.

Books.

Electric Ionization. By A. FRIEL, M.A., M.D. Bristol: J. Wright & Sons, Ltd.

The Coolidge Tube. By H. PILON. London : Bailliere, Tindall & Cox.

The Systematic Development of X-Ray Plates and Films. L. WENDALL, B.S., D.D.S.

The Radiography of the Chest. Vol. I., *Pulmonary Tuberculosis.* By WALKER OVEREND, M.A., M.D. London: Wm. Heinemann (Medical Books) Ltd.

Journals.

Archives d'Électricite Médicale et de Physiotherapie, Mar., 1920. April.

American Journal of Electrotherapeutics and Radiology, Feb., 1920.

American Journal of Roentgenology, Dec. 1919. Jan., 1920.

Bulletin et Mémoirs de la Société de Radiologie Médicale de France, Mar., 1920.

Bulletin of the Johns Hopkins Hospital, Jan., Feb., 1920.

Gaceta Medica Catalana, Dec. 31st, 1919. 15th Dec.

Hospitalstidende, Jan. 28th ; Feb. 4th, 11th, 18th, 25th ; Mar. 3rd, 10th, 18th, 24th, 1920.

Journals—*continued.*

Il Policlinico, Feb. 1st, 15th ; Mar. 1st, 1920.

International Journal of Orthodontia and Oral Surgery, Feb., 1920. Mar.

Journal de Medicine de Lyon, Mar. 5th, 20th ; Apl. 5th, 1920.

La Chirurgia degli Organi di Movimento, Feb., 1920.

La Radiologia Medica, Jan.-Feb., 1920.

Medical Journal of Australia, Jan. 24th, 31st; Feb. 7th, 14th, 21st, 28th ; Mar. 6th, 1920.

Medical Science, Abstracts, and Reviews, Apl., 1920.

Modern Medicine, Mar., 1920.

New York Journal of Medicine, Mar.,1920.

New York Medical Journal, Feb. 7th, 14th, 21st, 28th ; Mar. 6th, 13th, 27th ; Apl. 2nd, 1920.

Norsk Mag. for Lægevidenskaben, Apl. 1920. Mar.

Revista Medico-Quirurgica, Feb. 1st, 1920.

Revista Italiana di Neuropatologia, Psichiatria ed Ellettroperapia, Jan., 1920.

Surgery, Gynæcology, and Obstetrics, Mar., 1920.

Ugeskrift for Læger, Mar. 11th; Apl. 1st, 8th, 1920.

NOTICES.

ARCHIVES OF RADIOLOGY AND ELECTROTHERAPY is published monthly.

The index for each volume, which ends with the May number, is supplied with the June number of each year.

Communications to the Editors should be addressed to " ROBERT KNOX, M.D., 38, Harley Street, W. 1."

Communications and illustrations from American contributors may be sent to Messrs. REBMAN COMPANY, 141-145, West Thirty-sixth Street, New York City.

All radiographs and photographs must be originals, and must not have been previously published. Drawings should be supplied on separate paper.

Owing to the scarcity of paper the Publishers are reluctantly compelled to reduce the number of free reprints of Papers to twenty-five.

Annual Subscriptions, payable in advance, 30/- including postage. Single copies, 3/- (postage 2d.) Single numbers and back numbers can be supplied on application.

Vol. XXIV—No. 12   MAY, 1920   No. 238

ARCHIVES OF
RADIOLOGY AND
ELECTROTHERAPY

THE OFFICIAL ORGAN OF THE
BRITISH ASSOCIATION OF
RADIOLOGY AND PHYSIOTHERAPY

Editors.

ROBERT KNOX, M.D,. Hon. Radiologist, King's College Hospital.
E. P. CUMBERBATCH, B.M., M.R.C.P., Medical Officer in Charge, Electrical
  Department, St. Bartholomew's Hospital.
SIDNEY RUSS, D.Sc., Physicist to the Middlesex Hospital.

IN COLLABORATION WITH

A. E. BARCLAY (Manchester); BELOT (Paris); H. MARTIN BERRY (London); W. H. BRAGG (London);
N. BURKE (Woodhall Spa); J. BURNET (Edinburgh); W. J. S. BYTHELL (Manchester); J. T. CASE (Battle
Creek, U.S.A.); A. ST. GEORGE CAULFEILD (London); H. A. COLWELL (London); FOVEAU DE COURMELLES
(Paris); GUNZBURG (Antwerp); HALL-EDWARDS (Birmingham); HARET (Paris); HAUCHAMPS (Brussels);
F. HERNAMAN-JOHNSON (London); W. F. HIGGINS (Teddington); THURSTAN HOLLAND (Liverpool);
HURST (London); KLYNENS (Antwerp); LAQUERRIERE (Paris); LAZARUS-BARLOW (London); LEDUC
(Nantes); ALEXANDER MACKAY (Edinburgh); REGINALD MORTON (London); HARRISON ORTON (London);
W. OVEREND (St. Leonards-on-Sea); PFAHLER (Philadelphia); C. E. S. PHILLIPS (London); GEORGE
PIRIE (Dundee); HOWARD PIRIE (Montreal); A. W. PORTER (London); R. W. A. SALMOND (London);
WERTHEIM SALOMONSON (Amsterdam); S. SLOAN (Glasgow); SOMERVILLE (Glasgow); W. C. STEVENSON
(Dublin); W. J. TURRELL (Oxford); HUGH WALSHAM (London).

THE TREATMENT OF UTERINE CANCER BY RADIUM.

By HENRY H. JANEWAY, M.D., New York.

Attending Surgeon and Head of the Radium Department, Memorial Hospital.

[Reproduced, with permission, in part from Surgery, Gynecology, and Obstetrics, September, 1919,
pp. 242-265.]

DURING recent years an increasingly conservative attitude in the treatment of
cancer of the cervix uteri has been adopted in many of the large clinics.
Cancer of the cervix uteri, as regards its amenability to surgical treatment,
contrasts strongly with cancer of the fundus. The latter can be successfully
removed in a large percentage of cases without exposing an otherwise normal
individual to a serious risk, while the mortality after an adequately planned
operation for cancer of the cervix is high and the percentage of cures
disappointingly low.

  During the last five years of the past century, the low percentage of cures
produced by vaginal hysterectomy was generally recognised, and the extended
abdominal operation adopted by the more important operators. Wertheim has

earned the credit of perfecting the details of this operation, having published his description in 1898. His operation represents the widest removal of carcinoma of the cervix. In experienced hands it has given a generally considered high percentage of cures, based on a freedom from recurrence of three to five years. '

The percentage of cures in any series of cases is, however, dependent upon the favourable character of the cases selected for the operation, and the radical nature of the operation to which the patient is exposed. Thus we find that the most favourable statistics of cures accompanies, as a general rule, a low percentage of operability and a high primary mortality. In 1911, Jacobson collected statistics on the operability, primary mortality, and curability, as judged by the five-year standard, in 2,765 cases of uterine cancer, reported by 130 operators.

Twenty-eight operators recorded percentages of operability. These varied from 5 per cent. to 90 per cent.; seven less than 25 per cent., ten between 25 and 50 per cent., six over 75 per cent.

With some exceptions, a definite relation was found to exist between the percentage of operability and the mortality rate.

The primary mortality of the 2,765 operations was 19·45 per cent. The mortality of many operators was below this : in the case of Jacobs, 6·37 per cent.; Zweifel, 10·8 per cent.; Kline, 12·8 per cent.; Wertheim, 10 per cent. (last two hundred cases) ; Doederlein, 14·3 per cent.

If we accept Wertheim's conclusions that carcinoma of the cervix is twenty times as frequent as carcinoma of the fundus, it is possible to calculate on this basis the combined percentages for operability, mortality and curability of cancer of the uterus, i.e., including both cancer of the fundus and cancer of the cervix, by multiplying the percentages for carcinoma of the cervix by twenty, adding to the product the percentages for carcinoma of the fundus, and dividing by twenty-one.

Using this method the operability of carcinoma of the uterus is 37·61 per cent.; the mortality is 17·74 per cent.; the curability, based on the five-year standard for traced cases, is 36·63 per cent.; for cases operated on, 21·31 per cent.; for patients applying for treatment, 9·82 per cent.

A review of these tables indicates at first glance that the operative statistics, more certainly in the case of cancer of the fundus, but even for cancer of the cervix, are not unfavourable to this method of treatment. When, however, certain facts are considered in connection with these figures, the operative treatment of cancer of the cervix is far from satisfactory.

In the first place, while the immediate mortality in the most skilful hands is only 10 per cent., it is still 20 per cent. in skilled hands, and in the hands of even Wertheim, during the period of the development of his operation, in his first one hundred cases it was 30 per cent.

Such a high mortality restricts the usefulness of the operation to relatively few surgeons, entirely inadequate to meet the demands of the large number of patients having cervical cancer. .Nor does this high mortality tell the whole story. It leaves out of consideration entirely, first, the necessity for restricting the operation to a small percentage of the most favourable cases, and second, the suffering entailed by the operation itself and its sequelæ. Such sequelæ followed von Rosthorn's operations in no less than 42 per cent., and included ureteral and bladder fistulæ, secondary necrosis of the bladder, injury to the rectum, fistulæ of the intestine, and in one case a division of the obturator nerve with permanent paralysis of the leg. Weibel reports 6 per cent. of ureterovaginal fistulæ from the Wertheim Clinic.

Post-operative sequelæ, including suppuration of the abdominal incision, cystitis, peritonitis, ureteral fistulæ, vesical fistulæ, phlebitis, laceration of the rectum, pleurisy and rectovaginal fistulæ occurred in 22 cases of Clark's 36 patients, or in 73 per cent.

The majority of these post-operative sequelæ are, of course, temporary, but a sufficient number are permanent to constitute a real objection to the operative treatment of cancer of the cervix. These various unfavourable complications of the operation, the high mortality after an operation which is at all adequate, the by no means infrequent and unpleasant post-operative sequelæ, and finally, after a woman has faced all these risks, not to mention the discomfort of the operation itself, the rather small prospect that she will be permanently cured, that she will not be obliged to suffer a lingering and painful death, has caused many of the most prominent gynecologists to adopt a more conservative attitude toward the radical abdominal operation for cancer of the cervix.

This attitude is expressed in the concluding sentence of Schottlaender and Kermauner's book: "The time is not yet ripe for a review and criticism of the literature, many co-workers are yet necessary. . . . At present we can only say that we do not wish to underestimate or overestimate the importance of the abdominal operation. We are still at the beginning of its development." At the time he wrote he considered it to be the only way to meet demands of the carcinomatous process.

Clark voices the same dissatisfaction with the operative treatment of cancer of the cervix. He states: "If an operation or other therapeutic procedure is to have a permanent place in our armamentarium it must be sufficiently easy to make it available, not for a few skilled specialists, but for the great body of surgeons working in every quarter of this and other countries. In these days of low mortality percentages, attending nearly all the major operations, no operation can possibly gain headway which combines with it a shockingly high mortality and a large number of distressing and disabling sequelæ.

"Further, while the continental surgeon, with his large and overcrowded clinics, may ignore the question of mortality in working out a principle, the American surgeon as well as the American layman is so temperamentally constituted that the one cannot and the other will not disregard a high primary death rate. The effect upon the lay mind, therefore, must be taken into consideration, for while one may have over 50 per cent. ultimate cures, the effect upon the average intelligent citizen is abhorrent, if for this number of survivors there have been twenty-five deaths and for the other twenty-five a wretched existence attended by repulsive post-operative sequelæ followed by a painful and lingering death. It is possible that when we make a final summary of our combined experience we may have to accept the conclusion that a less radical operation, even though it save fewer cases, may be preferable when attended by a low surgical mortality and few or no operative sequelæ."

Peterson, I believe, sounds the same note. He states: "Unfortunately added experience has strengthened my belief that the extended operation for cancer of the cervix is an exceedingly dangerous operation, always attended by a high primary mortality. No one will be more glad to discard the radical abdominal method than will I, if I can be shown that more patients can be ultimately saved by less dangerous methods."

Since the above quoted expressions about the radical abdominal operation were written, another method of treatment of cancer of the uterus, its treatment by radium, has become prominent.

Wickham can be properly referred to as the father of the radium treatment of cancer. He began his work in 1906 and published the results of the treatment of a thousand cases of cancer in 1910 and 1913. Also as a pioneer, and working with Wickham, must be mentioned Dominici, who is responsible for the development of many technical improvements, particularly in the principles of filtration. Following these men many isolated reports have appeared: especially may be mentioned those by Caan in 1909, and Czerny and Caan in 1912, and Pinch in 1912, by Riehl, Ranzi, Schueller and Sparmann in 1913; in this country, Abbe, and finally the book by Paul Lazarus in 1913. It is just to give to Kroenig the credit of the most important introduction of the use of radio-activity in gynecology, but while he may have done the pioneer work in gynecology, it was Doederlein's and Bumm's reports before the *Deutsche Gesellschaft fuer Gynaekologie*, at Halle, in May, 1913, and the papers by Chéron and Rubens-Duval, Schauta, Schindler, Scherer, and Keley, and Latzko and Schueller, all in 1913, that furnished the great impetus to the treatment of cancer of the uterus by radium.

Doederlein reported one cure of an operable case of cancer of the cervix and excellent results in other cases. He presented microscopic sections proving the retrogression of cancer after the use of radium.

Bumm reported 9 cases of apparent clinical cure of patients with advanced cancer of the cervix by the use of mesothorium and X rays.

Chéron and Rubens-Duval reported 155 results, conservatively classified as improvements, of 158 patients with advanced cancer of the cervix. Forty-six of these improvements are probable cures. In two of the cases, both inoperable, the cure was proved, in one by autopsy, and in the other by histological section.

Schauta reported 11 clinical cures out of 16 patients with cancer of the cervix treated by radium and mesothorium. He believed that radium was the more effective of the two agents.

Schindler described some very favourable results in the treatment of cancer of the cervix by mesothorium and radium.

Scherer and Keley concluded that the treatment of 218 cases of cancer of the cervix by X-ray and radium gave 10·5 per cent. greater freedom from recurrence than operation alone formerly gave.

Latzko and Schueller reported 5 clinical cures of 7 advanced cases of cancer of the uterus.

In the succeeding year still more encouraging results were published.

Bumm then recorded 108 cases of carcinoma of the cervix treated by radium. Of these only 5 were operable growths. Among them there were only 15 recurrences to date, and a clinical cure had been produced in 10 inoperable growths.

Doederlein and von Suffert obtained a disappearance of all subjective and objective symptoms in 31 of 153 cases of cancer of the uterus, and 12 of the 31 were inoperable.

Kroenig recorded 254 cases of cancer of the uterus treated by X-ray and mesothorium. Sixty-four were treated prophylactically after operation and 150 entirely without operation. Nineteen have undoubtedly remained free from cancer. He concluded that in cases in which cancer was still localised to its primary site, the type of case usually termed operable, he was able to cause the complete disappearance of the cancer as far as could be recognised histologically. His longest cure, however, had been under observation for only two years. He had never been able to cure metastatic carcinoma, nor in those cases in which the disease had invaded the neighbouring tissues, deep invasion, for instance, of the broad ligaments, though remarkable retrogressions and temporary cessations of growth had followed the treatment of the latter.

Dobbert made, in many respects, the most important contribution in 1914. The results of the treatment of 44 cases of cancer of the uterus, of which 31 were cancers of the cervix, 18 inoperable and 6 operable, were so good that they justify him in concluding that it is permissible to treat early operable cancer of the cervix by radium alone. In many cases, when the invasion of the tissues around the site of origin was deep, an elimination of the growth might be expected. In still more advanced cases a condition temporarily approaching a cure could be obtained. In the very advanced cases he discouraged treatment.

Weinbrenner described 8 most successful results in the treatment of 32 cases of genital carcinoma by mesothorium.

Allman reported results on 85 patients with cancer of the uterus, treated with mesothorium. At the time of his report 15 of these patients were free from symptoms. These 15 patients either had recurrent growths or had refused operation. Twenty other inoperable cases became operable.

Legneu and Chéron reported a patient with an extensive, entirely inoperable, cancer of the vagina treated with radium, and two and a half years after the completion of the period of treatment the patient died after an operation for another trouble. An autopsy was obtained and the complete absence of cancer demonstrated. Other confirmatory reports, but of less definite character, have appeared from Morton, Dieffenbach, Foveau de Courmelles, Jacobs, Kroemer, Tate, Pozzi and Rouhier, Oertel, Seuffert and Klein.

In 1915 far more definite results were reported, many of which give information on the permanency of treatment by radium.

Doerderlein now reports 12 patients with inoperable uterine cancer treated by radium and well at the time of his report, more than a year from the time the treatment was given. He definitely advocates the use of radiotherapy for operable uterine cancer.

Flatau states that since December, 1913, a period of one and a half years, he has not operated upon a single case of cancer of the cervix, and has obtained a larger number of recoveries for an equal number of cases than he ever obtained by operation, though his mortality after operation was only 12 per cent.

Burrows reports that a disappearance of early cancer of the cervix and marked improvement in the more advanced lesions, after treatment by radium, is fairly constant.

Degrais reports a number of patients who had advanced cancer of the cervix treated by radium, who are in good health at the time of the report, four years after treatment.

Kelly and Burnam have made the most extensive use of radium in this country and have done so under very favourable conditions. They report the results on the treatment of 213 patients, 14 of whom were operable. Of these operable cases 4 were treated with radium alone and are all well, 2 for a period of two years and 2 for a period of one year after the treatment. The remaining 10 of the operable group were operated on first and afterwards treated with radium. All were well at the time of the report at intervals of six months to three years after the treatment. The authors consider that these results are suggestive, when it is considered that after operation alone there is a recurrence in 75 per cent. and in 60 per cent. of the cases in the first year. One hundred and ninety-nine patients treated were inoperable at the time of the treatment ; these included inoperable primary growths and inoperable recurrent cases. Fifty-three of this group are clinically cured and 109 markedly improved. Of 35 patients of this group, all primarily inoperable, 3 have remained well for four years, 2 for three years, and 17 for over one year. Eighteen primarily inoperable recurrent growths of this group are now clinically cured, 1 patient over six years, another over four years, 11 over two years, and 10 over one year.

In other words, 57 of 213 patients with cancer of the cervix, 4 operable and 53 inoperable, have been cured by radium ; that is, all of the operable cases and 26 per cent. of cases considered inoperable at the time of their treatment.

Baish reported that he has treated all cases of cancer of the uterus and vagina with mesothorium since February, 1914. At the time of his report he had treated 100 cases. The duration after treatment is from about twenty-one weeks to six months. He divides his patients into three groups. One group,

43 patients, were all inoperable, with definite parametrial infiltration. Many of these were benefited but only one clinically cured. In a second group of patients on the borderland of operability, 10, or 50 per cent., were clinically cured. The third group included 37 operable patients. Of these, 28, or 75 per cent., were clinically cured.

Adler reported a clinical cure in 9 inoperable cancers of the cervix, 2 inoperable cancers of the body of the uterus, and 1 of the vagina.

St. Clare recorded 2 cases in which radium was applied after incomplete operations for advanced cancer of the uterus. Fourteen months after the application in one case and a shorter interval in the other, both patients were, as far as could be ascertained, free from disease.

Fabre reported excellent results in 10 cases, the detailed histories of which were given.

Sir Thomas Oliver reported a very extensive recurrent cancer of the vagina apparently cured by a single application.

Von Graff, using the dosage recommended by Wertheim, and writing two years after a rather discouraging article by Wertheim on the radium treatment of uterine carcinoma, reported most encouraging results from the treatment of 102 cases of cancer of the uterus by radium. He concluded that radiumtherapy gives better results in the management of inoperable cases than any other method of treatment, and not a few cases thought inoperable have been so improved that the presence of carcinoma could no longer be demonstrated.

Miller also reported enthusiastically on the action of radium in advanced uterine cancer. He reported 6 cases, only one of which had gone one year from treatment. This patient presented, two years after operation, an extensive recurrence in the vault of the vagina. At the time of his report, one year after her treatment by radium, she was entirely free from symptoms.

Fueth and Ebeler reported results from the treatment of 56 patients with uterine cancer. Ten of these patients were operable and in each case retrogression had become complete, or nearly so, at the time of the report. Eleven other patients were treated prophylactically and six of the remaining number, all inoperable, were clinically cured. Other papers appearing in 1915, supporting the same conclusions, are by Bergonié and Spéder, Abbe, Kolischer, Turner and Ransohoff.

Schmitz, in a paper appearing in 1916, recorded his results in the treatment of 80 cases of pelvic cancer. Of these he has obtained a clinical cure in 11 of 35 cases of inoperable cancer of the uterus, in 7 of 12 operable patients, and in 4 of 15 recurrent cases, making a total of 22 clinical cures of 62 patients, or 35·5 per cent. The post-treatment interval varied from four to twenty-four months. This report is very significant when we consider that 50 of his 62 patients, or 80 per cent., were not operable.

In the past year several important papers have appeared which more than confirm previous reports.

Maiolo has treated 50 patients, all of whom were inoperable or recurrent after hysterectomy. Eight of these patients were recently treated, but of the remaining 42, 16 are anatomically and clinically cured for periods of one to two years.

Esquerido has treated 12 cases of uterine cancer ; of these 3 were operable and all completely retrogressed. Of the remaining 7 inoperable patients, 3 were apparently cured.

Bailey reported 16 patients apparently free from disease, of 120 patients with uterine cancer treated with radium. Of these the post-treatment period had been two years in 1 case and one and a half years to two years in 4 cases, six months to one year in 8 cases, and one to six months in 3 cases.

Myers reported three excellent results, though recent, in 3 patients out of 5 whom he had treated. Labhardt, Klatz, and Heimann also reported favourable results.

Two other papers of particular importance have appeared during the past year.

The first of these is by Recasens, of Madrid. Recasens at first used radium only upon those cases which were too advanced for operation, or in which operation was contra-indicated, but his uniform success makes him no longer hesitate to treat early cancer of the cervix with radium. He states that if in inoperable cancer in which an actual extension to the parametrium exists, so that the possibility of a cure by operation can no longer be entertained, one can obtain a cure by radium in 60 per cent. of the cases, it is only logical to believe that in early circumscribed cancer of the cervix a cure by radium is more certain. He contrasts the gravity of the Wertheim operation, with its primary mortality of 10 to 15 per cent. in the hands of the best surgeons, and its secondary mortality after the laspe of three to five years of 40 to 50 per cent., with the comparatively safe and simple procedure of treatment by radium with its "100 per cent. of cures" in this stage. His belief that 100 per cent. of the early cases are cured by radium is based on the fact that every one of 16 such cases, which he has treated, has undergone a complete retrogression, and a number of these have already completed three years since the treatment was applied.

In addition to these results in operable cancer he has treated 182 inoperable cancers of the cervix. Forty-seven of these were treated in the year 1914, and of these 29 were well at the time of the report. In 1915 he treated 79 patients, of which number 45 were well at the time of the report. He has not been so fortunate in cancer of the body of the uterus. Of 16 cases of cancer of the body, only 8 were clinically cured and 6 have died, 2 being still under treatment. He concludes that 70 per cent. of his inoperable cancers and 95 per cent. of those cases in which the growth was still limited to its site of origin have been cured by radium. Fifty per cent. of his cases of cancer of the fundus have been cured, but in this group he prefers operation, unless the woman is fat or possesses some other contra-indication to operation.

A second paper of equal importance is by Clark. He reports 100 patients with genital carcinoma treated by radium. Seventy-four of these were carcinoma of the cervix and 4 of the fundus. Fifty-five of these patients were alive and free from symptoms, two to thirty months after treatment, and in the case of 5 patients twenty-two to thirty months after treatment.

My own cases are few in number, being limited to patients referred to me for personal care. The majority of them are, from the standpoint of operability, border-line cases. They are in consequence important from the standpoint of radiumtherapy, and I wish to put them on record, first, because I believe that the results obtained in them illustrate what can be obtained by the use of radium, in place of operation, in early cancer of the cervix, a preference in treatment which is shared at present by very few surgeons ; second, because I believe that there is an advantage in using the method of treatment which has been employed in these cases and which has been the outgrowth of my use of radium in other portions of the body.

These cases, 30 in number, have a post-therapeutic period, varying from $3\frac{1}{3}$ years to 6 months, and comprise 17 carcinomata of the cervix, 4 recurrent carcinomata of the cervix, 4 carcinomata of the fundus, and 5 carcinomata of the vulva (labia minora and clitoris).

Of the 17 carcinomata of the cervix, the post-therapeutic period in one is $3\frac{1}{3}$ years, in another 3 years, and in a third $1\frac{3}{4}$ years. Nine of the remaining cases, all treated within the past year, have undergone the same continuous retrogression after a single treatment as the first three cases treated with the longer post-therapeutic period.

Five of the 17 carcinomata of the cervix have recurred after the first treatment and are again under treatment. The fact, however, that they have developed a recurrence is deemed a very unfavourable factor in their ultimate prognosis. In two of these cases a large portion of the vaginal wall was involved. Two others had bad symptoms of bleeding for many months before the radium treatment. The remaining case had a very advanced lesion, has been treated recently and is still under observation.

All four of the cases which developed a recurrence showed a primary retrogression which was complete for a short period in two cases and became almost complete in the other two. In all four of these cases the recurrence or renewed growth developed within four months from the time of the first treatment. The fifth case is still improving, but was so extensive at the time of treatment that a cure is not expected.

Of the four patients with carcinoma of the fundus, one, an old lady, died of intercurrent disease, two years after the radium treatment. She never had any return of her uterine symptoms. A second patient remained in perfect health for two years from the time of her first treatment. The third patient, treated $1\frac{1}{2}$ years ago, and the fourth patient, treated within the past year, are still free from symptoms.

Of the four recurrent cases, one patient treated first two years ago, is still free from any evidence of disease. Another, first treated a year ago, is free from evidence of disease. A third, treated two years ago, has recently required another treatment and at present shows symptoms of metastasis in the upper pelvic glands. The fourth case was not improved.

The greatest interest centres around the five cases of carcinoma of the vulva. In one of these the lesion involved the clitoris and in the other four the labia minora the urethral orifice, and anterior vaginal wall. In two of these cases a clinically complete retrogression followed treatment. One of these patients developed a recurrence which is at present satisfactorily retrogressing after a second treatment. The other has remained free from evidence of disease for 15 months since her treatment. In the third patient, wholly inoperable, the retrogression is at present so complete that a cure is expected.

A fourth patient with a very advanced lesion is still improving and under treatment. While none of these five patients can be classed as cures, it must be remembered that in all but one progressive improvement of over a year's standing and amounting to a fairly complete retrogression followed the radium treatment, a result which is better than that usually following operation for this form of cancer.

Of equal importance with the consideration of the results of the treatment of uterine cancer with radium is a consideration of the methods by which these results have been obtained.

The majority of radium therapeutists in gynecology use single tubes. These are inserted inside the uterus or within the cervical canal, or against the vaginal surface of the cervix, or in several of these locations, at the same or at alternate treatments.

The dosage generally used has been heavy, sufficient to cause extensive sloughing, and entirely too heavy for almost any other region of the body. Bumm, for instance, recommends a total dosage of 8,700 milligram hours to 15,000 milligram hours.

Chéron and Rubens Duval use the Dominici tubes, wrapped in gauze and placed in the vagina, and give 48 to 7,200 milligram hours, repeating this treatment when they deem it necessary.

Schauta recommends the use of 50 milligrams filtered by 2 millimetres of lead, applied for five days, or 6,000 milligram hours, and the repetition of this dose in ten days time, giving thus virtually 12,000 milligram hours. In eleven cases he has had two severe hæmorrhages, one vesicovaginal fistula and one rectovaginal fistula.

Schindler uses as small a quantity of radium carbonate as corresponding to 27 milligrams of pure radium bromide. This is enclosed in a lead capsule 1·3 millimetres thick and placed within the vagina for days.

Scherer and Keley filter through 1·3 millimetres lead and use a total dosage of 3,820 milligram hours.

Latzo and Schueler use the Dominici tubes of 0·5 millimetre silver covered with 1½ to 3 millimetre lead and a dosage of 15,300 to 16,800 milligram hours.

Doederlein gives 12,000 to 14,000 milligram hours, in divided doses in the course of 1 to 2 months.

Dobbert recommends 2,400 milligram hours, repeated every third day until 6,000 to 7,000 milligram hours have been given. He filters through gold and brass, rarely through lead.

Weinbrenner gives 8,004 to 13,680 milligram hours and filters through silver.

Allman uses 150 to 200 milligrams of radium bromide for 24 hours, 3,600 to 4,800 milligram hours, repeating the treatment at intervals of two to four weeks. He uses nickel plated brass filters. He had severe symptoms in a number of patients from overdosage.

Burrows uses a strong application within the cervix, 50 to 60 millicuries of emanation filtered through 1 millimetre of silver and simultaneously two to three needles containing emanation thrust into the broad ligaments and posterior lip of the cervix, left in place 24 to 48 hours.

This treatment is further reinforced by the application of varnish-plates over the abdomen.

Kelly and Burnam have not yet described their technique.

St. Clair has successfully used as small a quantity as 10 milligrams of radium, applied within the cervix and uterus, six times at intervals of 6 to 8 days, for 24 hours each time, a total dosage of only 1,440 milligram hours.

Sir Thomas Oliver obtained his excellent result from a single application of 24 hours duration, of a single tube of emanation, containing probably 50 to 100 milligrams of emanation, in other words, 1,200 to 2,400 milligram hours.

Von Graff reports severe effects from overexposure. He used at first 250 milligrams and later 40 milligrams for 24 to 48 hours. This is repeated once or twice at intervals of 2 to 3 days, and of a second series of exposures given in two to three weeks. This probably represents 1,000 to 2,000 milligram hours at each exposure. He reports no bad effects from his later weaker dosage.

Schmitz, who has furnished a very favourable report, uses 50 milligrams radium element for 40 to 48 hours, giving as a rule two treatments, 12 to 36 hours apart. This amounts to 2,000 to 2,400 milligram hours. The radium is filtered through brass 1·2 millimetres thick. It is divided into two tubes arranged tandem. These are applied within the cervix, and reinforced by cross-fire from a second application of two tubes, arranged side by side, and applied against the cervix. Thus the total milligram hours amounts to 4,000 to 4,800 milligram hours. This treatment is repeated in three weeks time, but only if there is no great change. If improvement occurs the consideration of further treatment is postponed for another three weeks. Schmitz also cites experiments on cutaneous nodules of breast cancer which demonstrated that the γ-rays from 50 milligrams of radium element, applied for 12 hours (600 milligram hours) will destroy carcinomatous tissue 1 centimetre distant.

Clark describes his dosage only in connection with uterine myomata, and here refers to 50 milligrams for 24 hours or 1,200 milligram hours, as a large dose for the interior of the uterus. We assume that he uses a similar dosage for cancer.

Bailey formerly used a dosage of 3,000 millicuries in the vagina applied to the cervix and filtered through 1 millimetre platinum. A tube of 600 millicurie hours is applied within the cervix, and 600 millicurie hours directed towards each parametrium. In addition to this, 3,000 millicurie hours is applied over the abdomen in three places, over the center of the abdomen, and over each inguinal region. He now uses 2,000 millicurie hours in one platinum tube placed in the cervical canal, and 3,000 millicurie hours from his bomb directed in fractions of 1,000 millicurie hours each in three different directions against the cervix, and a total of 18,000 millicurie hours applied externally at a distance of 4 centimetres from the spine over six different areas in a circle around the pelvis, *i.e.*, 3,000 millicurie hours over each area.

Recasens uses 70 milligrams of radium for 20 to 24 hours. He has used 130 milligrams for as long as four hours. In other words, 1,400 to 1,680, or even 6,240 milligram hours. This treatment is repeated after an interval of 8 days and again a third time after another 8 days. It is again repeated after 20 days and sometimes altogether six or eight applications are made, two months elapsing between the later applications.

Of these methods of treatment that of Schmitz corresponds more closely than the others with our own. We believe it important in the treatment, at least of cervical cancer, to cross-fire from within the cervical canal and from the surface of the ulcer. Moreover, we cannot understand the heavy dosage recommended by many of those whom we have quoted.

In our experience one treatment appears to be all that is required in many cases. The two cases which we here report having gone the longest time, one of them 3 years and 4 months and the other 3 years, have each received only one treatment.

For the average favourable case 6,000 millicurie hours in one treatment may be all that is necessary, while a repetition of this treatment at too soon an interval, or increasing it, may cause the patient much unnecessary discomfort, or produce fistulæ.

The radium should be divided equally among six tubes. These tubes may be the regular Dominici tubes of 0·5 millimetre silver, but we prefer tubes of 1 millimetre platinum. The tubes which we use are 2 centimetres long, with a central radium containing portion 1¼ centimetres long and walls 1 millimetre thick. Such tubes have the filtering power of 2 millimetres of lead and are less bulky.

While the Dominici tube filters out practically all the α- and β-rays it does not filter out many of the soft γ-rays. One millimetre of platinum or 2 millimetres of lead filters out also the softer γ-rays. One millimetre of platinum or 2 millimetres of lead permits, therefore, the use of a much larger percentage of deeply penetrating radiations, which are far more homogeneous. Radiations from radium filtered in this manner must be used for a longer period, and so used will exert a far more distant effect and a much better defined selective action.

For cancer of both the fundus and the cervix we advise the use of three of these tubes, containing 150 milligrams of radium, and inserted in the utero-cervical canal, arranged end-to-end in a long rubber tube. For cancer of the cervix three additional tubes are placed against the cervical ulcer. The tubes placed against the cervical ulcer should be distributed evenly over its surface, and the best method of retaining them in such a position is by embedding them within a mould of the cervical ulcer and vagina made of dental modelling compound. This compound is the preparation which dentists use for obtaining impressions of the teeth. Placed in hot water it becomes soft, like putty, and in this condition may be inserted into the vagina. Left there it cools to the body temperature, at which it becomes hard enough to retain its shape. It forms, therefore, a perfect mould of the interior of the vagina and may be easily removed and reinserted, and when reinserted it always finds the same position in the vagina. Upon this mould is an impression of the cervical ulcer. The three radium tubes may be embedded at equal distances from each other within the area of the mould, which shows the impression made by the cervical ulceration. When the mould then is reinserted into the vagina, these tubes come into accurate apposition and are evenly distributed over the ulcer. This mould serves an additional function in holding the vaginal walls, and with them the bladder and rectum, away from the cervix and the radium lying against it, and thus protects these organs from burning. If the radium is so placed that it comes into dangerous proximity to the bladder and rectum a piece of lead may be embedded behind it, in the opposite surface of the mould, thus still more completely insuring the protection of the bladder and rectum. An absolute protection of the bladder and rectum and overhanging vaginal walls is not desirable. Schottlaender and Kermauner have shown that in a definite percentage of cases of cancer of the cervix metastatic extensions are already present in the vaginal walls, at some distance from the cervix. It is, therefore, not desirable to protect the vagina too strongly when applying radium to the cervix.

Some protection is advantageous, because in its absence disagreeable bladder and rectal tenesmus and discomfort from burning in the vagina can follow strong applications to the cervix. The cervix itself is practically insensitive to strong treatment. I have found that the separation of the vaginal walls by the dental moulds is sufficient and yet allows a desirable amount of radiation of the vagina.

Special provision for directing strong radiations against the broad ligaments, with a comparative neglect of the anterior and posterior parametrium, is probably unsafe as compared to a uniform radiation of all the parametrial tissue.

Schottlaender and Kermauner have shown that the regions in front and behind the cervix are frequently involved by the direct extensions of the growth.

The distribution of the radiations should, therefore, be made as diffuse as possible around the cervical ulcer as a centre.

Attempts to supplement the internal treatment of uterine cancer for the purpose of more effectively reaching extensions into the uterus, broad ligaments and lymph nodes, by the application of heavily filtered radium over the abdomen, are of undetermined value.

Bailey, in his excellent work, uses such cross-firing through the abdomen in all his cases. Levine and Koernig have good results from cross-firing by X-ray radiations. My own experience in the treatment of epidermoid cancer in the deep cervical lymphatics, where the effects of the treatment can be followed with greater accuracy, and in a few advanced cases of uterine cancer, confirms the experience of these men and indicates that a definite additional impression is made upon the extensions of uterine cancer by cross-firing through the abdomen. We are not, therefore, justified in neglecting this accessory means of treating uterine cancer. Nevertheless, its importance must not be overrated, for there are some objections to its use. When the cross-firing is given by radium, and this is the agent of choice, because its radiations are more penetrating than the X-ray radiations, large quantities are needed. These quantities are only available in a few stations. Moreover, their use prevents the treatment of other patients. The X rays, which will be further improved in the future, are a more practical means of cross-firing uterine cancer through the abdomen, but even the use of these rays seriously complicates the treatment for many patients.

Until, therefore, the indications for the use of cross-firing through the abdomen are more thoroughly understood, until we know how much more it accomplishes than palliative improvement, a failure to be able to give it should not be regarded as a contra-indication to the treatment of uterine cancer by local applications alone.

It must not be forgotten that uterine cancer, when still limited to the regions of its primary appearance, is curable by these local applications alone. None of the cases, for instance, in this report has received any other treatment.

The dosage which I have found safe and efficient in cancer of the cervix, the radium being distributed as above described, is 6,000 millicurie hours, *i.e.*, divided into 3,000 millicurie hours within the uterus and 3,000 millicurie hours against the cervix ; in other words, it is recommended that the radium should be divided into 6 tubes for the treatment of cervical cancer, and, if each tube contains 50 milligrams, 3 of the tubes arranged end-to-end are placed in the uterocervical canal for 20 hours and the other 3 against the cervical ulcer for the same length of time.

One of these treatments may cause a complete retrogression, and a repetition of the treatment may not be necessary. In our experience the best results have been obtained when a repetition of the treatment was not necessary.

Theoretically this is so and should prove so practically, for just as the success of the removal of the cancer by operation is best when the removal is complete, so every effort should be made completely to destroy carcinoma of the uterus by one blow, when it is first seen, and, therefore, most limited around the site of origin. If repetitions of the treatment become necessary a long interval should elapse and much care used in making the second treatment, as the tissues will not bear the same dose a second time so well.

We believe there is some advantage in cervical cancer in the use of emanation enclosed within minute glass tubes, which are embedded in the tumour mass instead of the surface application of radium.

We recommend the use of 20 to 30 or 40 millicuries of emanation, according to the size of the tumour treated, distributed as evenly as possible throughout the tumour. Bagg has shown that 1 millicurie will produce a general necrotic effect through a sphere of tissue surrounding the tube for a distance of 1 centimetre. It is important, therefore, that the amount of emanation in each tube should be reduced to a minimum consistent with the avoidance of objectionable trauma, dependent on the introduction of too many tubes. The dose from 20 to 40 millicuries of emanation is 2,640 to 5,280 millicurie hours.

From our experience with unfiltered emanation in other regions of the body, the intense shower of β- and soft γ-radiations, having, it is true, a more limited radius of effectual activity, produces a more complete destruction of cancer than the more penetrating γ-radiations alone. These are more accurately applied and distribute the radiations more evenly through the cancer tissue, and subject the patient to less inconvenience than any other method of treatment.

A review of the cases reported in this paper does not, of course, prove that radium is, at the present time, the method of choice for treating primary carcinoma of the fundus or cervix uteri. Taken, however, in conjunction with the other reports in the literature above quoted, it suggests that in only a few years there will be ample proof that radium is the method of choice in the treatment of cancer of the uterus, at least of that most frequent form of cancer of the uterus and most difficult to manage by operation, cancer of the cervix.

The presentation of the evidence furnished by this report may, therefore, be premature in so far as operable cancer of the uterus is concerned. It is, however, conclusive for cancer of doubtful operability, but so strong for operable cancer of the cervix, that in the light of the other published observations the treatment of early cancer of the cervix by radium is, at the present time, justified.

More than this, it suggests that it is unjust to the women of the country to wait three to five years longer before the widespread distribution of radium throughout the country is planned for.

Each medical centre in the country should plan to own sufficient radium to care for at least the uterine cancers of its district. While it is desirable that sufficient radium should be purchased by each of these centres to permit the use of emanation, and this supply be placed under the care of a trained man, who can properly become responsible for its use by the physicians of the district concerned, yet for the treatment of uterine cancer alone the use of emanation is not an absolute necessity. The treatment used in the vast majority of the cases thus far reported, and in the author's earlier cases, those having remained well the longest, has not been by emanation and is quite within the power of the private owner of radium. This treatment has proved efficient. In the later cases the author has preferred the combination of filtered radium emanation with the embedding in the cervical ulceration of unfiltered emanation tubes. The advantages offered by this combination, at least in treatment of uterine cancer, may be sacrificed when the use of radium itself is only possible.   These facts are important because they make practical the treatment of cancer of the cervix generally throughout the country.

When we consider that at a conservative estimate 8,000 to 9,000 women die of carcinoma of the uterus each year in the United States [1] and that a search, as elaborate as can be made through the published reports, including, as these reports do, circular letters sent out by Cullen and Taussig, through the South and West in the United States, finds only 61 women operated upon five years prior to 1916 who have been cured of carcinoma of the cervix uteri, can any consideration justify the postponement of the general use of radium in the treatment of uterine carcinoma ?   While, of course, more than 61 women up to five years ago have been cured by operation of cancer of the cervix in this country, yet it is safe to say that this number indicates what a drop in the bucket the operative treatment of cancer of the cervix uteri is towards meeting the real demands of this malady upon the medical profession.   But, granting that the radical abdominal operation could cure 100 per cent. of the operable patients of cancer of the cervix applying for treatment, there are not in the country a sufficient number of capable surgeons to do the required work.

Contrasting with this record the record which radium has already made, however immature this record may be, the fact that it has produced cures of two to four years standing in cases too extensive for operation ; that it has produced cures of three years standing and over, in a larger percentage of early cases than operation has produced, one author claiming for it in this stage 100 per cent. of cures ; the fact that treatment by it in no way interferes with the patient's routine life and subjects her life to no risk ; the fact that it is a remedy capable of being used by any one possessing the simplest gynecological training, after receiving certain easily acquired technical instruction ; contrasting these facts with the operative records, is not the time ripe to urge each county medical society to make the effort to place a supply of radium in its district ?   Three hundred milligrams are sufficient for the treatment of one case every 24 hours.   Less may be successfully used, but if so the treatments must be longer and the number of cases treated less.

Aside from the relief in advanced cases, can there be any doubt that, if such a plan be carried out, more cases of cancer of the uterus would be cured than are now saved by operation, and a knowledge of this fact soon go further in inducing women to seek help in an early stage than are at present induced by the attractions of a radical abdominal operation ?

The strong argument for the radical abdominal operation has always been the fact that it is the only method by which lymphatic metastases may successfully be removed, and yet few of the cases with such metastases have ever been cured by operation.

Weibel, of the Wertheim clinic, states that 25 per cent. of all cases upon

---

1 The 17th annual report of the mortality statistics of the Bureau of Census for 1916 states that there were : 58,600 deaths from cancer that year, 8,898 deaths or 15·2 per cent. were from cancer of the female generative organs, divided as follows : ovary and fallopian tube, 544 ; uterus, 8,085 ; vagina and vulva, 218 ; unclassified, 51.

which he operated had cancerous glands and nearly all died of recurrences. In his whole series only ten such cases remained well five years.

Sampson reports one case cured in which a metastasis was found in the lymphatic gland.

Clark states that, if the higher pelvic lymphatic systems are the seat of metastases, it is scarcely possible for the widest and most painstaking dissection to completely eradicate it.

· None of Busse's cases in which the presence of carcinoma in the lymphatics was demonstrated ultimately recovered.

Hofmeier saved no case in which the removed glands contained carcinoma.

Schottlaender and Kermauner state, on page 456 of their book on carcinoma of the uterus, based on the 256 operations of von Rosthorn's clinic, that in the later years not much importance was attached to the necessity of removal of glands, and in the review which the author gave this book, he found no case which ultimately recovered in which the glands removed contained carcinoma.

We may conclude then that only isolated cures can be obtained by any method when the cancer has left its primary site, so that any error made in neglecting attention to the higher pelvic lymphatic glands is more than offset by higher mortality accompanying attempts to remove them.

Cancer of the cervix, in probably the majority of cases, displays a strong disposition to remain localised for a long period. Zweifel, for instance, records 23 operations for recurrent cancer of the cervix, of which 7 were free from further recurrence seven and a half years.

If cases with cancerous lymphatics can be cured, it is far better to attempt to do so by opening the abdomen after treating the primary disease with radium and embedding emanation in the enlarged glands. We have evidence in our work with radium in the mouth that its effect extends to the first set of regional lymphatics.

From the therapeutic standpoint, cancer of the uterus must be regarded as a local disease, and the most practical method of handling the disease at its site of origin must be adopted.

Our present evidence indicates that radium destroys the disease at this site to a greater distance than the knife is capable of removing it, and does this with no risk or inconvenience to the patient and only a small tax on the skill of the surgeon. Every effort should, therefore, be made to secure its general use throughout the country.

BIBLIOGRAPHY.

Abbe, R. "Uterine Fibroids, Menorrhagia and Radium.' *Med. Rec.*, 1915, lxxxvii, 379-381.
Adler. "Ueber Radiumbehandlung bei Gebaermutter Krebs." *Monatschr. f. Geburts. u. Gynaek.*, xli, 145.
Allmann. "Zur nicht operativen Karzinombehandlung." *Strahlentherapie*, 1914, iv, 625.
Bailey, H. "Radium in Uterine Cancer." *Surg. Gynec. & Obst.*, 1918. xxvi, 6, 625.
Baisch, K. "Erfolge der Mesothoriumbehandlung bei 100 Uteruskarzinomen." *Muenchen. med. Wchnschr.*, 1915, lxii, 1670.
Bergonie, J., and Spéder, L. "Le traitément du cancer utérin inopérable par la röntgen thérapie et la radium thérapie combinées." *Arch. d'élect. méd.*, 1915, xxiii, 140-148.
Bovée, J. W. "Statistics of Radical Operation for Cancer of Cervix Uteri." *Am. J. Obst.*, 1912, lxvi, 380.

Bumm. "Ueber die Erfolge der Roentgen und Mesothorium Behandlung beim Uteruskarcinom."
    Deutsche Gesellsch. f. Gynaek., Halle, 1913.
Bumm, E. "Weitere Erfolgerungen ueber Karcinombestrahlung," *Berl. klin. Wchnschr.*, 1914, lix, 193.
Bumm, F.   *Ztschr. f. Krebsforsch.*, 1920, x, 105.
Burrows. S "Radium Treatment of Cancer of the Cervix of the Uterus." *Am. J. Surg.*, 1915, xxix,
    296.
Busse W. V.   "Dauer resultate bei dem Operation des Uteruskarcinoma nach den abdominalen
    Methoden." *Monatschr, f. Gcburtsch. u. Gynaek.*, 1912, xxxv. 35.
Chéron, H., and Rubens-Duval, H. "Ueber den Wert der Radiumtherapie in der Behandlung der
    uterinen und vaginalen Krebse." *Fortschr. a. d. Geb. d. Roentgenstrahl.*, 1913, xxi, 229.
Clark, John G. "The Therapeutic Use of Radium in Gynecology." *Surg. Gynec. & Obst.*, 1918, xxvi,
    619.
Idem. "The Radical Abdominal Operation for Cancer of the Uterus." *Surg., Gynec. & Obst*, 1913,
    xvi. 255.
Cobb, F. "Cancer of the Uterus with Special Reference to the Possibilities of Cure by a Radical
    Abdominal Operation." *Boston M. & S. J.*, 1914, clxxi, 731.
Cullen, Thomas S. "Radical Operation for Cancer of the Uterus." *Surg., Gynec. & Obst.*, 1913, xvi,
    265.
Degrais, P. "Radium thérapie du cancer du col de l'utérus." *Ann. de gynéc, et. d'obst.*, 1915, xi,
    609; *Surg., Gynec. & Obst.* xxii, 3, 298.
Dent. *Gesellsch. f. Gynaek.*, Halle, 1913, May.
Dieffenbach, W. H. "Radium in the Treatment of Cancer." *Med. Rec.*, 1913, lxxiv, 1068-1072.
Dobbert, T. "Ergebnisse der Behandlung des Gebaermutter-Krebses mit Radium." *St. Petersb. m.
    Ztschr.*, 1914, xxxix, 97.
Doederlein. "Roentgen-Mesothorium Behandlung bei Myom und Carcinom des Uterus." *Surg.,
    Gynec. & Obst.*, 1913, xvii, 428.
Doederlein, A., and Seuffert, E. "Unsere weiteren Erfahrungen mit der Mesothorium Behandlung
    des Circinoms." *Muenchen. med. Wchnschr.*, 1914, lxi, 225.
Idem. *Zentralbl. f. Gynaek.*, 1915, xxxix, 12, 177.
Esquerido. "Resultadas de la application del radium en el cancer del utero." *Therapia*, Barcelona,
    1917, ix, 681.
Fabre. "Les indications de la radium thérapie dans le traitément du cancer de l'utérus." *Ann. de
    gynéc. et d obst.*. 1915, xi, 620.
Faure, J. L. "Traitément du cancer du col de l'utérus par l'hystérectomie abdominale." *Bull. et
    mém. Soc. de chir. de Par.*, 1913, xxxix, 1061.
Flatau, S. "Duerfen wir operable Uterus-Karcinome ausschliesslich Bestrahlen?" *Zentralbl. f.
    Gynaek.*, xxxix, 611.
Foveau de Courmelles (Paris). 1st part, "le rayons X"; 2nd part, "le radium en gynécologie."
    XXVII Internat. Congr. Med., Lond., 1913, viii, 79-96.
Fueth, H., and Ebeler, F. "Radiotherapy of Cancer." *Zentralbl. f. Gynaek*, xxxix, No. 14,217.
Graff, E. "Ueber die bisherigen Erfahrungen mit Radium und Roentgenstrahlen bei der Krebsbehand-
    lung." *Strahlentherapie*, 1915, v, 627.
Heimann, F. "Le traitément radio et radium thérapique des cancers utérins." *Arch. d'électricité
    méd.*, 1917, xxv, 530.
Hofmeier, M. "Zur operative Behandlung der Carcinoma colli uteri." *Ztschr. f. Geburtsh. u. Gynaek.*,
    1911, lxix, 453.
Jacobs. "Roentgen and Radium Therapy in Gynecology." Discussion. XXVII Internat. Cong. Med.,
    Sect. VIII (2), *Obst. & Gynæc*, Lond., 1913, 198.
Keene. "Radiotherapy in Gynecology." *Penn, M. J.*, 1917, xx, 469.
Kelly, H. A., and Burnam, C. F. "Radium in the Treatment of Carcinomata of the Cervix Uteri and
    Vagina," *J. Am. M. Ass.*, 1915, lxv, 1874.
Klein, G. "Roentgen and Radium Therapy in Gynæcology," discussion. XXVII International Cong.,
    Lond., 1913, viii, (2), 200.
Kolischer, G. "Modern Radiotherapy in Malignant Tumours and Localized Tuberculosis." *Lancet-Clin.*,
    1915, lxxiv, 287-289.
Koltz, R. "Economie d'énergie rayonnante dans le traitément du cancer inopérable." *Arch.
    d'électricité méd.*, 1917, xxv, 430.
Krinski, L. A. "Die operative Behandlung des Portio Carcinoms." *Verhandl. d. l. russ. Krebskong.*,
    St. Petersb., 1914; by *Zentralbl. f. d. ges. Gynaek., Geburtsh. u. d. Grenzgeb.*
Kroemer (Greifswald). "Roentgen and Radium Therapy in Gynecology." XXVII Internat. Cong.
    Med., Lond., 1913, viii (2), 193-195.
Kroenig. "Roentgen Rays, Radium and Mesothorium in the Treatment of Uterine Fibroids and
    Malignant Tumours." *Am. J. Obst.*. 1914. lxix, 205.
Labhardt, A. *Corres.-Bl. f. schweiz. Aerzte*, 1917, xlvii. 961-973.
Legneu and Chérou. "Guérison par radium therapie d'un cancer ureterovaginal inopérable." *J.
    d'urol.*, 1914, v, 3.

Maiolo, G. C. "Osservazioni cliniche sulla radium terapie ai 50 casi carcinoma uterino." *Ann. di ostet. e ginec.*, Milano, 1917, xli, 99.

Meyers. "Radium in the Treatment of Cancer of the Uterus." *Iowa St. M. J.*, 1918, viii, 296.

Miller, C. J. "Radium in the Treatment of Carcinoma of the Cervix." *Surg., Gynec. & Obst.*, 1916, xxii, 437.

Morton, Wm. J. "Radium for the Treatment of Cancer and Lupus." *Med. Rec.*, 1907, lxxii, 760-766.

Neel, J. Craig. "Results after the Wertheim Operation for Carcinoma of the Cervix of the Uterus." *Surg., Gynec. & Obst.*, 1913, xvi, 293.

Oertel, T. E. "The Present Status of Radium; Report of Cases Treated." *J. M. Ass. Georgia*, 1914, 180-181.

Oliver, Sir Thomas. "Radium and its Efficiency in Cancer of the Vulva." *Lancet.* 1915, 1, Feb. 6, 272.

Petersen, Reuben. "The Extended Operation of Carcinoma of the Uterus." *Surg., Gynec. & Obst.*, 1916, xxiii, 237 ; Tr. Am. Gynec. Soc., 1916.

Pozzi, S., and Rouhier, G. "De l'hystérectomie restreinte complétée par la radium thérapie dans les cancers de l'utérus." *Rev. gynéc. et chir. abdom.*, 1914-1915, xxiii, 209-264.

Prochownick, L. "Behandlung und Statistik des Gebaermutter Krebses." *Zentralbl. f. Gynaek.*, 1915, xxxix, 627.

Ransohoff, J. L. "Radium in the Treatment of Cancer of the Uterus." *Lancet-Clin.*, 1915, lxxiv, 289.

Sampson, John A. "Results of the Radical Abdominal Operation for Cancer of the Uterine Cervix." *Surg., Gynec. & Obst.*, 1913, xvi, 304.

Schauta. *Monatschr. f. Geburtsh. u. Gynaek.*, 1912, xxxvi.

Idem. "Radium und Mesothorium bei Carcinoma cervicis." *Monatschr. f. Geburtsh u. Gynaek.*, 1913, xxxviii, 503.

Scherer, A., and Keley, B. "Ueber die Behandlung des Uterus Krebses mit Roentgen und Radium-strahlen." *Versammt. deutsche Naturforsch. f. Aerzte.*, Wien., 1913.

Schindler, O. "Erfahrungen ueber Radium und Mesothoriumtherapie maligner Tumoren." *Wien. klin. Wchnschr.* 1913, xxvi, 1413, 1463.

Schmitz, H. "An Additional Contribution to the Therapeutic Value of Radium in Pelvic Cancer." *Surg., Gynec. & Obst.*, 1916, xxiii; 191.

Idem. "The Action of Radium on Cancer of the Pelvic Organs; a Clinical and Histological Study." *J. Am. M. Ass.*, 1915, lxv, 1879.

Schottlaender and Kermaunder. "Zur Kenntsiss des Uterus Karzinoms." Berlin : S. Karger, 1912.

Seuffert, E. Von. "L'état actuel, les problèmes et les limites du traitément radio et radium thérapique du cancer." *Arch. d'électricité méd.*, 1914, xxii, 552-571, 610 625.

St. Clair. R. "Radium Treatment of Malignant Tumours." *West M. Times*, 1915, xxxv, 89.

Tate, W. Discussion—"Roentgen and Radium Therapy in Gynecology." XXVII Internat. Cong. Med., Lond., 1913, viii (2) 199.

Taussig, Fred. "The Prognosis for Radical Abdominal Operation for Uterine Cancer." *Surg., Gynec. & Obst.*, 1912, xv, 147.

Taylor, Howard. "Operation for Carcinoma of the Cervix Uteri." *Surg. Gynec. & Obst.*, 1912, xv, 141.

Thaler. "Zur erweiterten vaginalen Karzin zu Operation." *Zentralbl. f. Gynaek.*, 1915, xxxix, No. 41.

Turner, Dawson. "Report on the Radium Treatment at the Royal Infirmary, Edinburgh, during the year 1915."

Weckowski. "Radium in Cancer." *Berl. klin. Wchnshr.*, li, No. 31, 1453.

Weibel, William. "Extended Abdominal Radical Operation for Cancer of the Uterus." *Surg., Gynec. & Obst.*, 1913, xvi, 3, 251.

Idem. "Die klinische Stellung des Carcinoma corporis uteri." *Arch. f. Gynaek.*, 1913, c, 153.

Weinbrenner, C. "Die Behandlung der Genital-carcinoma mit Mesothorium." *Monatschr. f. Geburtsh. u. Gynaek.*, 1914, xxxix, 181.

Wertheim. "Radium Behandlung des Gebaermutterkrebses." *Wien. klin. Wchnschr.*, 1913, xxvi, 1648.

Idem. Internat. Cong. Med., Lond., 1913.

Wickham, L., and Degrais, P. "Radium thérapie, cancer de l'utérus." Paris: 1912, 2nd ed·

Wilson. "The Results of Abdominal Operative Treatment of Cancer of the Uterus." *Med, Press & Circular*, 1914, xcviii, 302.

DENTAL RADIOGRAPHY.

By S. Gilbert Scott, M.R.C.S., L.R.C.P.

I. The Use of the Oblique Rays in Dental Radiography.

The practical radiologist makes use of various methods of his own which he has found to be of value by experience. These practical "tips," to use the term, are not as a rule included in books on radiology.

One is taught that the central ray should always pass through the part being examined in order to prevent distortion. This is perfectly correct in most cases, but one never hears a good word said for the oblique rays, which may be employed to advantage in overcoming difficulties by those who know how to use them.

I have been making use of the oblique rays for some years past and have found them of great practical value in examining various parts of the body.

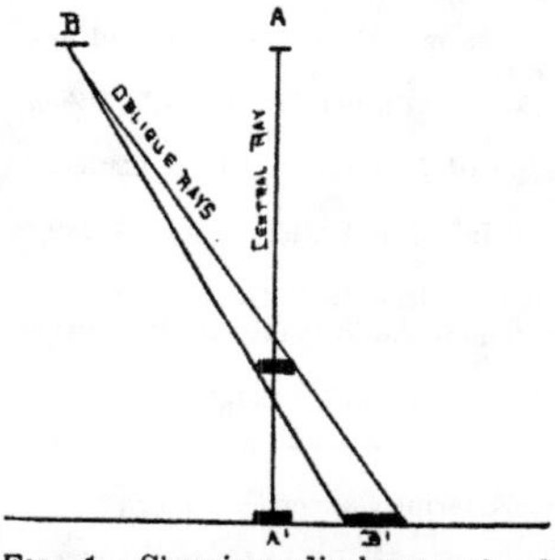

Fig. 1.—Showing displacement of shadow by oblique ray.

The radiographic examination of teeth in general is not always easy, and many radiologists dislike this "fiddling job," as they term it. Knack, experience and a good eye, used in conjunction with the oblique rays, are required to render the examination consistently successful. Many a film is wasted because on development the extreme tip of a root is found to have been missed altogether. If the oblique rays are used correctly, this elusive part of the root will be found to have been thrown well on to the film.

The method can be easily demonstrated by making use of the light given off from the spiral of a Coolidge tube. The tube is placed over the couch and a dried skull utilised. If, for example, we place the lower jaw on its side and displace the tube across its long axis, the shadow of the jaw nearest the tube will move in the reverse direction. In this way it will be noted that the shadows of both halves of the jaw are interposed when in the centre of the illuminated field, but clear of each other when the oblique rays from either hemisphere are utilised. Fig. 1 explains the method diagrammatically. Thus, in radiographing the lower jaw, it is necessary to centre the tube on a spot well below the level of the jaw itself and rather behind its angle. In order to get a correct idea as to the exact position in which the tube should be placed, it is not a bad plan to watch on the screen the displacement of the shadows produced by the movement of the tube and tilting of the part under examination.

The same method is utilised for displacing the shadow of a tooth on to the film placed in the mouth, but owing to the fact that the distance between the tooth and the film is small, the displacement is proportionately less, although at the same time this will be found sufficient to show the whole tooth, where the lower half would probably have been missed.

In actual practice one should visualise what one is aiming at. Thus, in order to throw the shadow of a tooth lying in the upper jaw downwards on to the film, the central ray must fall somewhere on the frontal bone, and in the case of the lower teeth it would be quite six inches below the lower jaw. If one works with the tube above, the limit of one's field must be known, otherwise it may be found that in the effort to make full use of the oblique rays, the film has been placed outside the illuminated area. The tilting of the tube is unnecessary and frequently defeats one's object.

The best position for the head can only be found out by experience, and depends on the part of the jaw under examination.

It might be expected that distortion of the image would result from using the oblique rays as described, but this is negligible so long as the film lies more or less in the same plane as the tube.

I have only given a very rough outline of this method, and it must be understood that it is necessary to use one's ingenuity to obtain its full practical value. I think, however, sufficient has been said to indicate how the oblique rays may be made use of, and I must leave it to each one's ingenuity to work out their practical application.

II. The Uses of a Quarter Plate in Dental Radiography.

The point of the chin and the floor of the mouth are not easy regions to radiograph satisfactorily. A few words as to the technique used to overcome certain difficulties may, I hope, be found of practical value to the radiologist. In describing the following method I am taking it for granted that the tube is above the patient. The operation may be divided into three stages :—

1. Placing of the patient's head.
2. Insertion of a quarter plate into the mouth.
3. Placing of tube.

1. The patient lies on his back and a large sand-bag is placed under the shoulders, so that the head is thrown back as far as possible.

2. The next stage is the placing of a quarter plate with its envelope inside the mouth—at any rate, half of it. To many this may sound impossible, and if one compares the narrowest side of the plate to one's own mouth, this doubt may appear well founded. But the adult mouth is very elastic, and the making a mouthful of a quarter plate is easily accomplished with a little coaxing and lubrication. Needless to say, it is hardly a becoming operation, and if tried on oneself it is some time before the feeling of the artificially-produced grin wears off. It is unnecessary to cover the plate with waterproof, and in the case of children, where the insertion is necessarily more difficult, but in most cases possible, the outer black envelope may be discarded, the inner red one being carefully fastened down right up to the corners. Those plates sold already done up in double wrappers are the best, as they fit tighter and so lessen the

breadth of the mouthful. A little vaseline smeared on the long edges of the
plate and in the corners of the mouth will ease things considerably.

The fingers should be used as miniature shoe-horns assisting the first part

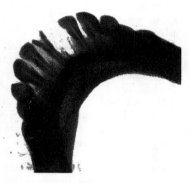

Quarter plate in mouth.
No. 1.—Lower jaw. Chin.

of the operation and the plate gently pushed home. The amount of plate that
disappears into the mouth is rather astonishing. Remember to place the film
downwards.

3. Now see that the patient's head is as far back as it will go and tilt the tube
so as to bring it into the same plane as the plate, or as nearly so as possible.

It is hardly necessary to say that the sooner the operation is over the better
will the patient be pleased.

The method has only been described in detail for examining the lower jaw

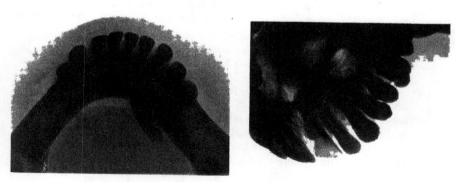

No. 2.—Calculi in Wharton's duct.   Quarter plate in mouth.
                                         Right side.   Upper jaw and roof of mouth.

and floor of the mouth, but it will be readily seen that it can be equally applied to
the upper jaw, and if skilfully used by one with a good eye—most of the teeth of
one side can be shown altogether on one quarter plate with little or no distortion.

CASE OF FRACTURED SESAMOID IN FOOT, WITHOUT HISTORY OF TRAUMA.

By Francis Hernaman-Johnson, M.D.

Cases of fractured sesamoid are not very rare ; the interest in this case lies in the fact that there was no history or external trace of injury. The patient, a boy of 12, felt his foot a little sore one morning in school, and had some difficulty in walking home, a distance of one mile. He was sent to me for a

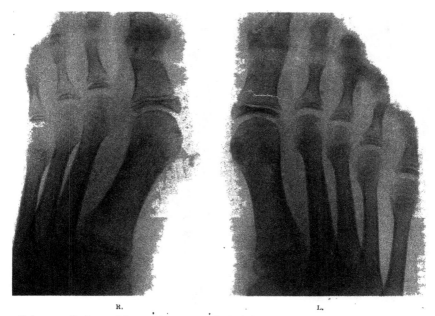

R.   L.

Note crescentic shape of fragment seen in profile, and absence of the greater part of the normal sesamoid shadow (R.).

diagnosis, and I made the plate shown, and also a lateral view. I gave a diagnosis of fractured sesamoid, as the X-ray evidence seemed to be clear. However, this was doubted, owing to the lack of history. Fortunately for me, if unfortunately for the patient, the place suppurated and had to be opened. Fragments of bone were extracted, which undoubtedly represented a broken sesamoid.

I have not seen any report of a case exactly similar to this, but the fracture of metacarpals in marching soldiers, without definite trauma—as described in the ARCHIVES some time ago—would appear to be analogous.

A NOTE ON TWO CASES OF SCHLATTER'S DISEASE.

By *F.* Shillington Scales, M.A., M.D., B. Ch. (Cantab).

Hon. Physician in charge of X-ray and Electrical Department, Addenbrooke's Hospital, Cambridge.

It may be of service to call attention to this complaint, as it is less rare than is usually supposed, but is, I believe, frequently not recognised. It affects the tubercle of the tibia in growing boys and girls, though much more frequently in boys, coming on about the age of puberty, generally before the ossification of the epiphysis. It is stated to occur sometimes as the result of

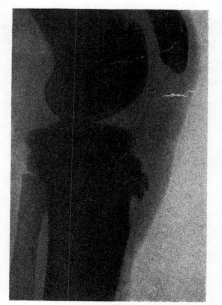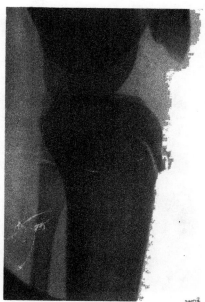

Schlatter's disease. Boy, æt. 14.

a blow and to have been described by Dr. Barrett, of Southport, as "Rugby knee," but in both the cases illustrated here there was no definite history of injury, though the patient complained of pain, tenderness, and swelling in front of and below the tubercle of the tibia. The ligamentum patellæ was more prominent than usual, there was no redness, and the clinical condition, without X-ray examination, might be wrongly diagnosed as tubercular, as delayed rickets, or as bursitis.

The normal tubercle in young people shows in a skiagram as a tongue-shaped projection hanging down, and is often developed from an independent centre, but in Schlatter's disease it will be noted (provided ossification has not taken place) that there is an irregular outgrowth which is quite characteristic.

A skiagram taken from front to back shows no abnormality, and the condition could therefore easily be overlooked.

The disease generally yields to rest and the use of a back splint, with general or local treatment, but severe cases, according to Tubby, require trephining or removal of the epiphysis.

The best short account of the disease is to be found in Tubby's "Deformities," Vol. I, page 316 (2nd edition), where two characteristic X-ray photographs are shown, very similar to those accompanying this note, and several references given.

A CASE OF SPONDYLITIS DEFORMANS.

By R. M. BEATH, B.A., M.B., BCH. (Belfast), M.B., B.S. (London).

Radiographer Ulster Hospital for Women and Children, and Assistant to Physician in charge of Electrical Dept., Royal Victoria Hospital, Belfast.

This case appeared to be of interest radiographically, owing to the very definite changes seen in the spinal column in the plates, and clinically owing to the early age of onset.

The patient, T.W., aged 27, a farmer, was admitted to the surgical wards of the Royal Victoria Hospital, Belfast, under the care of Mr. A. B. Mitchell, suffering from pain and rigidity of the spine.

His History was as follows : No evidence of any previous illness could be elicited. At the age of 17 he began to suffer from pain in his right hip and down the upper part of the anterior aspect of the right thigh, and this still continues. Six years later he began to feel stiffness and pain in his chest, and this gradually extended up to the neck, which was reached about a year ago.

Present Condition.—There is absolute rigidity of the spinal column and of the lower limbs. He looks healthy in face and is fairly well nourished, but there is definite wasting of the back muscles, especially of the rhomboids, and the serratus anterior.

The sacrospinalis muscle is contracted and hard on palpation. There is slight wasting of the leg muscles. The rigidity of the spine is very marked and it is practically straight—a regular " poker-back."

X-Ray Examination.—The most marked changes are seen in the lumbar region. Here definite bridges of bone are seen connecting the bodies of adjacent vertebræ and suggesting ossification of the lateral ligaments. These are well marked on the left side between the 12th dorsal and 1st lumbar, and between the 1st and 2nd lumbar vertebræ, and on the right side, between the 2nd and 3rd, and the 3rd and 4th lumbar vertebræ.

There appears to be also destruction of the cartilage and ossification between the 4th and 5th lumbar vertebræ.

The cervico-dorsal region was examined stereoscopically and showed an earlier stage of osteo-arthritis, with decided narrowing of the intervertebral spaces and irregularity of the articular surfaces of the body.

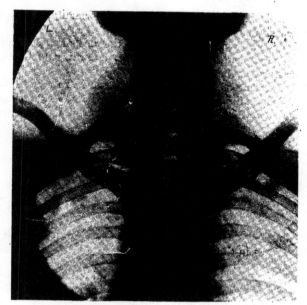

Cervical and upper dorsal region.

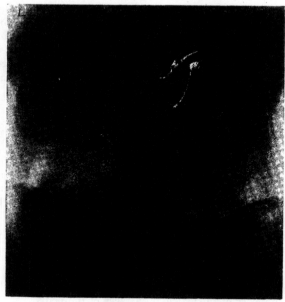

Lumbar region.

A " stippled " appearance is seen in the intervertebral spaces, suggesting ossifying changes beginning in the spinal ligaments.

The costo-vertebral articulations also show evidence of arthritic changes.

The pain in the hip and thigh is presumably due to the pressure of the bony bridges on the nerves as they pass through intervertebral foramina.

There are two points specially worthy of notice in this case :—

(1) The early age of onset—17 years.

(2) The absence of any of the usual antecedent causes—trauma, rheumatic fever, gonorrhoea.

I am indebted to Mr. Mitchell for permission to publish this case.

NEW TECHNIQUE.

DEVELOPING TANK STOPPER.

By I. S. TROSTLER, M.D., Chicago, Ill.

A VERY satisfactory and highly efficient plug or stopper for top of the developing tank may be made of a piece of rubber inner tube. This should

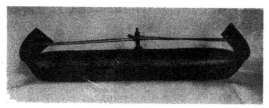

Tank Plug.

be the size of the cross diameter of the tank, and about 6 or 8 in. longer than the long diameter of the top of the tank.

Have a small (bicycle) valve fitted into the middle of this tube, and the ends sealed and carefully vulcanised, so that the two ends of the air space so made will be square and about $\frac{1}{8}$ in. longer than the long diameter of the tank opening.

Inflate this short balloon with a small pump until snugly full and the stopper is complete.

If this plug is forced down into inside of tank to the level of the fluid an almost airtight seal is made. By its use I am always able to use the developer so preserved until the chemicals are exhausted. The solution does not oxidise and become dark-coloured as before using this stopper.

I have passed a loop of twine through the ends of the vulcanised parts of the plug so as to hold these ends at, or nearly at, a right angle with the hollow part of the tube (see accompanying photo).

REVIEW.

The Principles and Practice of Roentgeno-logical Technique. By I. SETH HIRSCH, M.D., Director X-Ray Departments, Bellevue, Fordham, Harlem and Gouverneur Hospitals, New York City. American X-Ray Publishing Company, New York, 1920. (pp. xvii. + 244, with 343 illustrations and 22 tables.)

Part I deals with the principles of technique. Starting with the elementary principles of electricity, the author leads up to apparatus, with which he deals in a thoroughly up-to-date way, as seen by the inclusion of an aeroplane radiological unit.

The discovery of X rays is described, also the evolution of the various forms of gas tubes.

The hot cathode tube is fully discussed, including the Lillienfeld tube. The properties of X rays, their production and measurement are each the subject of well illustrated chapters.

Part II deals with the application of these principles in technique and methods of examination. Fluoroscopy and radiography are dealt with, and the control of the Coolidge tube is clearly set forth. A very large portion of Part II is devoted to standard positions, which are profusely illustrated and explained.

The difficult subjects of exposure and of dark room technique are discussed, and finally the organisation and equipment of the X-ray department.

The text is clear, full of interest and systematically arranged, and one notices with pleasure that the lengthy American nomenclature is not adhered to. This work can be confidently recommended, not only as a book of reference, but also for those reading for the Diploma of Radiology and Electrology.

REPORTS OF SOCIETY.

SOCIÉTÉ DE RADIOLOGIE MÉDICALE DE FRANCE.
Séance du 9 Mars, 1920.

Du voile des sommets pulmonaires dans les anévrysmes de l'aorte, par le Dr. LEBON.—Dans tous les cas d'anévrysme de l'aorte on constate une diminution parfois trés prononcée de la transparence de l'un ou de l'autre des deux sommets pulmonaires. Ce voile apical peut provenir d'un refoulement du parenchyme pulm. par la poche anevrysmale qui remonte jusqu'à la région sous-claviculaire où les battements sonttperceptibles. Mais, et c'est ce qui arrive lorsque l'aorte est simplement élargie, sans ectasie véritable, l'obscurité plum., l'obscruites des sommets est bein plus souvent due à une compression de la trachée ou des grosses bronche et du nerf pneumogastrique. Si les anévrysmes de l'aorte ont leur cachexie comme la tuberculose, ils peuvent faire croire à une lésion tuberculeuse ancienne ou récente limitée aux sommets.

Radiographies de lésions osseuses, par les Drs. GARCIN et AUBOURG.—Les A. présentent les clichés et les observations cliniques ; 1° d'exostoses ostéogéniques multiples coexistant avec un mal de Pott cervical trés accentué ;

2° d'une tumeur osseuse du radius à aspect alvéolaire, probablement de nature tuberculeuse ; 3° de corps vertébraux détruits par un anévrusme de l'aorte.

Note sur le radiodiagnostic et certaines affections osseuses chroniques, par le Dr. COLANERI.—L'A. présente quelques clichés concernant des ostéomyélites chroniques de l'humérus, du fémur, et de l'os iliaqee ces lésions classés sous la même étiquette clinique présentaient, au point de vue radiologique des lésions d'aspect très différent.

Examen radioscopique du gros intestin dans un cas de pericolite sigüe avec sténose du celon descendant, par le Dr. LAURENT-MOREAU.—L'A. relate l'observation d'un malade qui, au cours d'une pericolite sigüe, fut examiné à l'écran, apréslavement bismuthé ; On trouva une sténose de le moitié supérieure du colon descendant, coincident avec un empétement diffus de cette région. Les phénoménes inflammatoires ayant disparu, on fit un nouvel examen qui montra la complète disparition de cetta sténo.

La durée d'évacuation du sulfate de baryte ; la micro-rétention, par la Dr. SPECKLIN.—

L'observation porte sur plus de 500 examens gastriques, L'A. conclue que le repas baryté est évacué en moins de 4 h.; lorsque cette évacuation a une durée plus longue, il s'agit de cas pathologiques. A un premier degré de retard, c.-à-d. lorsqu'on trouve 4 h.; aprés le repas une petite cupole opaque dane le fond de l'estomac, L'A. propose le nom de micro-rátention; il faut songer dans ces cas à un ulcus gastre-duedénal (dans 2/3 des cas): il a trouvé, en effet 40 ulcus (diagnostic confirmé par l'opération) sur ce sujets présentant ce symptême.

Lèsions sous-diaphragmatiques reconnues à l'examenradiologique chez un malade tuber-culeux, par le Dr. LEBON.—Ches un malade prés atant des lésions multiples de l'appareil pleuro-pulmouaire à cardio-pericou-diques, avec conformation défectueuse du thorax datant de la premiére enfanee, l'examen radiologique a montré l'existence de lésions sousdiaphragmatiques d'explication difficile. Il existait au dessous de la voute diaphrag-matique du coté droit un espace triangulaire séparant le foie du diaphragme, et du coté gauche une bride fibreuse très nette se dirigeant de haut en bas et de dehors en dedans vera la colonne lombaire.

Utilisation de deux tubes Coolidge-Baby sur le transformateur dit Goolidge, par le Dr. SALEIL.—Le Dr. BELOT présente un dispositif imaginé par le Dr. SALEIL qui pernet d'actionner à la fois deux tubes Baby-Coolidge avec le marériel transformateur pour Coolidge. Ce dispositif présente de l'interêt au point de vue de la meilleure utilisation de ce matériel et simplifiera la réalisation de la radiostér-éoscopie.

Séance du 9 Mars, 1920.

(Suite).

Un nouveau cas de radiographie positive de calculs du cholédoque, par les Drs. PIERRE-DUVAL et HENRI BECLERE.—Il s'agit d'un homme de 63 ans petit de taille et du poids de 72 kil., donc relativement corpulent, alcoolique et hépatique de longue date. Le malade est examiné radioscopiquement au sujet d'une affection présumée de l'estomac. L'examen à l'écran révèle la présence, un peu au dessus de la créte iliaque droite d'une ombre anormale, en demi lune. La radiographie monte qu'il s'agit de calculs biliaires dans une vésicule distendue. Le cliché montee en plus la présence de cinq petits calculs très nets dans le canal cholédoque. Un nouvel examen eut lieu quelques jours aprés. Dans l'intervalle, le malade présenta toute une série de crises hépatiques avec finalement brusque cessation des douleurs. Le nouvel examen, pratique dans le décubitus abdominal, montra dans cette position, un groupement étalé des calculs de la vésicule. Le canal cholédoque contenait, à ce moment? calculs très distincts. La radiographie avait pu saisir le résultat des que venaient de se produire et l'évacuation dans la voie biliaire principale de nouveaux calculs. L'intervention chirurgicale confirma le diagnostic radiologique. L'examen chimique des calculs, pratiqué par M. GRIGAULT donna 25% de sels de chaux.

Présentation d'un châssis-table pour examen radioscopique, par M. DUTERTRE.—Cet ap-pareil, grâce à une manœvure très facile, peut être utilisé pour l'examen debout ou couché.

Le Secrétaire Général: Dr. HARET.

NOTES AND ABSTRACTS

Can Lead be used as a Filter in Radio-therapy?—DISSEZ (*Arch. d'Élect. Méd.*, May, 1919).—The author describes experiments from which he concludes that lead filters of 1/10 to 4/10 mm. thickness permit the passage of rays of the value of 9 Benoist and upwards. Under the conditions of the experi-ments the epilation dose was obtained in 2 min. 15 secs., without filter, in 18 min. through 1/10 mm., and in 4 hours 10 min. through 4/10 mm. A lead filter of 1/10 mm. is equivalent to 100/10 of aluminium. As the power of tubes increases, it may be con-venient to use thin lead filters instead of thick aluminium for treatment of deep or large tumours or other conditions requiring very hard rays. The result of these experiments also indicates the need for serious precautions for the protection of both patient and radiologist during long exposures to highly penetrating rays.   N. B.

Pedunculated Malignant Growths of the Stomach.—G. W. HOLMES (*Amer. Jour. of Roent.*, June, 1919, pp. 279-283, with 2 skiagrams and 3 figs.).—The author records two cases of the above. In both cases the peristaltic waves passed over the involved area of the stomach without evidence of break, such as is seen in lesions which involve the stomach wall. When the gross pathology of these growths is considered, there is no reason to expect that the wave would be obstructed.

The appearance of the bismuth-filled stomach in a case of pedunculated growth is most suggestive of the appearance when there are large masses of food present, or of advanced carcinoma. Food can be ruled out by repeated examinations. Gastric cancer, as a rule, involves the wall of the stomach sufficiently to prevent the free passage of the peristaltic wave.   R. W. A. S.

Destructive Action of X Rays on Blood Cells.—H. D. TAYLOR, W. D. WITHERBEE, and J. B. MURPHY (*Jour. of Exper. Med.*, Jan., 1919, pp. 53-82).—As (*a*) it is not possible to estimate the dosage employed in most of the older experiments concerning the effect of X rays on the blood, because gas tubes were used, (*b*) only a few blood counts have been published in these cases, and their significance has not been adequately explained ; (*c*) X rays are now being used with increasing frequency in therapeutics ; it seemed important to obtain accurate information regarding the response of the blood to X rays. With this object the following results are recorded by these observers.

X rays in large doses affect the lymphocytes before any of the other circulating cells. There is a sharp fall in the total number of circulating lymphocytes, which is complete forty-eight hours after the treatment. Following the immediate decrease there is a primary rise, followed by another fall, which in turn is followed by a permanent rise of these cells to normal.

The effect of X rays on different species of animals varies considerably, but in those studied, cat, monkey, guinea pig, rabbit, rat, mouse, and pony; the selective action on the

lymphocytes was in all instances apparent. When several animals of the same species are given the same dose the effect on the circulating lymphocytes seems to be quantitatively parallel when determined by blood counts.

The polymorphonuclear neutrophilic leucocytes, when affected at all, increase in number immediately after the administration of X rays and then tend to decrease below their normal level. This decrease is followed by a return to normal many days before the lymphocytes reach their original level. The other cells of the blood follow the neutrophilic curve.

Percentage figures, as determined by differential blood counts, do not give an accurate indication of the effect of X rays. It is only when these are multiplied by the total white blood count that a figure, representing the total number of cells of the series per c.mm. of blood, is obtained, which varies to the stimulus in a constant manner, the variations being practically quantitative.   R. W. A. S.

White Ink for Marking Glass (*Topical Therapy*, April, 1919). — Mix one part of barium sulphate with three parts of sodium silicate solution (water glass). The silicate solution should be of the consistency of glycerine. Applied with an ordinary steel pen, the ink will dry in 15 minutes, and will withstand water. It can be readily removed by scraping with a knife.   R. W. A. S.

Influenza and Bronchopneumonia.—J. A. HONEIJ (*Amer. Jour. of Roent.*, May, 1919, pp. 226-238, with 14 skiagrams).—The X-ray changes found in the chest of cases during the recent epidemic show a very early and marked active congestion of the parenchyma and bronchial tissues. There is also a marked lymphatic and glandular congestion and reaction, as seen by changes in the hilus area, and a diminution in pulmonary function, as shown by the increased convexity of the diaphragm. The heart shows a slight dilatation of the right auricle.

When bronchopneumonia supervenes the first changes seen, after those described above, are apparently bronchial in character. There is a greater irregular diffuse peribronchial thickening. Then there occur small, more or less localised areas, most visible in the middle of the lung. These areas next spread out and become confluent. Resolution may now take place but more often the process progresses, the bronchial outline becoming no longer visible and the pulmonary changes more extensive. The hilus shadow becomes increased in size and density from an early stage. Two interesting associated changes occur early in these cases, acute dilatation of the right auricle and also dilatation of the pulmonary area, and the diaphragm becomes more dome-shaped and higher in position. R. W. A. S.

Notes on Diathermy Apparatus.—C. M. Dowse and C. E. Iredell (*Proc. Roy. Soc. of Med.*, June, 1919, Sect. of Electro-Therapy.).—

In view of the use of X-ray coils as a source of current for the production of diathermy, this paper is of interest for the comparison of the two main forms of apparatus in general use, both as regards their practical use and suggested technical improvements.

R. W. A. S.

Diathermy in Abdominal Disorders.—C. E. Iredell (*Proc. Roy. Soc. of Med.*, June, 1919, Sect. of Elect-Therap.).—

This observer records good results in several cases, and believes that the diathermy current has a definite action on the movements of the intestinal canal, both in producing peristalsis and in checking vomiting and diarrhœa. R. W. A. S.

Removing Pyro Stains (*Topical Therapy*, June, 1919).—

A fluid drachm or two of strong sulphuric acid is added to half a pint of a 25 per cent. solution of sodium sulphite. Half an ounce of this solution is diluted with four or five ounces of water for use. The stained fingers are dipped into it, and pumice stone used if desired. R. W. A. S.

Diathermy in Gynæcology.—C. E. Iredell, A. D. Marston, and G. Bellingham Smith (*Proc. Roy. Soc. of Med.*, June, 1919, Sect. of Electro-Therap.).—

In many cases of inoperable cancer of the cervix, diathermy can temporarily check the pain, bleeding, and discharge. The amount of constitutional disturbance on the day after the operation is in proportion to the amount of breaking down of tissue produced by the heat. For this reason it is advisable first to scrape the growth. It is stated that the constitutional effects can be partly prevented by the 24 hours application of 10 or 20 mgr. of radium suitably protected.

The risks attaching to the operation by diathermy are apparently small.

R. W. A. S.

Lung Abscess and Bronchiectasis.—H. Wessler (*Amer. Jour. of Roent.*, April, 1919, pp. 161-174, with 31 radiograms).—

This well illustrated article is based on a clinical and radiological examination of 100 cases. The great value of consecutive X-ray examinations is pointed out, and by its means large cavities may be seen to disappear in a few weeks, and it is said that such rapid return to the normal is characteristic of the healing of lung defects when the infection has subsided. Apparently a large pneumonic infiltration and cavity can regress as readily as a small one, the only prerequisite being the sloughing out of the gangrenous area.

In cases of long standing, however, the persisting irritation soon leads to fibrosis, which leads to rigid membranous cavity walls that will not collapse.

It is pointed out that before a lung abscess can be stated to be cured, the clinical symptoms and signs and all X-ray evidence of disease must have disappeared.

In detecting a cavity, an examination in the lateral recumbent position may disclose a cavity not otherwise visible. Upright oblique views will also at times do the same. The existence of a cavity cannot safely be excluded from a single examination. It may only become visible after it is partly emptied by expectoration, or after a removal of the overshadowing pneumonic process.

Wessler says that one of the more striking symptoms of lung abscess is hæmorrhage, as it occurs in almost every case at some stage; in fact, it is a more constant sign than is hæmorrhage in pulmonary tuberculosis.

R. W. A. S.

Notes on the Internal Use of Radium and its Emanation.—G. and D. Bardet (*Bull. Gén. de Thérap.*, Sept., 1919, pp. 653-659).—

Colloidal metals, it is stated, act in a physical manner rather than a chemical. The metallic granules, being charged with electricity, are carriers of energy. Accordingly, the authors believe that radio-active preparations should act in like manner.

From their experience they think that when a physician is faced with a serious septicæmia, large doses of radium injection should be tried.   R. W. A. S.

A Note on the Chemical Testing of Barium Sulphate for Use in X-ray Diagnosis.— H. PRIESTLEY and H. G. McQUIGGIN (*Med.*

Jour. of Australia, May 10th, 1919, p. 383).— Qualitative and quantitative tests for the presence of soluble barium salts, and the presence of other heavy metals, are given.

Tests from Merck's Annual Report for 1912 are also quoted.   R. W. A. S.

PUBLICATIONS RECEIVED.
Books.

Atlas for Electro-Diagnosis and Thera-peutics. By F. MIRAMOND LAROQUETTE, M.D. London : Bailliere, Tindall & Cox.

Diathermy in Medical and Surgical Practice. CLAUDE SABERTON, M.D. London : Cassell & Co., Ltd.

Journals.

Archives de Medicine et de Pharmacie Militaires. March-April-May, 1919.

British Journal of Dermatology, March, April, 1920.

British Journal of Surgery, April, 1920.

Bulletins et Mémoirs de la Société de France, April, 1920.

Bulletin of the Johns Hopkins Hospital, March, 1920.

Gaceta Medica Catalana, Jan. 15th, 31st, 1920.

Hospitalstidende, March 31st; April 7th, 14th, 21st, 1920.

Journals—*continued.*

Il Policlinico, March 15th, 1920.

Journal de Radiologie et d'Electrologie, Jan., 1920.

Journal of the Röntgen Society, April, 1920.

Medical Journal of Australia, March 13th, 20th, 1920.

Medical Science Abstracts and Reviews, May, 1920.

New York Medical Journal, April 10th, 17th, 1920.

New York State Journal of Medicine, April, 1920.

Norsk Mag. for Lægevidenskaben May, 1920.

Quarterly Journal of Medicine, April, 1920.

Surgery, Gynæcology, and Obstetrics, April, 1920.

Ugeskrift for Læger, April 15th, 22nd, 29th ; May 6th, 1920.

NOTICES.

ARCHIVES OF RADIOLOGY AND ELECTROTHERAPY is published monthly.

The index for each volume, which ends with the May number, is supplied with the June number of each year.

Communications to the Editors should be addressed to " ROBERT KNOX, M.D., 38, Harley Street, W. 1."

Communications and illustrations from American contributors may be sent to Messrs. REBMAN COMPANY, 141-145, West Thirty-sixth Street, New York City.

All radiographs and photographs must be originals, and must not have been previously published. Drawings should be supplied on separate paper.

Owing to the scarcity of paper the Publishers are reluctantly compelled to reduce the number of free reprints of Papers to twenty-five.

Annual Subscriptions, payable in advance, 30/- including postage. Single copies, 3/- (postage 2d.) Single numbers and back numbers can be supplied on application.

CPSIA information can be obtained
at www.ICGtesting.com
Printed in the USA
LVHW05*1434041018
592408LV00012B/206/P